"This remarkable resource – an American Group Psychotherapy Association publication – is an outstanding blend of accrued clinical wisdom and state of the art science. Written by an international cadre of leading clinician – scientist group therapists, this text illuminates how structured client assessment and preparation, combined with ongoing measurement of group process and client progress improves client access to high quality, effective and inclusive group therapy. All contemporary group psychotherapists will find great value in this excellent text."

Molyn Leszcz, MD, FRCPC, CGP AFPA-DF, *Professor of Psychiatry, University of Toronto, Past President, AGPA*

"This outstanding resource will change the way group practitioners approach their group work. By applying advancements in measurement-based care to group practice, the authors have laid an important foundation for improving group work through consistent client feedback. Well-written, comprehensive, and accessible: this will be the go-to book for guidance on tracking processes and outcomes in group therapy."

Nathaniel Wade, Ph.D., CGP, *Professor of Psychology, Iowa State University*

"This volume, like its predecessor, constitutes another crucial step towards advancing measurement-informed care that is evidence-based and culturally responsive. These chapters together offer a coherent and systematic approach that transcends international and cultural boundaries to the unfolding process within the therapy group. I am confident this book will set the stage for an intriguing dialogue among group psychotherapy educators and practitioners, and for an exciting pipeline of research studies in the decade to come."

Eric Chen, Ph.D., *Professor of Counseling Psychology, Fordham University*

Group Psychotherapy Assessment and Practice

Group Psychotherapy Assessment and Practice is the definitive guide to assessment in group therapy, offering the reader a means to understand and implement group therapy screening, process, and outcome tools.

Geared to group psychotherapists as well as academics, this state-of-the-art text provides the reader with a framework to support and augment clinical judgment as part of routine clinical practice. It demonstrates how utilizing measurement-based care collaboratively with clients can help maximize therapeutic processes and mechanisms of change. This book shows how measures can improve the detection of client worsening and prevent premature dropout—two factors that contribute greatly to our duty to client care. Leading experts in the field provide examples of new measures that can enhance multicultural training and group leader cultural sensitivity, illustrating how awareness of diversity can enhance clinical practice and provide more contextually responsive treatment. Examples of cross-cultural adaptations of measurement are also included that place group therapy assessment within an international framework.

This modern guide provides practical tools such as handouts, measures to aid in member selection, and methods of tracking progress and outcome to strengthen the group leader's effectiveness.

Rebecca MacNair-Semands, Ph.D., CGP, AGPA-F is a Co-Chair of the Science to Service Task Force for the American Group Psychotherapy Association (AGPA). She recently co-authored *The Ethics of Group Psychotherapy: Principles and Practical Strategies*.

Martyn Whittingham, Ph.D., CGP, AGPA-F is a licensed psychologist at Whittingham Psychological Services, Cincinnati, Ohio, United States. He is the founder of *Focused Brief Group Therapy (FBGT)*.

AGPA Group Therapy Training and Practice Series

Series Editors: Les Greene and Rebecca MacNair-Semands

The American Group Psychotherapy Association (AGPA) is the foremost professional association dedicated to the field of group psychotherapy, operating through a tri-partite structure: AGPA, a professional and educational organization; the Group Foundation for Advancing Mental Health, its philanthropic arm; and the International Board for Certification of Group Psychotherapists, a standard setting and certifying body. This multi-disciplinary association has approximately 3,000 members, including psychiatrists, psychologists, social workers, nurses, clinical mental health counselors, marriage and family therapists, pastoral counselors, occupational therapists and creative arts therapists, many of whom have been recognized as specialists through the Certified Group Psychotherapist credential. The association has 26 local and regional societies located across the country. Its members are experienced mental health professionals who lead psychotherapy groups and various non-clinical groups. Many are organizational specialists who work with businesses, not-for-profit organizations, communities and other "natural" groups to help them improve their functioning.

The goal of the AGPA Group Therapy Training and Practice Series is to produce the highest quality publications to aid the practitioner and student in updating and improving his/her knowledge, professional competence and skills with current and new developments in methods, practice, theory, and research in the group psychotherapy field. Books in this series are the only curriculum guide and resource for a variety of courses credentialed by the International Board for Certification of Group Psychotherapists. While this is the series' original and primary purpose, the texts are also useful in a variety of other settings including as a resource for students and clinicians interested in learning more about group psychotherapy, as a text in academic courses, or as part of a training curriculum in a practicum or internship training experience.

For more information about this series, please visit https://www.routledge.com/AGPA-Group-Therapy-Training-and-Practice-Series/book-series/AGPA.

Books in this Series:

Core Principles of Group Psychotherapy: An Integrated Theory, Research, and Practice Training Manual *Edited by Francis J. Kaklauskas, Les R. Greene*

The Ethics of Group Psychotherapy: Principles and Practical Strategies *by Virginia Brabender and Rebecca MacNair-Semands*

Group Psychotherapy Assessment and Practice: A Measurement-Based Care Approach *by Martyn Whittingham and Rebecca MacNair-Semands*

Group Psychotherapy Assessment and Practice

A Measurement-Based Care Approach

**Edited by
Rebecca MacNair-Semands and
Martyn Whittingham**

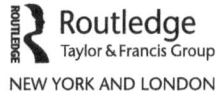

Routledge
Taylor & Francis Group

NEW YORK AND LONDON

Designed cover image: © Getty Image

First published 2023
by Routledge
605 Third Avenue, New York, NY 10158

and by Routledge
4 Park Square, Milton Park, Abingdon, Oxon OX14 4RN

Routledge is an imprint of the Taylor & Francis Group, an informa business

Access the Support Material: www.routledge.com/9781032186337

Library of Congress Cataloging-in-Publication Data
Names: Whittingham, Martyn, editor. | MacNair-Semands, Rebecca, editor.
Title: Group psychotherapy assessment and practice : a measurement-based care approach / edited by Martyn Whittingham and Rebecca MacNair-Semands.
Description: New York, NY : Routledge, 2023. | Includes bibliographical references and index. |
Identifiers: LCCN 2022059869 (print) | LCCN 2022059870 (ebook) |
Subjects: LCSH: Group psychotherapy. | Cultural psychiatry.
Classification: LCC RC488 .G695 2023 (print) | LCC RC488 (ebook) |
DDC 616.89/152--dc23/eng/20230414
LC record available at https://lccn.loc.gov/2022059869
LC ebook record available at https://lccn.loc.gov/2022059870

ISBN: 978-1-032-18634-4 (hbk)
ISBN: 978-1-032-18633-7 (pbk)
ISBN: 978-1-003-25548-2 (ebk)

DOI: 10.4324/9781003255482

Typeset in Baskerville
by Taylor & Francis Books

Rebecca dedicates this book to Steve MacNair-Semands and Allison Semands and the late Jack Corazzini, a teacher and mentor, whose passion for group therapy lives on in all the people he touched.

Martyn dedicates this book to his family and to Rex Stockton, a wise and kind mentor.

Contents

Figures

Tables

About the Editors

Rebecca MacNair-Semands, Ph.D., CGP, AGPA-F, is a licensed psychologist and a fellow of both the American Group Psychotherapy Association and Division 49 of the APA. In 2017 Dr. MacNair-Semands was named Group Psychologist of the Year by the American Psychological Association (APA)'s Society of Group Psychology and Group Psychotherapy. She is currently in her ninth year as a Co-Chair of the **Science to Service Task Force for the American Group Psychotherapy Association**. She recently retired as the Senior Associate Director of the UNC Charlotte Counseling and Psychological Services Center, where she was employed for over 25 years. In addition to coordinating the clinical and group services for the center, she delivered more than 40 national and international professional presentations. She has published 30 articles and book chapters, as well as the first edition of *The Ethics of Group Psychotherapy*. She recently co-authored the book *The Ethics of Group Psychotherapy: Principles and Practical Strategies*.

Dr. Martyn Whittingham, Ph.D., CGP, AGPA-F, is a licensed psychologist in Ohio. He is the founder of *Focused Brief Group Therapy (FBGT)*, a transdiagnostic, measurement-based care approach to reducing interpersonal distress in less than eight sessions. He is a Fellow of the American Group Psychotherapy Association (AGPA) and Division 49 (Group Psychology and Group Psychotherapy) of the American Psychological Association and a former President of Division 49. He currently serves on AGPA's Science to Service Task Force, APA's Health Care Financing Advisory Group, the National Health Service (United Kingdom) Advisory Board on Group Training Standards and on the Editorial Board of the International Journal for Group Psychotherapy. Dr. Whittingham has been the recipient of two national awards for group therapy: the Association for Specialists in Group Work, *Group Practice Award, 2010*, and American Psychological Association's Society for Group Psychology and Group Psychotherapy, *Group Dynamics Teacher of the Year, 2021*.

Contributors

Rachel Arnold is a graduate student in the Clinical Psychology doctoral program at Brigham Young University, United States. Her research focuses on therapy effectiveness and factors that make therapy work, with group psychotherapy being a specific theme throughout the majority of her research.

Gary M. Burlingame is a professor of Psychology, Brigham Young University, United States and researcher of small group treatments and measurement. He has contributed over 70 books, manuals and chapters and some 160 articles. He has served as a consultant to federal, state and private entities with awards recognizing his contributions from national and international associations.

Les R. Greene is on the clinical faculty of Yale University School of Medicine where he teaches and supervises group and couples psychotherapies. He is a past President and distinguished fellow of the American Group Psychotherapy Association and has served as editor of the International Journal of Group Psychotherapy. He has received the Alonso Award for Excellence in Psychodynamic Group Theory several times, most recently for his coedited work "Core Principles of Group Psychotherapy".

Paul L. Hewitt is a Professor in the Department of Psychology and a Member of the Psychotherapy Program at University of British Columbia, Canada. He is the recipient of the Donald O. Hebb Award for Distinguished Contributions to Psychology as a Science and published more than 300 research papers, books, and chapters.

Anthony S. Joyce is a registered psychologist and clinical professor in the Department of Psychiatry at the University of Alberta in Edmonton, Canada. As a principal member of the Edmonton Psychotherapy Research and Evaluation Unit, Dr. Joyce has been actively involved in treatment intervention and outcomes research investigations.

Martin Kivlighan is an Associate Professor in counseling psychology at the University of Iowa, United States. His research interests are in psychotherapy process and outcome, group psychotherapy, multicultural orientation (MCO), and psychotherapy training.

Shi Min Liew is a Singapore based Clinical Psychologist and a Certified Group Psychotherapist with America Group Psychotherapy Association. In addition to a decade of clinical practice in public hospitals, she is also an Associate Faculty at the Singapore University of Social Sciences, Singapore.

Cheri L. Marmarosh is a Research Professor at Divine Mercy University, the Director of the International Center for the Psychology of Spirituality and Mental Health, and a Professor of Clinical Psychology at the George Washington University, United States, where she studies how attachment relates to individual and group psychotherapy. She has published more than 70 empirical and theoretical articles and is the lead author of two books: *Attachment in Group Psychotherapy* and *Groups: Fostering a Culture of Change.*

Joseph R. Miles is a Professor of Psychology at the University of Tennessee, Knoxville, United States. His research and teaching focus on the process and outcome of group interventions and multicultural and social justice issues. He is Associate Editor for the *International Journal of Group Psychotherapy* and *Group Dynamics: Theory, Research, and Practice.*

Bernhard Strauss is a Full Professor of Psychotherapy and Medical Psychology with a psychodynamic, psychoanalytical and group training, head of the Institute of Psychosocial Medicine and Psychotherapy, and Psychooncology, University Hospital, Friedrich-Schiller-University Jena, Germany. Past president German College of Psychosomatic Medicine (DKPM), German Society for Medical Psychology (DGMP), and Society for Psychotherapy Research (SPR).

Giorgio A. Tasca is a Professor in the School of Psychology University of Ottawa, Canada, director of the Psychotherapy Practice Research Network (www.PPRNet.ca), and editor *Group Dynamics.* He is a Fellow of the American Psychological Association (APA) and received the 2016 Group Psychologist of the Year Award from APA Division 49.

Martyn Whittingham is a licensed psychologist at Whittingham Psychological Services, Cincinnati, Ohio, United States. He is the founder of *Focused Brief Group Therapy (FBGT)*, a research-informed, integrative interpersonal approach to reducing interpersonal distress that utilizes measurement-based care to enhance and inform all aspects of therapy. He is the recipient of two national awards for group therapy.

Preface

The use of assessment in group psychotherapy represents not only cutting-edge practice but also the future of the field. Recent changes in payment and regulatory models in the USA are foreshadowing a movement toward accountability and measurement in psychotherapy, while in other countries, such as Australia and the United Kingdom, it is already a required part of practice. This will eventually become a core requirement of practice as the USA moves toward value based care—a system that measures outcomes for all health conditions and rewards based on recovery. However, the need for assessment in group therapy is clear, regardless of incentives or national mandates, and encompasses not only outcome measurement but also selection/pre-group preparation and process.

As the authors will be outlining throughout this edited work, assessment can add considerably to clinical judgment, and in ways that are particularly important to the effectiveness of treatment. The argument for measurement is not a dry, research-based one, but rather a case based on helping clients in real time. Not only does the research support using assessment this way—transparently and collaboratively to help make adjustments as therapy progresses—but therapists can also add to their clinical judgment across a range of factors important to group therapy.

Groups are, by their nature, complex. Adding more people to a therapy approach increases its level of complexity exponentially. A dizzying number of variables exist to pay attention to, some of which can result in client worsening or client dropout. Leaders may ask: Which factors will predict a referral to group not showing up for the first group? What factors predict group members dropping out early in its life? What factors might mean someone has improved or worsened? Does one pay attention to excessive anxiety, avoidance of work, how cohesive the group is, conflicts, dramatic incidents, or some other variables? When a group is finished, how does the leader determine if it went well? Does seeing members looking happy and expressing wishes that group would continue actually predict good outcomes? Can we even trust that a "good group" that expresses happiness and positivity about their experience does not contain members who are unwilling to contradict the consensus by expressing it did not work for them?

Assessment is helpful in that it can identify variables specifically connected to desired process-outcome variables that impact the quality of care. Many of the instruments showcased in this volume draw on research specific to group therapy. That is, they track variables of interest to groups, such as group cohesion and the working alliance, which are well supported in the group literature. This is important for group leaders to understand.

It is not always obvious in a group when it has achieved appropriate cohesion levels or whether some members feel it and others do not. Clients sometimes display outward signs of distress, lack of engagement or disinterest, but they may just as often be unwilling to disclose how they are feeling in a group or may be motivated to disguise their true reactions. For example, while a conflict is taking place, some members may be reveling in the drama, while others feel frozen and wish to leave. Factors such as interpersonal style, cultural values, personality differences and situational factors such whether a client feels that they have allies in a group, can all impact their reactions to a conflict. The group leaders are also bringing their own personality and cultural variables to bear, albeit often unconsciously. If they are uncomfortable with conflict or conversely seek to engender it between group members due to their theoretical orientation, they may risk missing the internal experiences of each member and can end up being surprised by a group member leaving.

Assessment gives clarity to what is actually happening in the group. Since it is based on self-report, it offers a window into key concerns related to entering a group and working through group processes and outcomes. Even the most skilled clinicians stand to benefit from either having their hypotheses confirmed (thus enabling the therapist to intervene with more certainty) or discovering new information that helps them to shape their interventions to maximize positive outcomes. As will be mentioned multiple times during this book, assessment can aid and improve clinical judgment – it is not intended to supplant it.

Assessment is also not context-free. Diversity, Equity, and Inclusion (DEI) issues are rightly at the front of therapists' minds in the USA. The increased attention to multicultural awareness and cultural humility are more in focus now than they have ever been. This book places particular emphasis on this movement, with attention given to the impact of diversity on everything from the validity of instruments to how to adapt measures or questions to be culturally relevant. There is also a focus throughout the book on the role of group leaders' attitudes, values, and willingness to embrace diversity, as well as barriers to effective functioning in this area.

Equally, cross-cultural issues in group are increasingly coming to the fore as the internationalization of psychotherapy increases. With group assessment now being used in places such as China, Singapore, and Australia, issues like validity and reliability of instruments for different cultures has never been more important. The field as a whole is in a transition phase with respect to adoption vs. adaptation of instruments; this book will give an honest appraisal of where gaps remain, what works need to be done and how to utilize best practices to bring the benefits of assessment to different cultures while simultaneously creating awareness around possible drawbacks. It is a challenging process and one that requires skilled clinicians being able to consider the relative strengths and demerits of each instrument—appraising the potential clinical benefits of instrument usage against any possible risks.

Chapter 1, ***Assessment in Group Therapy: An Introduction and Overview***, by Martyn S. Whittingham, Rachel Arnold, and Gary M. Burlingame is an overview of the book, contextualizing the chapters with descriptions of measurement-based care (MBC), constructs related to assessment and exploring how to decide to combine measures to maximize client gain. It also outlines the differences between measurement-based care and using assessment to measure overall program quality, providing an overview of some of the important statistical means for doing so. The chapter also explores factors such as how to balance the positive value of assessment against factors such as therapist and client fatigue, explaining how careful selection and timing of assessment to maximize gain can promote therapeutic gains while minimizing burnout. It also considers the role of important therapeutic constructs, foreshadowing the work in the other chapters by contextualizing the evidence-based factors related to selection, process and outcome. The chapter is intended to clarify for practitioners how to choose measures in combination; for example, combining selection/pre-group preparation measures with process and outcome tools while preventing client assessment fatigue and ensuring multicultural sensitivity remains a paramount concern.

Chapter 2, ***Group Selection, Group Composition, and Pre-Group Preparation***, by Anthony S. Joyce and Cheri L. Marmarosh gives consideration to how assessment can inform selection of clients for groups and pre-group preparation. It is not easy to select clients who are likely to be successful in group, but there are many evidence-based factors that can serve to better predict the likelihood of a successful referral, leading to a positive group experience. Use of measures can be a vital aid in separating the useful information that then requires intervention to ensure a referral "sticks," to the interesting information that has less relevance. Separating the metaphorical wheat from the chaff allows therapist to narrow their focus in a pre-group preparation meeting to either enhance the working alliance and prevent premature dropout or to help a client who is unsuited to group to find another type of treatment where they may find more success and satisfaction. In this chapter, the authors outline relevant measures, highlighting ones that are most utilized and based on group research. They also offer suggestions around new and promising approaches that require more research before they are fully implemented. They offer case studies to illustrate the complexities of pre-group preparation.

Chapter 3, **Process Measures**, by Joseph R. Miles, Bernhard M. Strauss, and Les R. Greene outlines the world of group process. It provides an in-depth guide into the assessment of key constructs, first outlining the "grey" areas and conceptual complexity before narrowing down the constructs into those that are most helpful in organizing the group leader's thinking. They showcase assessment tools that have been intentionally designed to measure group process, ranging from "classic" measures to more recent instruments that are empirically validated and have analytics that flag potential client worsening or dropout. This chapter gives the practitioner considerable guidance in how to begin to think about process and to link it to outcome. It serves as a primer for both assessment tools and constructs contained within them. Case studies demonstrate the evolution of group process. Lastly, they also highlight measures used to amplify and understand the role of diversity in group leadership and process. In particular, they explore how group leader attitudes toward diversity can influence group process – an important concept in the training of group leaders.

Chapter 4, **Assessing Outcomes in Group Psychotherapy**, by Martin Kivlighan and Giorgio A. Tasca explores the well-developed world of outcome measures, with aims to help clinicians select psychometrically sound measures to assess client change in group. Unlike the previous two chapters, most of the outcome measures they discuss are used in individual as well as group therapies. The chapter outlines reasons for routinely assessing outcomes in group psychotherapy and provides recommendations for selecting measures for clinical use with a specific focus on multicultural issues. Recommendations for identifying outcome measures for group practice include using measures that are a) brief and user-friendly; b) valid and reliable for diverse populations; and c) provide clinical cut-off scores and reliable indices of meaningful change based on normative and clinical data. The chapter provides an overview of outcome measures based on this recommended criterion. Finally, the chapter closes with two clinical case examples to illustrate the application of routine outcome monitoring in clinical group practice and multicultural group work.

In Chapter 5, **Enhancing Group Therapy Outcomes with Measurement-Based Care: Two Case Examples**, by Paul L. Hewitt and Shi Min Liew gives two detailed case examples of how assessment can be integrated into group therapies. Liew uses an example from a Singaporean hospital, explaining her concerns about using assessment. She incorporates a description of diversity within Singapore and how her own cultural identity needed exploring as a part of this conceptualization. She then explains how a model of therapy was used within the outpatient unit and where she adopted it as designed and provided rationale as to how she adapted it to improve its applicability to local populations' norms and preferences. Hewitt gives an example of a transdiagnostic group running in Canada, showing how assessment can be interwoven into the therapy at all stages. He provides a deidentified case study of how group leadership is informed by assessment and how it is used to advise clinical judgment. Both examples offer thoughtful application of the processes outlined in the prior chapters. They show how assessment can be woven into group therapy in a comprehensive manner to both improve client well-being while also providing accountability for outcomes to administrators.

Organization and Selection of Measures

It is important to note that this book was not intended to be a comprehensive detailing of every measure available. Rather, the authors of each chapter were invited to offer some examples of measures currently in use in the field. These would then serve as exemplars of the kind of instruments available while also showing how they might be used. This is also the case with the appendices, where some but not all of the measures mentioned in the chapters are featured. In some cases, these measures are replicated in their entirety and in other cases, copyright holders gave their permission for reproduction of select items. Therefore, not all measures mentioned in chapters are in the appendices.

With respect to copying measures that are printed in this book, significant care must be taken. In some cases, measures are entirely free and in the public domain and so can be copied from this book and used in practice. However, in many cases, permission needs to be sought or measures are proprietary and a fee must be paid to the publisher. If seeking to use a measure, it is incumbent on the reader to check carefully in our tables (and on the links provided within those tables) to determine whether the measure is proprietary or non-proprietary and to follow ethical and legal requirements in terms of appropriate credit and/or payment.

We hope that this book becomes a useful resource for beginning conversations around measurement-based care in group psychotherapy. It contains examples, encouragements and cautions that can all progress the conversation about how to move the field forward and improve client care.

Acknowledgments

We would like to express our gratitude to the American Group Psychotherapy Association and Marsha Block for extending to us the invitation to write this edition of *Group Psychotherapy Assessment and Practice: A Measurement Based Care Approach*. We wish to thank Angela Stephens and Katarina Cooke for their ongoing support of this project. We feel privileged to engage in co-editing about such an important subject, about which we have both been enthusiastic for many years, together with some of the most accomplished authors and practitioners in this global field. We also have much appreciation for the mentors in the field who helped to shape our passion and often shared the knowledge about group psychotherapy across the globe, leaving important legacies for the training of such intimate work that happens in group. Contributing immensely to this project have been the comments and recommendations of our three reviewers: Les R. Greene, Ph.D., CGP, AGPA-DLF; Eric Chen, Ph.D., and Nathaniel Wade, Ph.D., CGP. We also wish to thank Molyn Leszcz, MD, FRCPC, CGP, AGPA-DF, who has been a strong supporter with generous spirit throughout the book series. From Routledge, we would like to acknowledge the competent efforts of Amanda Savage, Katya Porter, and John Maloney.

Gratitude goes to our wonderful families who provided the loving support and enthusiasm for this project along the way. Specifically, we thank our spouses, Steve (RMS), Felisa (MW) and our children, Allison (RMS) and Felisa Iris (MW). We are so thankful for all the ways in which you contributed to help things go smoothly at home during the busy times and to help us celebrate the final product.

1 Assessment in Group Therapy

An Introduction and Overview

Martyn Whittingham, Rachel Arnold and Gary Burlingame

The American Group Psychotherapy Association (AGPA) has had an interest in utilizing *measure-informed care* in group therapy for several decades, which involves the use of measurement data to inform treatment and assess the effectiveness of therapy. This longstanding interest is demonstrated through the history of the CORE battery, which began in the 1980s when AGPA appointed a research committee chaired by Roy MacKenzie and Robert Dies to formulate the original clinically-oriented research evaluation or CORE battery. This original CORE was comprised of just six measures in total, which aimed at evaluating group therapy effectiveness. Then, in the late 1990s and early 2000s, leaders within AGPA—including Harold Bernard, Marsha Block, and Robert Klein—created a taskforce of renowned group researchers and clinicians to identify the best available group therapy outcome and process instruments. Their goal was to revise the CORE battery to reflect current empirical research and to support group leader efforts in starting a group, assessing critical group dynamic processes, and tracking group member outcomes, with the CORE-Revised (CORE-R) being the end result in 2006. At the time of the revision in 2006, the authors noted that regulatory bodies, funding sources, and professional associations were advocating for the use of objective measures by clinicians to document the effectiveness of treatment.

Since that revision in 2006, the landscape has changed significantly in terms of use of objective assessment instruments to inform therapy (Barkham, 2016; Fortney et al., 2017). Previously, assessment use by practitioners was seen as aspirational and few therapists or agencies saw the need to add seemingly burdensome tools that they perceived added little value to clinical observation and served as a potential threat to their self-perceptions of competency (Beecher, 2008). Since then, the field and society have shifted considerably, with changes occurring at multiple levels, ranging from how measurement in therapy is understood and defined (Lewis et al., 2019) to an increasing evidence base (Burlingame & Strauss, 2021; Mellor-Clark et al., 2016), national movements to promote accountability for outcomes (Burgess et al., 2015) and a growth in models of group therapy that integrate assessment into treatment (e.g., Hewitt et al., 2020; Tasca et al., 2013; Whittingham, 2018). Altogether, these developments have engendered a stronger interest in and commitment to measurement, and, as a result, measure-informed treatment has become a part of daily practice in the past 15 years.

The present revision is sensitive to these advancements in the zeitgeist and research surrounding measure-informed care, and it seeks to build upon the present attitudes on the use of assessment in group therapy. The purpose of this revision is therefore to support efforts to engage in formal measurement by providing recommendations for the most empirically supported tools in group treatment at this time. In doing so, this revision works to uphold the standards of evidence-based practice. There are various definitions of evidence-based practice, with one definition concerning the use of population-specific treatment protocols

DOI: 10.4324/9781003255482-1

that have garnered empirical support, and yet another definition involving the development of practice guidelines that offer treatment recommendations. However, the branch of evidence-based practice we will be exploring in this book is *the use of standardized measures to enhance group selection, pre-group preparation, process and outcomes*. There is no doubt that these goals are worthy of pursuit, as it has become clearer over time that measurement can improve clinical practice by providing clinicians with valuable data about clients, which has made it possible to enhance outcome and prevent treatment failure (Shimokawa et al., 2010). Thus, as we endeavor to once again identify and recommend the most empirically supported measures in group treatment, we hope to aid clinicians in maximizing their effectiveness in group therapy.

Purpose of the Revision

Authors were charged to examine the CORE-R and retain or delete instruments from the prior editions based on the extant research. In some cases, instruments were utilizing outdated constructs that have fallen out of use, while in other cases, instruments were updated or new ones added. As with the prior edition, authors were invited to add instruments that met the criteria of being empirically sound—that is, instruments that are reliable, valid, sensitive to change and normed against representative samples (Barkham et al., 2021). This effort also included a goal to explore multicultural factors in the development and implementation of assessment tools, ranging from norm group representativeness to cultural considerations in administration and scoring. The authors were invited to contribute based on their experiences with either research, practice or both for their respective chapters. Several of the authors have group models that utilize assessment collaboratively with the client, while other authors conduct research and practice integrating assessment. The authors represent several different countries, ranging from the USA and Canada to Germany and Singapore. This emphasis on cross-cultural implementation is an important one and the perspectives of those working outside of the American mental health care system offer a wider perspective on adaptation of models to different populations.

There are also major societal and paradigm shifts that are addressed in this edition that contextualize the use of assessment. For instance, the increased focus on multiculturalism and diversity (Buchanan & Wiklund, 2020) and the increased internationalization of psychotherapy practice (Fatemi et al., 2019) are important evolutions in the field. These two strands receive greater focus in this update, with additions to each chapter on diversity, multiculturalism and cross-cultural adaptations. Each chapter discusses these as part of their remit and case examples are used to provide context. It is also important to root this book in current paradigm shifts in world health economics. Since accountability for outcomes requires measurement of change, the role of assessment in therapy is inevitably going to broaden. However, the case for assessment is not just driven by economic forces. It is also driven by increasingly clear research that shows assessment brings significant added benefit to therapy when integrated thoughtfully into practice.

Introduction to Measurement-Based Care

Recent efforts have sought to increase the use of measurement in group therapy, with assessment having the capacity to contribute to clinical decisions in several impactful ways. One of the most obvious applications is symptom tracking and outcome evaluation, with the clinician tracking clients' symptoms over time to assess whether clients are improving over the course of therapy. However, measurement can also be used to gauge perceptions of the therapeutic relationships, understand client expectancies regarding therapy, appraise client satisfaction, as well as performing other important functions. Thus, there are both outcome and process measures that can enhance therapy. Measurement data is preferably collected through psychometrically sound instruments, which typically involve client self-report. Armed with this data, clinicians are better equipped to work with clients who are not showing a favorable outcome trajectory, attend to ruptures in therapeutic relationships, address negative expectancies, and to address other factors of therapeutic relevance.

The purpose of this book is to support the implementation of measurement-based care in group therapy. To do this, the book will introduce measurement-based care and discuss group selection and group preparation methods (Chapter 2), process measures (Chapter 3) and group outcome measures (Chapter 4). This book will also explore how to enhance group therapy outcomes with measurement-based care using two case examples (Chapter 5). Within chapter one, we will discuss research on measurement-based care, barriers to implementation, purposes of assessment, components of measurement-based care, and multicultural considerations. Furthermore, we will explore how to select measures, analyze data, and evaluate a practice or program. This chapter will additionally explore the logistics of assessing outcome and introduce important concepts in measurement-based care such as reliable change and benchmarking. The content of this book places a special focus on group therapy, with the intent of specifically aiding group therapists in utilizing measurement-based care in their clinical practice. Measures in each chapter were selected as exemplars of the kind of measures used in group therapy assessment. Therefore, this book does not provide an exhaustive list of all possible measures but rather shows how correct selection and application of measures can enhance therapeutic processes and outcomes.

The Case for Assessment

The case for using assessment tools in group therapy is now unequivocal. Meta-analytic research has found statistically significant improvements on a range of variables including symptom reduction and percentage of deteriorated cases, while dropout was also found to be reduced (de Jong et al., 2021; Duncan et al., 2021; Lewis et al., 2019). The effects of therapists and clients receiving feedback have been shown to be particularly important for those clients identified as being at risk of treatment failure. Research has shown that this type of feedback has the potential to enhance client outcomes while reducing potential treatment failures (Shimokawa et al., 2010). Other research has shown findings that when the same therapists integrated assessment into therapy, over two thirds showed improved outcomes for clients compared to those not utilizing feedback from formal assessment (Lambert et al., 2018). These effects have also shown to be impactful across a wide range of groups, such as youth (Tam & Ronan, 2017); clients with eating disorders (Tasca et al., 2013); ethnic minorities (Connors et al., 2022); and individuals diagnosed within the autism spectrum (McFayden et al., 2021). Careful and well thought-through use of assessment as a routine part of treatment can also promote effective treatment by improving the attention paid to evidence-based common factors that are predictive of success in group therapy, such as the working alliance, group cohesion and attending to diversity (Wampold & Imel, 2015), which are discussed toward the end of this chapter. Thus, assessment not only provides data on client progress and outcome, but also can be used to evaluate therapeutic processes that contribute to outcome.

Research has also consistently found that regardless of training level (whether novice or expert), clinicians were poor at noticing treatment worsening and predicting premature dropout (Walfish et al., 2012). Given the potential for clients to suffer adverse outcomes from failing at group treatment that was supposed to cure their hopelessness, this is an alarming finding (Yalom & Leszcz, 2020). Therefore, it is no surprise that articles (e.g., Muir et al., 2019) are now discussing the ethical imperative to utilize assessment in therapy. The benefits of assessment use are clear and the risks of failing to conduct it can be deleterious for clients.

Barriers to using Assessment during Treatment

As Trauer et al. (2009) point out, there are many barriers to implementing measurement in treatment. These include therapist beliefs in the sufficiency of their own clinical judgment, perception of a lack of time to administer and score instruments, organizational restrictions (paying for instruments, little time for training, scheduling time to take them, competing tasks etc.) and concerns about confidentiality. Other reasons for hesitation include concerns that payers and administrators do not know how to interpret results, the belief that clients will find it onerous and worries about software use and associated costs (Mellor-Clark et al., 2016). Some clinicians fear that assessments might interfere with the formation of the therapeutic alliance (Youn et al., 2012). However, there is a lack of evidence supporting this notion (Boswell et al., 2015). In fact, when clinicians fully embrace and integrate the use of measures into treatment, leaders may be able to deepen engagement as they begin sessions by reviewing measurement data and allowing members to discuss their own experiences as well as the group's (Burlingame et al., 2003).

Arguably the most significant of the reasons is that practitioners are not convinced that assessment adds enough to their clinical judgment to invest the extra time and effort. Why would a therapist invest extra time, money and effort into a set of procedures they feel are not adding to client welfare? Yet group therapy is a highly complex undertaking and therapeutic mistakes are inevitable. Some of these mistakes, either of commission (for example, making a comment that is perceived as a microaggression) or omission (failing to address a rupture in the group that continues to fester) can lead to alliance ruptures, premature dropout and client worsening (Lo Coco et al., 2019). Assessment can catch significant amounts of missed information and provide a different perspective which may strengthen or challenge the therapist's views. Group therapists are only human and can benefit from adding data that they might otherwise miss, which they can use to supplement (rather than supplant) clinical wisdom. When measurement data conflicts with their perceptions, clinicians are then afforded the opportunity to explore that difference and what it means. Learning from mistakes, professional and personal humility, and confidence in one's ability are uneasy bedfellows. As Mellor-Clark et al. (2016) point out, clinicians often misjudge their effectiveness and can fall victim to the normal human trait of self-serving bias when making sense of treatment failure. Assessment offers considerable value in off-setting these tendencies and helping group leaders to become even more responsive to client needs. Group leaders can think of assessment like a lab test (Burlingame et al., 2017), which offers valuable data that can inform clinical practice and build upon clinical wisdom. How this assessment is conducted is also linked to its purpose.

Purposes of Assessment Use

The purposes of assessment use in psychotherapy are manifold and the strategies for collecting and analyzing data tend to follow from those objectives. These purposes can vary depending on the agency or practice, but range from closely integrating them into client care in real time, to conducting summative program evaluation. Therefore, two main dimensions aligning with the purposes are: 1) how closely they involve the client in the assessment; and 2) at what level (individual, group or agency?) the assessment is targeted.

For example, at one end of the spectrum is Measurement-Based Care (MBC, addressed at length in the next section), which involves transparent and collaborative use of assessment with the client in real time. At the other is a summative report presented to an administrator or payer to justify and explain results on a yearly basis. The same tools may be used for both levels, but different strategies are utilized to conduct the analyses. Examples of each will now be explored (and examples given in Chapter 5 of each), with the more individualized approaches explored first. To begin this process, it is first important to understand some definitions of these different types of care.

Definition of Measurement-Based Care

There are currently many terms used in the field to describe the utilization of assessment in therapy and the field is currently striving to come to a consensus. These terms include but are not limited to: Practice Based Evidence; Routine Outcome Monitoring; Feedback Informed Treatment, Patient Focused Research, Patient Level Feedback, Progress Monitoring and Assessment-Informed Therapy (Lewis et al., 2019). As Lewis et al. note, these terms are used so interchangeably that making sense of the differences in terminology can be a challenging task. They express a preference for the term Measurement-Based Care (MBC) based on it being explicit about the means (measurement) and goal (care) within its name. This term has also been adopted by APA's Practice Directorate (Wright et al., 2020) and in calls for professional practice guidelines (Boswell et al., 2022) demonstrating that MBC as a term is consistent with the language utilized for nationwide psychological practice.

It is important to define what MBC is and is not. MBC focuses on treatment of clients using assessment collaboratively to inform therapy. As Lewis, (2019) states, MBC is defined as "the systematic evaluation of patient symptoms before or during an encounter to inform behavioral health treatment" (p. 324). As such, it represents the most thoroughly integrated and collaborative use of assessment into direct client care. According to the authors, to be considered MBC, the intervention must satisfy the following components: 1) be routine, involving assessment of a symptom, an outcome, or a process preferably before each session or at very regular intervals; 2) involve therapist review of data to inform treatment; 3) include patient review of the data and 4) promote collaborative review of the data in which the client and therapist discuss the results to inform treatment and clinical decisions (Lewis et al., 2019).

1 Must be Routine

Routine assessment use can be as often as before or after every session or can be more intermittent. When deciding on the frequency of measure administration, therapists must carefully consider the balance between the utility of an assessment and any potential negative reactions from over-use. For example, to prevent dropout or client worsening a lengthier assessment may be used more regularly, but there is also the possibility of clients experiencing assessment fatigue from filling out instruments every session and irritation about measurement's intrusion into therapy; thus, the clinician must seek a balance. However, the assessment must be conducted regularly otherwise it risks missing important data points regarding the process of therapy. For example, choosing to use an outcome measure every session is particularly important in catching client worsening or potential dropout. Too long a gap between administrations can run the risk of missing the impact of a critical incident or deleterious process, that if allowed to fester, can lead to premature dropout. A routine use of measures allows the therapist to catch possible ruptures before they become a source of withdrawal or lead to confrontation for which the therapist is unprepared (Lo Coco et al., 2019), therefore helping the therapist to predict and prevent premature drop-out in real time while also ensuring therapy is on track.

2 Therapist Review

The second criterion is that the assessment be reviewed by the therapist in ongoing, regular intervals. Reviewing the findings from an assessment tool allows the therapist to integrate that information into their clinical judgment and to enhance their decision-making skills. In many cases, the findings can provide powerful evidence that affirms the clinicians' decision-making, providing increases in confidence for the group leader that they are accurately perceiving what is happening and intervening effectively. This review process allows the therapist to add more data to enhance their clinical judgment. It also enables the therapist to identify client deterioration as it is taking place and which otherwise might have been missed. This allows the group leader a chance to repair and remediate in a way that would not be possible if they were to explore the data long after it was collected.

It is also important to remember that reviewing instruments is an exercise in clinical judgment in and of itself. The therapist should take considerable care to integrate instrument findings with other clinical observations and to consider contextual and cultural factors (e.g., whether specific items are a good cultural fit). Instruments can often reveal important data that is often outside the group leader's awareness such as the potential for dropout, augmenting the therapist's clinical judgment.

3 Client Review

It is not only therapist review of data that is crucial. Client review of the data fosters client empowerment and offers rich potential to engage the client in their own care, thereby promoting a sense of agency. For example, a screening, process or outcome measure offers the opportunity for the client to self-reflect and discuss the issues with a therapist in real time. Client review also allows the client to learn more about themselves. For instance, clients may learn that a construct such as perfectionism (see more on this in Chapter 5) applies to them. This can provide a sense of relief that their problem has been named, which serves to 1) validate their experience; and 2) offers a therapeutic opportunity for the therapist to instill hope that change is possible. Absent this kind of insight, some clients remain unaware of the causes of their problems and therefore hopeless about a solution. Review of assessment can also help the client gain insight into their current feelings about therapy—for example, when realizing that they are in fact, quite ambivalent about group therapy. This allows them to consider the issue and to discuss this with the therapist. Altogether, the inclusion of a client review can add significantly to treatment. However, without collaboration with the therapist, a client may misinterpret or misunderstand the findings in the assessment.

4 Collaborative Review Between Therapist and Client

MBC assumes a collaborative approach between client and therapist. Research emphasizes the additional benefits of clients being involved in the review of data and highlights the need for *sharing and discussing the data* (De Jong et al., 2014). A collaborative review of screening, process and outcome results (either as a whole group or individually, depending on the purpose of the review) can shed light on issues and processes that may be outside the client's conscious awareness. This can then serve to promote insight and increase the likelihood of enhanced working alliance, emotional climate, and group cohesion—all evidence-based constructs linked to outcome in group therapy (e.g., Alldredge et al., 2021; Arnold et al., 2022; Burlingame et al., 2018; Wampold & Immel, 2015). Furthermore, collaboration can aid in shaping a more accurate interpretation of the assessment data. While assessment tools can be highly illuminating, they should be compared and contrasted with the clinical judgment of the therapist and insights from the client. To repeat a message from the last edition of this book (Burlingame et al., 2006) and from earlier in this chapter, *assessment should augment and not replace clinical judgment.* Therapists should hold onto hypotheses lightly until they incorporate information gleaned from the client.

It is also important to note that MBC does not explicitly cover other uses for assessment, such as program evaluation for the purposes of supervision and quality improvement or for reporting to third party payers or other stakeholders. These other uses will be addressed in this chapter, using the term "program evaluation." It is also important to note that many programs and therapists primarily use assessment in non-transparent, non-collaborative ways, with the therapist merely reviewing the results and incorporating them into treatment without informing the client. We contend that integration of assessment into therapy has uses at many levels. While it may be optimal to use an MBC model, and we recommend thoughtful application of this with group therapy, the practice of doing so requires training, thought and consultation on the optimal means to do so. Therefore, each therapist should consider how to build competency in implementing MBC, a case made by Boswell et al. (2022).

Implementing Measurement-Based Care: Clinician Skills

MBC requires skill on behalf of the clinician. Poorly trained therapists risk oversimplifying results, treating assessment findings as objective truth, and failing to account for client meanings, motivations, and contexts, including factors such as multicultural or cross-cultural variables that can impact results. While it is often easy to think of assessment as revealing an immutable truth about a client or clients, the reality is far more complex. For example, a measure of depression might illuminate for client and therapist that a client is feeling more than just a momentary lapse into sadness. In fact, it may represent a diagnosable, pervasive clinical issue in need of treatment. Equally, a screening measure for group therapy might reveal a hesitancy on the part of the client that is worthy of discussion when in a pre-group meeting. In both of these cases, the therapist and client discover something together that enhances treatment in real time.

In other cases, the assessment tools can reveal something that is more nuanced. For example, the Inventory of Interpersonal Problems (IIP-32) (Horowitz et al., 2000) is a self-report tool that measures total interpersonal distress, and also highlights what particular type of interpersonal distress is most impacting them (e.g., social inhibition or being too eager to please others). However, this instrument may be capturing an underlying style (e.g., rigidly trying to please everyone and ultimately feeling resentful as others fail to reciprocate), a context issue (e.g., working in a service industry where the client feels abused by the clientele), a diversity issue (e.g., moving from a culture where people help each other out to one where people tend to be less forthcoming with offers of help) or some combination of those factors. In other words, the therapist should be careful to elicit information that is more nuanced and comprehensive rather than accepting a single possible explanation for a result.

Collaboration with the client on assessment also involves using assessment transparently, albeit with therapeutic sensitivity. An assessment tool should be used to illuminate, help, guide and inform a variety of therapeutic processes that aid the process of therapy, and transparently sharing data with clients can facilitate these aims. To illustrate, Chapter 3 explores the notion that a group therapy process measure could be used in real time to inform the therapy itself. For example, a measure that uncovers problems with group cohesion could be used to bring that issue to the group. A group session in which a therapist shares the process measure data in a nonjudgmental way to explore why members are struggling to feel connected to each other could prove fruitful on multiple levels. Since group cohesion is a well-established construct linked to both reducing dropout and improving outcomes (Burlingame et al., 2018), focusing on problems with cohesion offers rich therapeutic potential. In all, collaboration between the client and the therapist has many benefits such as promoting better outcomes, informing interpretation of data, and guiding the therapeutic process.

Selection of Measures: Creating a Meaningful and Clinically Useful Battery

As demonstrated above, there are compelling reasons to integrate MBC into clinical practice. However, an essential aspect of MBC is utilizing measures that will be the most beneficial. As will be laid out more fully in each chapter, there is sufficient evidence to suggest that *group therapists should consider employing screening / pre-group preparation, process, and outcome measures in combination with tracking individual member attendance.* These measures may alert and even prevent member premature dropout, reducing inadequate screening and tailoring pre-group preparation to an individual member's concerns. Both of these practices may alert therapists to potential dropouts during the group and ensure appropriate outcomes are being delivered. In other words, this is not measurement for its own sake, but rather it is *intentionally targeted at the constructs and processes that create successful group programming.*

The means to achieve this success is also predicated on therapists being able to adequately evaluate which measures to select. This requires some skill in itself. The measures in this volume have already been evaluated for their psychometric properties: validity, reliability, norm groups and sensitivity to change. The group therapist must still make thoughtful choices that take into account the benefits of assessment, including clinical utility, program evaluation, information for supervision or consultation, and learning opportunities for both students and professionals. However, group leaders must also consider cultural applicability, client fatigue, therapist fatigue and time to complete, among other factors, when selecting instruments.

The combination of instruments should carefully consider what is the *optimal number and type of instruments that accomplishes the most clinically, while not exhausting or irritating the client or therapist.* It is a delicate balance, and one that is addressed in chapter five with case examples. Careful attention needs to be paid to the role of *construct overlap* (e.g., Johnson et al., 2005). Some measures capture exactly the same constructs, others have significant overlap. As an example, attachment style and interpersonal style, discussed in Chapter 2, are roughly equivalent constructs (Whittingham, 2017). Using several attachment and interpersonal measures for the same client may be interesting in academics and in research projects, but is likely to feel onerous for clients when used routinely in practice. Therefore, measures with considerable overlap should only be used when there is a clinically purposeful reason for doing so that is immediately useful and meaningful to both the client and therapist. Therefore, selection of measures should include *consideration of the utility of an instrument but also whether it adds value above and beyond an instrument that is already being used.*

Selection of Measures to Optimize Evidence-Based Processes

The link between evidence-based group processes and outcome is now clear (Alldredge et al., 2021; Lo Coco et al., 2019; Wampold & Imel, 2015). For example, client-rated alliance with the group leader is clearly linked to outcome and, furthermore, is significantly related to *change* in outcome over time (Arnold et al., 2022). Research findings construct a compelling narrative about the importance of therapeutic relationships in group therapy, highlighting the utility of tracking relationships through MBC (e.g., Alldredge et al., 2021; Arnold et al., 2022; Burlingame et al., 2018). This will be covered in more depth in Chapters 2, 3 and 4. Therefore, mobilizing these factors and selecting measures that capture them in real time can be powerful tools in promoting outcomes.

Clinicians should select measures that align with evidence-based constructs related to the purpose of the measure. For instance, in the work of pregroup preparation and screening, instruments to assess motivation (MacNair-Semands, 2002) or expectancy (Burlingame et al., 2012) are useful since these concepts have been shown to be related to outcome. The Group Readiness Questionnaire (GRQ) (Burlingame et al., 2012) provides an example of an expectancy item, which is as follows: "If I participate in a group, I expect to feel quite a bit better when we are finished." If a client scores low on this expectancy item, they can be flagged for a pre-group preparation intervention around expectancies. More specifically, a group leader might see low scores as an opportunity to set a data-based expectation for likely improvement. If, for instance, a client is starting a depression group, the group leader could share data on the average improvement from depression groups using findings from meta-analyses (e.g., Janis et al., 2021) as a means to instill hope. This practice can foster reasonable expectations of improvement.

Measures must be carefully selected to optimize consideration of these empirically researched constructs, thereby simultaneously providing the therapist with guidelines on what should be a focus for clinical attention. This entails selecting measures that cover the variables offering the greatest possibility of augmenting clinical judgment with evidence-based constructs. As part of this, the clinician must be aware of how evidence based-constructs are represented differently according to the measure being used. For example, the Group Climate Questionnaire (GCQ; MacKenzie, 1981) and Working Alliance Inventory (WAI; Horvath & Greenberg, 1989) are alike in the sense that they both measure alliance, yet there are important differences in the levels at which they measure alliance. In particular, the GCQ captures more group level data while the WAI assesses the client-therapist relationship (see Table 1.1). Therefore, combining them has some overlap, but the WAI captures content about the working alliance between members and the group leader(s), whereas the GCQ measures content related to group climate and group cohesion.

Group Therapy Evidence-Based Constructs: Levels of Analysis

As group leaders gather information through the process of MBC, there are various levels at which they can then evaluate the data: within-person, between-person, and between-group. This reflects how there are different ways of looking at clients as a clinician. For one, they may take note when one member has a relatively low score compared to scores they have shown historically (i.e., a within-person comparison). An example of this level of comparison is illustrated through Figure 1.1, which shows a group member (Mary) having her outcome tracked on a session-by-session basis using the Outcome Questionnaire-45.2 (OQ) (Lambert et al., 2013). As she completes the OQ, her scores naturally fluctuate from session to session. Ideally, her OQ scores will decrease over the course of the group, indicating a decrease in distress.

When these scores are averaged, she has a mean total OQ score of 59.2. A within-person analysis would explore those session-to-session differences that deviate from Maria's overall mean score of 59.2. As can be seen in Figure 1.1, Maria's score first drops to 62 but then increases at sessions three and four, indicating an increase in distress. It then begins to drop

Table 1.1 Group Process Measures and Process Component-Perspective Combinations

Measures	Bond Relationship Therapist	Bond Relationship Group	Working Relationship Therapist	Working Relationship Group	Negative Factors Therapist	Negative Factors Group
WAI						
Bond	✓					
Tasks			✓			
Goals			✓			
GCQ						
Engagement		✓				
Conflict				✓		
Avoidance						✓

Note: WAI = Working Alliance Inventory; GCQ = Group Climate Questionnaire

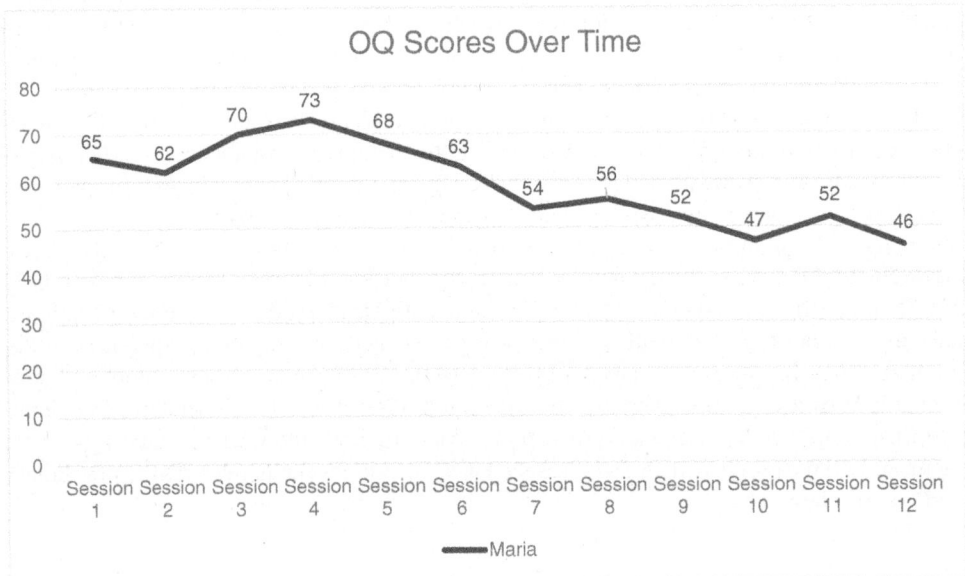

Figure 1.1 OQ Scores for Maria Over Time: Within-Person Difference

again at session five. Noticing this data, the group leader then must determine whether these changes are due to something happening within the therapy group, more to do with something occurring outside the therapy group (for example, a worsening romantic relationship) or both? Pairing this with process measures could also indicate whether these fluctuations may be connected to something happening in the group. For example, if process measures (not shown) demonstrated evidence of poor alliance, low cohesion and poor climate at sessions three, four and five, it might suggest a need for intervention that strengthened her relationships with both the group and group leaders.

It would also be possible to compare group members to one another—a between-person comparison. Like Maria, overall mean OQ scores could also be calculated for Jamal, Susan, Enrique, and Don, who also have their OQ scores tracked at each session (illustrated in Figure 1.2). When averaging their scores across individual group sessions, Jamal's average

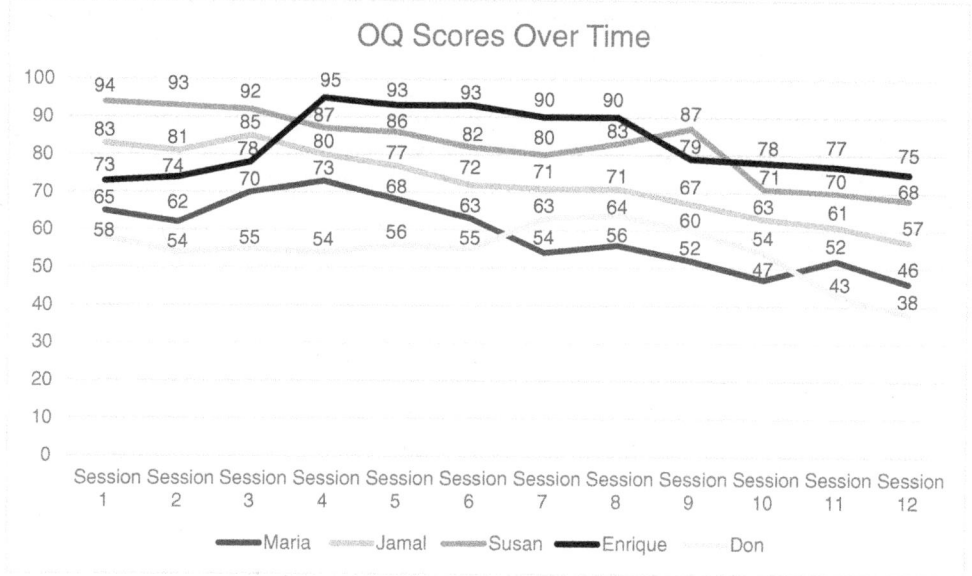

Figure 1.2 OQ Scores Over Time: Within-Group Difference

OQ score is 72.3, Susan's is 82.8, Enrique's is 82.9, and Don's is 54.5. A between-person analysis considers how Maria's overall mean score differs from these other group members' mean scores.

Traditionally, a between-person analysis comes from statistical modeling of group member means. However, we can take the underlying principle of comparing members and use it clinically by comparing members' session scores across time. An example of this can be seen from this graph. Maria starts out with lower distress in session one than Jamal, Enrique, or Susan and slightly higher distress than Don. However, early in the life of the group, Maria gets worse before she gets better, whereas Susan has a difficult week in week 9. Enrique shows the most concerning pattern, with a significant increase in distress between sessions 3 and 4 that remains at a high level before slowly coming down.

As the therapist takes note of these varying patterns among group members, they must determine if client worsening is due to the group, factors in the client's life, or some combination of those. This can be demonstrated through Enrique's pattern of scores. Certainly, the increase in Enrique's score at session 4 is worthy of clinical attention from the group leader and may increase the risk of dropout. Adding process measures can help clarify whether this is an alliance rupture or something outside of the group. For example, if the group is highly cohesive, they might give considerable solace and support in navigating through what appears to be a crisis in his life. However, this also depends on whether Enrique discloses and receives the help he needs. Group members will not always make clear to the group or to the leaders that they are in distress. Sometimes this is due to factors related to interpersonal style (e.g., social inhibition and difficulties in sharing or conversely a style marked by high assertiveness and an unwillingness to show "weakness"). In other cases, factors such as a lack of time (a critical incident occurring toward the end of the group or the focus being on other members) can lead to similar unexpressed distress. Given the possibility of Enrique not disclosing, MBC can help the therapist become aware of increases in distress that Enrique may not otherwise make explicit. Indeed, Chapman et al. (2012) found that group therapists were unable to accurately predict treatment deterioration.

In an alternative scenario, the change in scores is accompanied by a reduction in Enrique's experience of cohesion and alliance, reflecting a rupture with the group which he perceived the group leader not protecting him from. MBC helps to make this explicit, as group therapists also tend to be poor predictors of how clients perceive the group relationship (Chapman et al., 2012). The assessments provide information about significant events that can add to clinical judgment and suggest interventions. If it were to be shown to be related to a rupture, the leader then has an opportunity to repair this in future sessions.

This level of analysis is useful insofar as it allows understanding of growth within a group dynamic. If the whole group is progressing and one member is not, that suggests a different intervention than if the group as a whole is not progressing as expected. One client's scores relative to other clients' scores can inform interventions by helping the therapist understand an individual within a group dynamic. Therefore, the scores of one client relative to another are important to understanding client outcomes.

Lastly, between-group analyses allow the leader to compare group performance from one group to another. In this instance, the leader becomes a local clinical scientist, whereby they can clinically compare the performance of one group to another group. For example, a leader may use all group members' scores to calculate an average OQ score for the group as-a-whole. Then, the group leader can compare this average score to the scores of other groups that they have led.

As a note, the concepts of within-person, between-person, and between-group comparisons are also relevant in the research literature, with researchers having the ability to statistically assess outcomes at different levels. The level of analysis is important to consider, with research showing that the type of comparison can have an influence on the results. As an example, Arnold et al. (2022) tested the relationship of client outcome with alliance, cohesion, and climate at all three levels: within-person, between-person, and between-group. *Cohesion and climate consistently showed significant relationships with outcome at all three levels.* This adds further evidence to support the need to *focus on common mechanisms of change in group*s such as the working alliance and group cohesion.

Foundational Concepts to Measurement-Based Care

Much of the value of Measurement-Based Care (MBC) lies in its ability to show client change. *Change scores* are the currency of outcome evaluation. How a client improves from admission to discharge is the goal of any treatment and in most (but not all) clinical cases this can be captured with pre-post assessment of change. However, the trajectory of change scores can be impacted by a number of factors, such as:

- initial severity of the diagnosis
- chronicity of the diagnosis
- prognosis based on complexity or external factors
- the typical change pathway of a specific diagnosis
- effectiveness of the treatment
- the skill of the practitioner

and many other factors. Change in outcome can be assessed in several ways. These include reliable change indices, cut scores, and clinical significance. We will now address each of these methods in turn.

Reliable Change Index

Reliable change indices (RCI) (Jacobson & Truax, 1991) are a commonly used metric that statistically classifies significant *client-level change* into one of three categories—improved, no change, or deteriorated. This index of change that is created through the RCI method is sensitive to and accounts for measurement error along with normal variability in symptoms over time. Analytic tools and online calculators can significantly ease the clinician burden in conducting such analyses. This method allows for greater understanding of client change at different levels. At the individual level it is possible to see how a single client improved. For a therapy group it is possible to see how all the members progressed. The advantage of this system of measurement is that it allows a therapist to simultaneously monitor both individual clients and the group together. It can also provide summative data at the end of the year.

For example:

Table 1.2 Reliable Change Indices Among Group Members

Client	Pre	Post	Difference score	RCI*	RCI Change Category
Joe	76	57	19	-5.82	Improved
Mikayla	71	67	4	-1.23	No change
Lang	67	47	20	-6.14	Improved
Sarah	76	83	7	2.15	Deterioration
Eden	73	70	3	-0.92	No change

Note: *RCI = Reliable Change Index

As can be seen from Table 1.2 (using de-identified data and names), Joe and Lang showed positive change from pre and post and met criteria for reliable change (as can be seen from the Reliable Change Scores). Eden and Mikalya showed no reliable change. Sarah deteriorated. That is, her scores went from bad to worse and the amount of that change was reliable. This is consistent with research using RCI's—a percentage of clients will deteriorate and measuring that allows for the possibility of reengaging the client around continuity of care.

Another way of representing these scores would be to show them as percentages. For example, for this group:

Table 1.3 Change Among Group Members

	Improved	No change	Deterioration
Number of clients who changed (and percentage)	2 (40%)	2 (40%)	1 (20%)

As can be seen from this example in Table 1.3, the small sample size (n=5) must be taken into account when assessing success or failure. For this group, one person deteriorating represents 20 percent of the total group, whereas if only one person deteriorated in a group of ten people, then it would represent 10 percent deterioration. Thus, it is important to assess scores individually and as a group and to consider this in relation to the size of the group overall. Percentages must take into account the number of people in the group overall.

These patterns of reliable improvement and deterioration are important feedback for therapists, providing sufficient care is taken to analyze the data. This gives the therapist an opportunity to reflect on whether their clinical judgment is accurate (for both clinical successes and clinical failures) while providing a means to explore more deeply what may have worked or not worked with a client. In other words, these results become a starting point for therapist reflection and an opportunity to consider how to grow and learn from the experience, whether that was from the positive outcomes or those that showed deterioration.

Cut Scores

Another way to measure client change is through the use of a *cut score*. A cut score is a line that signifies the difference between one type of population or level of wellness and another. Jacobson and Truax's (1991) original formulation had a cut score that distinguished between a "dysfunctional" population and a "functional" population. They acknowledged that there would be some overlap between these two populations since the cut score reflected the 50th percentile between the means of the two populations. Its application with different measures might include more than two populations (e.g., inpatient, outpatient, normal), but Figure 1.3 depicts the original formulation. Cut scores provide valuable information regarding how a client's level of functioning changes over the course of treatment, which can add information to clinical decision making. However, they should not be used to replace clinical judgment or to make decisions about level of care. They serve as a data point that can add to an overall clinical picture but that in some cases may be misleading about a specific case. Cut scores are a useful approximation but still represent a "best guess" of level of care and therefore should be used judiciously and with care to identify those who do not fit neatly into categories.

Clinical Significance

Cut scores not only provide information about the client's current functioning, but they can also be used to determine whether a score change is clinically significant. In Jacobson and Truax's (1991) original formulation, clinically significant change required a client's score to move from one population (e.g., clinical) to another population (e.g., normal), thereby crossing the cut score.

In addition, clinically significant change also required the change score to meet or exceed the reliable change index. Thus, a client moved from one population to another and showed reliable change.

To properly understand these figures requires an understanding of how test developers set levels of statistical significance and also where the cut scores fall. Programs with analytics sometimes provide this as part of their output. In this book we also indicate whether analytics are a part of the assessment tool and what output they provide.

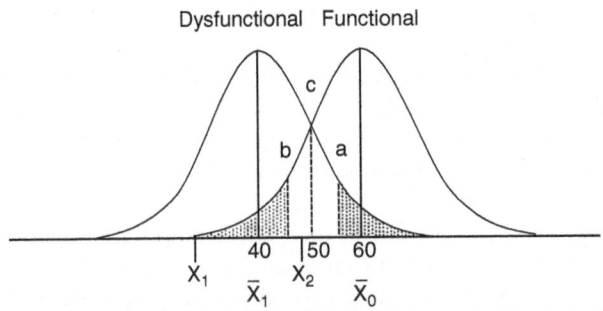

Note: This figure is modified from Jacobson and Truax (1991).

Figure 1.3 Jacobson and Truax (1991) Clinically Significant Change

Evaluating a Practice or Program

Measurement can also be applied to programs as a way of providing feedback for the purposes of supervision, consultation and quality improvement while also serving to address the oversight of stakeholders. Stakeholders might range from management at a hospital to third party payers such as insurers who are seeking to create accountability and to ensure programing is high quality. To be useful and to allow for accurate benchmarking later, the process of evaluating a practice can only take place using reliable and valid tools that are sensitive to change and normed against the population of interest; otherwise, results are likely to be flawed at best and highly misleading at worst.

The above terms can be very helpful in program evaluation. In terms of *reliable change indices*, it is possible to aggregate scores to see how all groups combined performed or how all cases at an agency or practice changed. For example, a practice might show that at the end of the year, 50 percent of clients statistically improved, 35 percent showed no significant change, and 15 percent deteriorated. These figures can then be compared against benchmarks to determine if this is acceptable performance as an agency or for an individual practice.

When conducting continuous quality improvement (involving running a program, learning from successes and failures, modifying and then retrying) and program evaluation, there are other important metrics to consider that do not fall into the realm of the chapters outlined in this book. However, they are no less important. Benchmarking and attendance are crucial to any efforts to develop high quality group programming within an agency. Patient satisfaction is also an important consideration.

Benchmarking

A common request from those engaged in program evaluation is how their change profile compares to similar clinical populations and settings? For instance, a community mental health center program for children and adolescents may wonder if their aggregate change profile matches similar agencies. One child and adolescent outcome measure (Youth-Outcome Questionnaire (Y-OQ) (Burlingame et al., 2022) provides the average intake and posttreatment scores that have been reported by studies performed in community mental health centers (see Table 1.4). When combining data from multiple studies, the overall average Y-OQ intake score is 78.62 and the average posttreatment score is 56.18. Table 1.4 also provides data on the percentage of clients in community mental health centers who recover, reliably improve, show no change, and deteriorate on average. This enables a community mental health agency using the Y-OQ to compare their change profile with published benchmarks.

Benchmarking against realistic outcomes is important for program evaluation. Without an understanding of normal dropout rates, typical levels of client improving or worsening and expected outcomes based on treatment dosage, clinicians can end up in 'apples to oranges' comparisons as they compare the clinical populations they treat to different populations (e.g., comparing client outcomes in a university counseling center to outcomes in a residential facility, which may have very different types of clients). There are also differences within and between settings based on the variables of interest.

Altogether, the benefits of benchmarking are clear. However, benchmarking is a difficult undertaking and is currently far from exact. Some methods involve proprietary information while others like the YOQ example above used published information. It is also important to note that benchmarks also vary by setting and are impacted by initial severity. Therefore, care should be taken when interpreting. Benchmarking is in its infancy in the USA and

Table 1.4 YOQ Community Mental Health Center Benchmarking

Community Mental Health Center Sample

Name	N	Intake		Posttreatment		RCI Data (%)			
		$\bar{x}$	SD	$\bar{x}$	SD	Recovered	Reliable Improvement	No Change	Deteriorated
Dunham (2010)	91	61.0	39.7	40.9	32.6		59.4%		
Henderson (2013)	407	70.6	34.3	59.6					
McClendon (2009)	134	91.7	29.7			14.7%	39.7%	30.2%	15.4%
Packard (2020)	339	87.8	35.5						
Salisbury (2015)	138					50%		32%	18%
Warren (2010)	936					16.8%	27.5%	31.6%	24.1%
Total N/Mean	**2045**	**78.62**	**34.68**	**56.18**	**32.6**	**16.5%**	**31.4%**	**31.5%**	**22.4%**

Note: This is drawn exactly from Burlingame et al. (2022). Permission to reuse will be needed from Outcome Measures.

currently relies either on the instrument developers to have determined their own bench-marks or on practitioners to find equivalent settings with which to compare. Currently, this only exists in piecemeal form but is a logical next step if systems and smaller practices are to understand and contextualize their performance relative to their peers.

Patient Satisfaction

Patient satisfaction is an important metric in USA health care as it is a measured carefully by hospital systems and reported on to regulators as part of their checks on quality. Yet few systems measure patient satisfaction in *mental* health. There are many explanations for this, ranging from mistaken beliefs that people with mental health issues may not be able to accurately report their own satisfaction, to the possibility that administrators in larger health systems may be worried that poor patient satisfaction scores in mental health (reflecting poor quality of care after years of neglect and siloing) might bring down their system scores overall. For inpatient and outpatient units that are part of large hospital systems to be brought into the light of accountability, patient satisfaction needs to be a part of the measurement strategy.

However, the evidence is mixed for the relevance of patient satisfaction to quality of care. For example, research by Aimola et al. (2019) suggested that although patient satisfaction was somewhat important, self-reported patient outcome was more relevant to measures of overall quality of care. Certainly, more detailed and nuanced research is needed to under-stand the meaning of patient satisfaction and to determine its causes and correlates. None-theless, it will remain the lingua franca of hospital systems for the foreseeable future and, as such, needs attention from clinicians and researchers alike. Since group therapy appears most frequently in hospitals and agencies, this is of particular importance to the field. Patient satisfaction measures are also addressed in Chapter 4 on outcomes.

Attendance

The inclusion of how to measure attendance is an extremely important one. The difference between those who a program or model has *intent to treat* compared to who actually *completes* treatment is a vital data point to determine the success of therapy and therapy programs. Intent to treat can mean different things based upon the setting. For example, if an inpa-tient setting has twenty patients and only 50 percent of them ever show up for therapy, then this reporting of attendance is based on potential treatable clients in the setting. This can be an important metric for those overseeing therapeutic services, since *the efficacy of any treatment is only potent if patients actually engage in it.*

However, this is a slightly different problem than if a group leader accepts ten people into an outpatient treatment group and only eight people show up on the first day. Thus, how attendance is counted is an important metric with considerable nuance and implica-tions for training. For example, if referrals to a group screening session have very low follow through then this suggests a need for in-house training on how to make an effective referral. If clients are making it to the screening and are accepted into the group but have low rates for starting to attend, then that suggests more training is needed on how to build a strong working alliance during the screening/pre-group preparation session. If clients drop out once the group has started then more attention needs to be paid to leadership skills in developing cohesion, managing alliance ruptures and other variables that can lead to pre-mature dropout.

The question of what constitutes premature treatment dropout is clinically important. What constitutes premature dropout is a complex formula that requires: (1) an assessment of dose-effect for that therapy; (2) the expected mechanisms of change and where those mechanisms occur in the therapy; (3) how and why the client leaves; and (4) whether they experienced the therapy as successful. We suggest the formula proposed by O'Keeffe et al. (2019) who noted that the most widely used measure of dropout is based on the *therapists' judgment* that the client ended treatment *prematurely and without the agreement of the therapist*. However, this presupposes a combination of clinical judgment and awareness of the literature regarding dose-effect, typical treatment pathways and benchmarking for that specific population.

Logistics of Assessing Outcome

It is also important to consider the *logistics* of scoring. These can impact the degree of success a program has in translating scores into usable data. Recent research has been undertaken on the use of online systems to do so. Naturally, clinicians who are hoping to implement MBC within their practice may have concerns about the ease of doing so. However, advancements in technology have made it possible to rely on online systems to largely manage outcome measurement. Using technology for the purposes of collecting, scoring, and interpreting data has a number of benefits. Gual-Montolio et al. (2020) note that using information and communication technologies (ICT) makes it possible for therapists to "evaluate and receive patient progress feedback in real time, thus minimizing patient recall bias" and obtain "objective data of patient changes in natural settings" (p. 2). In reviewing how ICT is used for MBC, Gual-Montolio et al. conclude that such practices are feasible and acceptable. Furthermore, they report that "technology in MBC was found to be effective and cost-effective, particularly for not-on-track patients" (p. 18). However, while technology is a wonderful tool that can allay the burden of tracking and scoring outcome measures, clinicians should also be willing to consider hand-scored measures, especially in instances where desirable measures are not available in an online format or when costs are prohibitive for practitioners. When reading the other chapters in this book, it is important to consider which instruments can be administered online and which have analytics that can translate the results. This can be a powerful time-saving device that can prove helpful in helping the therapist manage their time effectively.

Drawbacks of Self-Report Assessments

In assessing outcome, clinicians should be aware of differing options and their associated concerns. Hill et al. (2013) provide a thorough review of outcome measurement and explore some of these options, such as self-report. Self-report questionnaires constitute a large portion of outcome measurement tools. However, Hill et al. identify a number of concerns and challenges related to the use of self-report measures. Clients may respond differently to questionnaires depending on the context (e.g., after experiencing therapy and coming to understand questions differently), meaning that changes in scores may not truly reflect actual psychological change. Yet another challenge is that clients may respond defensively on questionnaires, leading to inaccurate reporting of symptoms. It is also important to be wary of "faking good" and "faking bad" motivations, which can lead to a client intentionally responding in a way that suggests better or worse functioning than is true for them. For instance, patients who are involuntarily hospitalized may be motivated to "fake good" to convince their treatment team that they are ready for discharge. In all, clinicians should be aware of the limitations of self-report measures and always use clinical judgment rather than take questionnaire results at face value. As an example, a common medical practice is for the doctor to ask their patients to rate their pain on a 1 to 10 scale. These ratings suffer from the same limitations of self-report (i.e., they are subjective), but are still commonly used in medical practice.

Hill et al. (2013) additionally consider the use of qualitative versus quantitative methods of assessing psychotherapy outcome. As the above paragraph demonstrates, there are considerable issues with quantitative methods. Qualitative methods are able to offer a number of benefits, with Hill et al. explaining:

> "With a qualitative approach, participants are not constrained by predetermined items on a specific measure that may or may not relate to them personally, but rather can respond in a way that allows them to reflect deeply about their experiences."
>
> (p. 72)

They highlight how qualitative methods provide a greater view of context, multiple realities, and unique perspectives. Hill et al. state that ideal study "combines both quantitative and qualitative methods (p. 68)"; they emphasize how such a "multimethod, multi-perspective approach" could "paint a rich picture of outcome, being aware that different measures provide different answers to the outcome question" (p. 75). This can also apply to clinicians. A mixture of qualitative and quantitative items can illuminate both underlying constructs while also capturing nuance and client experience.

Working within a Multicultural Framework

In using routine measurement, it is essential to thoughtfully and sensitively consider how to work effectively within a multicultural framework and engage in cross-cultural assessment. At a national level, therapists in the USA should be sensitive to cultural differences as well as systemic racism that plays out in therapy, with a disproportionate number of therapists and other mental health gatekeepers being white and with white individuals holding a large amount of influence, resources, and power. Further, on a larger scale, international accountability for outcomes is rapidly becoming a movement within both health care and psychotherapy. Panels such as the International Consortium of Health Outcomes Measurement are emerging to recommend instruments (Krause et al., 2021) and this trend is rapidly disseminating throughout the world. MBC is also proving effective in cultures other than the USA. Studies (e.g., Guo et al., 2015; Burgess et al., 2015) are increasingly showing that the utility of MBC is universal. Thus, the need for competence to work within a multicultural framework is becoming clear.

Cultural Attitudes Towards Assessment

One aspect of working effectively within a multicultural framework involves being sensitive to cultural attitudes towards assessment, with attitudes potentially differing both between and within cultures. In the USA, some clients may complain about assessment that is not immediately used and they may balk at the idea of homework. However, as Chapter 5 points out, some other cultures value the addition of instruments, seeing it as adding value for their money and therefore a good use of time. Other cultures may reject the notion of assessment altogether, and when this is the case, it is beholden to the therapist to approach this with cultural humility and to seek to learn why (Hook et al., 2017). Therefore, when using MBC in therapy, clinicians should consider cultural background and beliefs about what therapy is and is not, and about the role of assessment. This can in turn shape their approach to measurement, including how many measures they use and how they introduce MBC to their clients.

Cultural Appropriateness of Instruments

In addition to being sensitive to cultural views on assessment, it is also essential to be attentive to the cultural appropriateness of the instruments being used. This involves becoming familiar with psychometrics and norm populations, and then using that knowledge to inform instrument selection, administration, and scoring. The Association for Specialists in Group Work (ASGW) (Bennett et al., 2021) recently published recent standards of care for assessment in group work, in which they note that therapists should be "...aware of the assessments' norm population and that results may be skewed or biased toward the population with which the instrument was normed, and therefore score results with caution" (p. 241). In an ideal situation, all measures should be tested for validity, reliability, and sensitivity to change and should be normed against the population being studied. Being aware of the demographics within the norm group allows the therapist to evaluate whether the instrument is sufficiently generalizable to norm groups other than the majority. Unfortunately, this is seldom easy to determine, since few instruments are clear about the demographic qualities of the norm group. Further, even if they do report demographics, it can be unclear whether particular aspects of clients' intersectional identities are represented. Some items or even whole measures may be invalid for certain clients if they are not properly attuned to the client's cultural background. For example, a client identifying as Latinx woman who immigrated from Central America and has English as a second language might have different responses to the same instrument than a Mexican-American woman from Los Angeles with English as a first language. Thus, even the notation on an assessment tool that "Hispanic" or Latinx" is included as part of the population norm group does not guarantee the validity of the instrument or specific items within it.

Therefore, until researchers are able to cross-validate, refine and test measures in each culture, practitioners should carefully weigh the cost-benefit analysis of utilizing existing instruments when psychometric and demographic data is unavailable. Appraisal, selection and modification of instruments should be conducted thoughtfully, considering the impact of either changing or not changing items and with clear understanding of the potential impact on the clinical usefulness and reliability of outcomes.

Notably, there is limited utility in understanding instrument norms and psychometrics when the clinician is unfamiliar with the cultural background of their clients. Thus, when becoming familiar with psychometric and demographic properties of measures, it is important for therapists to inquire about a client's self-reported most salient, multiple identities and then use that knowledge to assess instrument appropriateness. For example, the Group Therapy Questionnaire-Short Form (GTQ-S) group screening tool has been revised and now states:

> "Are there any aspects of your identity that you would like to share with the group, or that might be challenging to discuss/explore? Aspects of identity that might be discussed include race, ethnicity, language, nationality, sex, gender identity, sexual orientation, religion, ability, and socioeconomic status."

> (MacNair-Semands, 2014)

Questions such as this are essential to include in *any* assessment battery. *We recommend the use of this, or an equivalent question, as an essential part of screening and pre-group assessment.* Such questions help therapists to be aware at the outset of important cultural identities that their clients might have and might want to talk about. Further, such questions can act as a to signal to clients with minoritized identities that the group leader is willing and able to address issues of culture. Without this data, the therapist risks missing out on important variables that could impact not only the relationship between client and therapist but also the validity of items or the entire measure.

Other concepts that are pertinent to cultural appropriateness include Cultural bias, Comprehension bias, and Translation bias (the CCT procedure), which were each identified by Bader et al. (2021) as three potential sources of problems in using assessment tools in different cultures. Cultural bias, sometimes referred to as measurement invariance or measurement equivalence, relates to the possibility that a construct or variable of interest may change in small or large ways depending on the culture. Important differences may exist in cultural definitions or meanings of a psychological construct, making measurement of that construct more complex. While in some cases, there may be extreme examples where a construct is completely invalid, in many cases, the cross-cultural generalizability is more nuanced. For example, researchers (Benitez et al., 2019) looked for bias in the General Health Questionnaire (GHQ-12) (Goldberg & Hillier, 1979), a World Health Organization assessment of global functioning, using a Spanish speaking sample from different backgrounds (European Spanish speaking compared to Central/South American). They found some differences on items related to questions about feelings and on items that were double-barreled (i.e., questions involving two issues but only allowing for one answer). Most of the items were valid across cultures, but several items were not. Interestingly, they found that items that had a negative valence or spoke about feelings ("…feeling depressed") did not hold up as well. They cautioned that anyone using the instrument cross-culturally should be cautious in using it to compare cross-cultural groups since those specific items may not be valid for some of those groups. Chin et al. (2015) also found some issues with the measure with a Malaysian population, finding that the Chinese version tended to underestimate symptom severity. Since the measure is a screener for psychological distress, it would therefore need significant modification and re-norming, per the authors' recommendations. Therefore, item analysis and how it relates to the reliability and validity of scoring is an important part of cross-cultural assessment.

Other types of bias include translation bias and comprehension bias. If an instrument is incorrectly translated, nuances of meaning can be missed. Accurate translation processes involve not only an initial translation but also a back translation. Back translation involves the first translator completing the initial translation (for example from English to Spanish) and then another translator must translate the measure back into the language it was first created in (From Spanish back to English) to see if the translation still captures the original meaning.

Meanwhile, comprehension bias involves determining whether the local test-taker truly comprehends what the item or items are asking for from the respondent. For example, if a respondent does not understand what "depressed" means, since this is a culturally informed concept, then responding to the question may yield results that deviate from the expectations of the instrument when constructed.

To mitigate the effects of cultural bias, translation bias, and comprehension bias, it is helpful to communicate to clients about how they understand items; this builds upon the notion that assessment informs but does not replace clinical judgment, with the idea that clinical judgment includes multicultural and cross-cultural discussions to better understand the client's system of meanings. This is particularly important with items that may have poorer cross-cultural generalizability. The clinician must be thoughtful about how they interpret overall results in light of those items potentially being invalid. Further, they must consult and collaborate with the client to develop an understanding of their idiographic meanings. Chapter 5 addresses how this worked in Singapore when adapting instruments to fit that culture.

As a final note on the importance of determining instrument appropriateness, clinicians should be aware of how cultural appropriateness can engender stronger alliance. The working alliance's three components: (i.e., bond to the therapist, goal agreement and task agreement; Castonguay et al., 2006) are enhanced only when there is a good fit between the choice of instrument, client readiness, cultural appropriateness and how assessment is used thoughtfully to enhance each aspect. For example, a client may experience a greater *bond* from being invited to discuss their intersectional identity variables, feel a heightened sense of *goal agreement* from an instrument that measures a variable they feel is important to them (e.g., perfectionism), and sense *task agreement* when the therapist explains what is expected of them in group and they feel it is realistic and achievable. However, as they do this, it will be important that they use measures that are culturally appropriate.

In all, working within a multicultural framework necessitates effort on the part of the clinician to be sensitive to the cultural appropriateness of instruments, which should then shape instrument selection, administration, and scoring. This can ensure that the measures used are valid and can aid in the development of alliance. Instrument selection must strike a balance between being cautious about what interpretations are possible and being sensitive to the possible clinical benefits of its use. Clinicians must avail themselves of the current literature and be cautious when using instruments cross-culturally, making sure that they understand (1) which specific items are generalizable and which are not; and (2) what the impact might be on the results. Since these findings will be used in therapy, it may prove to be important to discuss the meanings the client ascribes to certain items, so that any clinical inferences are accurate.

Clinician Knowledge and Learning

When engaging in MBC, another multicultural consideration pertains to the clinician's own knowledge and thoughtfulness, with a need to be conscious of cultural variables and to engage in a continued process of learning. The ASGW assessment document (Bennett et al., 2021) makes the case that when interpreting, the therapist must "consider other contextual variables (e.g., culture, society, identities) that may influence assessment results" (p. 76). In many cases, therapists are unaware of what they do not know in terms of data about cultural groups. Thus, Ridley et al. (2000) note that they must always be working to increase their knowledge of nomothetic data (what we can know about different cultures) while also pursuing idiographic understanding (how does this particular client experience their own multiple identities). The therapist must be in a constant process of learning about culture and also remaining open minded to how the client experiences themselves and their relationship to identity variables and wider cultures. This process of learning can help protect against issues of intolerance, prejudice and inequity that can be detrimental to the assessment process. This can prevent issues such as systematic bias in interpretation of assessments, therapists over-diagnosing or over-pathologizing, and errors of understanding about a cultural variable that can lead to therapeutic decision-making mistakes with deleterious outcomes.

As previously discussed, clinicians must be careful to elicit information that is nuanced and comprehensive. Collaboratively seeking to understand a client's history, meanings, intersectional identities and relationships to power and privilege can provide a more complex and layered view of the client while strengthening the alliance. In doing so, this can protect against the therapist relying on stereotypes and categorization as the sole lens through which to view the client. Therefore, this can also help protect against the influence of stereotyping, which is connected to the stigmatization and devaluing of identities (Remedios & Snyder, 2018). To discover the nuances requires using the assessment tool as a starting point to discuss, ask further questions, and work with the client to gain a full understanding of their multiple, intersectional identities. This necessitates the implementation of clinical judgment and

1) the ability to listen to the client; 2) ask elaborative questions; and 3) invite discussion and to be prepared to learn from the client with genuine cultural humility (Hook et al., 2017).

Language Considerations

Lastly, working within a multicultural framework entails efforts to communicate in culturally sensitive ways. The ASGW document on assessment with a sociocultural focus (Bennett et al., 2021) states that group leaders should "use person-first, culturally-sensitive, and non-stigmatizing language (see Goodrich et al., 2017; Singh et al., 2012)" (p. 77). The working alliance can fail to form, or be ruptured by difficulties arising from clients feeling unheard, disrespected or misunderstood, and thus language should be used carefully when collaboratively working on administering, scoring, reporting back on and collaborating on assessment.

In all, it is ethically necessary for practitioners to be attentive to multicultural issues when engaging in MBC. This includes (but is not limited to) being aware of cultural attitudes toward assessment, understanding instrument appropriateness as it pertains to various cultural groups, engaging in continued efforts to learn about cultures, being cautious of bias, considering different variables that may influence results, and using non-stigmatizing language. Chapters throughout this book will discuss the implications for diversity awareness and measurement in detail, relative to the purpose of that assessment. Chapter 3 will also spend significant time discussing the implications of diversity for both leadership and cross-cultural dialogue groups.

Leadership

The impact of multicultural awareness on implementation of assessment in therapy has also been accompanied by an increase in the focus on group therapy leadership attributes. Implementation of evidence-based models and evidence-based practices of group therapy is only as effective as the skill of the leader. As several chapters discuss, measures are now available, such as the Group Leader Self-Assessment (GLSA) (Barnes et al., 2017), that provide insight into group leadership skills and capacities. The need for leaders to develop attitudes, skills and techniques in working with diverse groups is also a new focus in the literature and is reflected throughout this book.

Structure of the Book

This text has been divided into sections covering three main types of group therapy assessment and a final chapter giving more elaborated case examples. These chapters mirror the structure of the CORE-R as they are divided into sections on selection and pre-group preparation, process measures and outcome measures. Joyce and Marmarosh first discuss how to integrate selection and pre-group preparation materials to facilitate focus on inclusion and exclusion criteria while promoting the working alliance. Strauss, Miles, and Greene then discuss the importance of process, including evaluation of leadership skills and diversity awareness. Kivlighan and Tasca then consider outcomes, broadening the criteria to include not only international measures but also consideration of commonly used instruments that are becoming increasingly utilized in health care. Finally, Hewitt and Liew illustrate how measures can be combined. Using examples of implementing different models within two distinctly different international regions and cultures—Canada and Singapore— they explore how assessment can be used as MBC while also serving as program evaluation within a multiculturally and transculturally sensitive framework.

Multipurpose Assessments

In terms of the structure of this book, it is also important to understand that although we have divided this text into chapters organized by assessment type, some assessments could fit into several chapters, depending on how they are used. This particularly applies to measures of attachment and interpersonal style, which might be used to help understand screening and pregroup preparation issues, group process and outcome. For example, the IIP-32 (Horowitz et al., 2000) could be used to help screen for interpersonal distress types that may be predictive of early self-sabotage (which would be helpful in screening and pregroup preparation in chapter two) as well as to predict into how members might interact with each other in the group dynamic (a part of chapter three), while also serving to measure interpersonal outcomes pre-post (something that would be germane to chapter four on outcomes). Therefore, it may be that some instruments can function in multipurpose ways.

Value to a Society: National and International Trends toward Accountability

As can be seen from this chapter, there are many reasons to consider using assessment tools in group therapy. Many of the reasons given were related to the leader needing to consider the therapeutic value of integrating MBC into care. However, the need to utilize assessment in therapy is also driven by *external forces*, and in particular current national and international trends in healthcare finance toward greater accountability. Across the globe, health care costs continue to rise, and as a result countries are focused on providers who successfully manage costs while providing superior health outcomes (Rosen et al., 2012). Thus, nations are becoming more attentive to the need for cost-efficient treatment that provides improvements in population health (Porter & Teisberg, 2006). To show improvement, governments are increasingly seeking greater accountability from health care providers (see Burgess et al., 2015). This requires documentation of evidence of changes in conditions, which means *measurement* becomes crucially important.

Several countries are currently engaging in efforts to increase accountability for mental health outcomes. In Australia, the government has already moved toward greater accountability and outcome assessment for mental health as a national policy (Burgess et al., 2015). Equally, the English National Institute for Health and Care Excellence (NICE) model also targets outcomes under its Quality and Outcomes Framework (McCrady, 2013), seeking to reward good performance and ensure evidence-based practices are taking place, while tracking clinical outcomes and indicators. In England, assessment of therapy outcome is *required* and evaluation is conducted every session. Meanwhile, the USA is also engaging in efforts to promote more consistent implementation of measurement informed care, with a push to shift from *fee-for-service* (i.e., being paid for every visit and insurance companies regulating and restricting access) to *value-based care* in which providers are incentivized to improve outcomes for patients by tying specific outcomes to increased payment (Bao et al., 2017).

This value-based care payment system for physical health is still under development in the USA and remains only partially implemented in health care systems. *Mental* health accountability has thus far moved slowly, with data suggesting that less than 20 percent of practitioners currently utilize therapy assessment in the USA (Lewis et al., 2019) and only around 30 percent of agencies use outcome assessments for their groups (Whittingham & Arlo, 2019). However, there is now increasing attention being paid toward mental health and value-based payment. For example, in Patient-Centered Medical Homes (i.e., a type of primary care doctor's office) physicians are required to prove reductions in depression based on assessment tools (Bogucki et al., 2020). Equally, the Joint Commission, the main regulatory body for USA hospitals, now requires inpatient psychiatric units to administer outcome measures that capture change throughout treatment. A recent rule (CTS-03.01.09) now mandates three steps for those under its regulatory aegis, namely 1) using standardized instruments chosen from their list of approved measures; 2) requiring analysis of the data to inform treatment objectives and goals; and 3) assessing outcomes (see Outcome Measures Standard for Behavioral Health Accreditation | The Joint Commission). As can be seen this requires three pillars of assessment that will feature throughout this book: 1) selection of valid measures; 2) integration of those measures to enhance treatment; and 3) measurement of outcomes. In 2019 the US government also opened the Merit-based Incentive Payment System (MIPS) system to psychologists and mental health providers (American Psychological Association, 2019). This system provides enhanced payment for clinicians who can show clinical improvement on clinical and outcome measures and reduced payment for those underperforming on those metrics. Although this program is currently one that practitioners only opt-in to, this may represent an initial testing of the waters by The Centers for Medicare and Medicaid Services (CMS) to promote accountability for outcomes.

In all, the movement toward measuring client progress is one that is inexorably moving forward in the USA. While it remains short of its full potential, this movement toward implementation of assessment in therapy has significantly increased since the last edition of this text. The inevitability of what will become a requirement for payment for therapeutic services is likely to dramatically change the field's stance toward assessment over time, requiring therapists to become conversant with the nomenclature and practice of integrating assessment into treatment. It will also require practitioners to become adept at considering the logic behind selection of measures and choice of measurement strategy.

Conclusion

Measurement in group therapy is becoming increasingly relevant to clinical practice. Whether it is being used to promote accountability and to aid supervision, as measurement-based care to enhance clinical judgment in real time, or both, it is clear that is adds considerably to the quality of clinical practice. Screening and pregroup preparation, process and outcome measures can all be used to enhance but not replace clinical judgment. Equally, clinicians can now find added value in measures that help assess group leadership skills and multicultural skills and attitudes.

References

Aimola, L., Gordon-Brown, J., Etherington, A., Zalewska, K., Cooper, S., & Crawford, M. J. (2019). Patient-reported experience and quality of care for people with schizophrenia. *BMC Psychiatry*, 19 (1), 1–6. doi:10.1186/s12888-018-1998-y.

Alldredge, C. T., Burlingame, G. M., Yang, C., & Rosendahl, J. (2021). Alliance in group therapy: A meta-analysis. *Group Dynamics: Theory, Research, and Practice*, 25(1), 13–28. doi:10.1037/gdn0000135.

American Psychological Association. (2019, January 10). CMS adds psychologists to the Merit-based Incentive Payment System: What psychologists need to know about Medicare's new reimbursement program. www.apaservices.org/practice/reimbursement/government/cms-psychologists-system.

Arnold, R. A., Burlingame, G. M., & Olsen, J. A. (2022). The relationship of alliance, cohesion, and climate with outcome among college counseling populations. *Journal of Counseling Psychology*. Advance online publication. doi:10.1037/cou0000613.

Bader, M., Jobst, L. J., Zettler, I., Hilbig, B. E., & Moshagen, M. (2021). Disentangling the effects of culture and language on measurement non-invariance in cross-cultural research: The culture, comprehension, and translation bias (CCT) procedure. *Psychological Assessment*, 33(5), 375–384. doi:10.1037/pas0000989.

Bao, Y., McGuire, T. G., Chan, Y. F., Eggman, A. A., Ryan, A. M., Bruce, M. L., Pincus, H. A., Hafer, E., & Unützer, J. (2017). Value-based payment in implementing evidence-based care: the Mental Health Integration Program in Washington state. *The American Journal of Managed Care*, 23(1), 48–53. www.ncbi.nlm.nih.gov/pmc/articles/PMC5559616.

Barkham, M. (2016). Patient-centered assessment in psychotherapy: toward a greater bandwidth of evidence. *Clinical Psychology: Science and Practice*, 23(3), 284–287. doi:10.1111/cpsp.12163.

Barkham, M., Lutz, W., & Castonguay, L. G. (Eds). (2021). *Bergin and Garfield's handbook of psychotherapy and behavior change* (7th ed.). John Wiley & Sons.

Barnes, M. A., Marfeo, E., Schwartzberg, S. L., & Bedell, G. (2017). Group Leader Self-Assessment (GLSA): Reliability and Validity. *The American Journal of Occupational Therapy*, 71(4, Supplement 1), 7111500016p1–7111500016p1.

Beecher, M. E. (2008). A clinician's take on evidence-based group psychotherapy: a commentary. *Journal of Clinical Psychology*, 64(11), 1279–1283. doi:10.1002/jclp.20530.

Benitez, I., Adams, B. G., & He, J. (2019). An integrated approach to bias in a longitudinal survey in the United Kingdom: Assessing construct, method, and item bias in the General Health Questionnaire (GHQ-12). *Assessment*, 26(7), 1194–1206. doi:10.1177/1073191117739979.

Bennett, C., Blount, A., Gerlach, J., Schroeder, K., Ausloos, C. D., Bloom, Z., Goodrich, K. M., Hollenbaugh, K. M. H., & Taylor, J. (2021). Standards for care for assessment in group work. *Counseling Outcome Research and Evaluation*, 12(2), 73–78. doi:10.1080/21501378.2021.1962117.

Bogucki, O. E., Williams, M. D., Solberg, L. I., Rossom, R. C., & Sawchuk, C. N. (2020). The role of the patient-centered medical home in treating depression. *Current Psychiatry Reports*, 22(9), 1–12. doi:10.1007/s11920-020-01167-y.

Boswell, J. F., Kraus, D. R., Miller, S. D., & Lambert, M. J. (2015). Implementing routine outcome monitoring in clinical practice: Benefits, challenges, and solutions. Psychotherapy Research, 25(1), 6–19. doi:10.1080/10503307.2013.817696.

Boswell, J. F., Hepner, K. A., Lysell, K., Rothrock, N. E., Bott, N., Childs, A. W., Douglas, S., Owings-Fonner, N., Wright, C. V., Stephens, K. A., Bard, D. E., Aajmain, S., & Bobbitt, B. L. (2022). The need for a measurement-based care professional practice guideline. *Psychotherapy*. Advance online publication. doi:10.1037/pst0000439.

Buchanan, N. T. & Wiklund, L. O. (2020) Why clinical science must change or die: Integrating intersectionality and social justice. *Women & Therapy*, 43(3–4), 309–329. doi:10.1080/02703149.2020.1729470.

Burgess, P., Pirkis, J., & Coombs, T. (2015). Routine outcome measurement in Australia. *International Review of Psychiatry*, 27(4), 264–275. doi:10.3109/09540261.2014.977234.

Burlingame, G., MacKenzie, K., & Strauss, B. (2003, February). Evidence-based group practice [Workshop]. Annual Meetings of the American Group Psychotherapy Association, New Orleans, LA, United States.

Burlingame, G., Strauss, B., Joyce, A., MacNair-Semands, R., MacKenzie, K., Ogrodniczuk, J., & Taylor, S. (2006). *CORE battery: A revision and update.* American Group Psychotherapy Association.

Burlingame, G., Davies, D., Cox, D., Baker, E., Pearson, M., Beecher, M., & Gleave, R. (2012). *The Group Readiness Questionnaire manual.* OQ Measures L.L.C.

Burlingame, G. M., Gleave, R., Beecher, M., Griner, D., Hansen, K., Jensen, J., Worthen, V., & Svien, H. (2017). *Administration and scoring manual for the group questionnaire OQ-GQ.* OQ Measures L.L.C.

Burlingame, G. M., McClendon, D. T., & Yang, C. (2018). Cohesion in group therapy: A meta-analysis. *Psychotherapy*, 55(4), 384–398. doi:10.1037/pst0000173.

Burlingame, G. M. & Strauss, B. (2021). *Efficacy of small group treatments: Foundation for evidence-based practice.* In M. Barkham, W. Lutz, & Castonguay, L. G. (Eds), *Bergin and Garfield's handbook of psychotherapy and behavior change* (pp. 591–631). Wiley.

Burlingame, G. M., Arnold, R. A., Rands, A., Wells, M. G., & Lambert, M. J. (2022). *Administration and scoring manual for the Y-OQ 2.01.* Unpublished manual.

Castonguay, L. G., Constantino, M. J., & Holtforth, M. G. (2006). The working alliance: Where are we and where should we go? *Psychotherapy: Theory, Research, Practice, Training*, 43(3), 271–279. doi:10.1037/0033-3204.43.3.271.

Chapman, C. L., Burlingame, G. M., Gleave, R., Rees, F., Beecher, M., & Porter, G. S. (2012). *Clinical prediction in group psychotherapy. Psychotherapy Research*, 22(6), 673–681. doi:10.1080/10503307.2012.702512.

Chin, E. G., Drescher, C. F., Trent, L. R., Darden, M., Seak, W. C., & Johnson, L. R. (2015). Searching for a screener: Examination of the factor structure of the General Health Questionnaire in Malaysia. *International Perspectives in Psychology: Research, Practice, Consultation*, 4(2), 111–127. doi:10.1037/ipp0000030.

Connors, E. H., Arora, P. G., Resnick, S. G., & McKay, M. (2022). A modified measurement-based care approach to improve mental health treatment engagement among racial and ethnic minoritized youth. *Psychological Services*. Advance online publication. doi:10.1037/ser0000617.

de Haan, A. M., Boon, A. E., de Jong, J. T. V. M., Hoeve, M., & Vermeiren, R. R. J. M. (2013). A meta-analytic review on treatment dropout in child and adolescent outpatient mental health care. *Clinical Psychology Review*, 33(5), 698–711. doi:10.1016/j.cpr.2013.04.005.

De Jong, K., Timman, R., Hakkaart-Van Roijen, L., Vermeulen, P., Kooiman, K., Passchier, J., & Van Busschbach, J. (2014). The effect of outcome monitoring feedback to clinicians and patients in short and long-term psychotherapy: a randomized controlled trial. *Psychotherapy Research*, 24(6), 629–639. doi:10.1080/10503307.2013.871079.

de Jong, K., Conijn, J. M., Gallagher, R. A. V., Reshetnikova, A. S., Heij, M., & Lutz, M. C. (2021). Using progress feedback to improve outcomes and reduce drop-out, treatment duration, and deterioration: A multilevel meta-analysis. *Clinical Psychology Review*, 85, Article 102002. doi:10.1016/j.cpr.2021.102002.

Delespaul, P. A. E. G. (2015). Routine outcome measurement in the Netherlands—a focus on benchmarking. *International Review of Psychiatry*, 27(4), 320–328. doi:10.3109/09540261.2015.1045408.

Duncan, B. L., Reese, R. J., Lengerich, A. J., DeSantis, B., Comeau, C. V., & Johnson-Esparza, Y. (2021). Measurement-based care in integrated health care: A randomized clinical trial. *Families, Systems, & Health*, 39(2), 259–268. doi:10.1037/fsh0000608.

Dunham, J. B. (2010). Examining the effectiveness of functional family therapy across diverse client ethnic groups (Publication No. 3380076) [Doctoral dissertation, Indiana University]. Proquest Dissertations & Theses Global.

Fatemi, A., Stewart, A., & Nghiem, K. (2019). Counseling psychology faculty's contributions to the internationalization of counseling. *International Journal for the Advancement of Counselling*, 41(1), 61–72. doi:10.1007/s10447-018-9346-y.

Fortney, J. C., Unützer, J., Wrenn, G., Pyne, J. M., Smith, G. R., Schoenbaum, M., & Harbin, H. T. (2017). A tipping point for measurement-based care. *Psychiatric Services*, 68(2), 179–188. doi:10.1176/appi.ps.201500439.

Freckelton, I. (2008). *Trends in regulation of mental health practitioners. Psychiatry, Psychology and Law*, 15(3), 415–434. doi:10.1080/13218710802480785.

Goldberg, D. P. & Hillier, V. F. (1979). A scaled version of the General Health Questionnaire. *Psychological Medicine*, 9(1), 139–145. doi:10.1017/S0033291700021644.

Goodrich, K. M., Farmer, L. B., Watson, J. C., Davis, R. J., Luke, M., Dispenza, F., Akers, W., & Griffith, C. (2017). Standards of care in assessment of lesbian, gay, bisexual, transgender, gender expansive, and queer/questioning (LGBTGEQ+) persons. *Journal of LGBT Issues in Counseling*, 11(4), 203–211. doi:10.1080/15538605.2017.1380548.

Gual-Montolio, P., Martínez-Borba, V., Bretón-López, J. M., Osma, J., & Suso-Ribera, C. (2020). How are information and communication technologies supporting routine outcome monitoring and measurement-based care in psychotherapy? A systematic review. *International Journal of Environmental Research and Public Health*, 17(9), Article3170. doi:10.3390/ijerph17093170.

Guo, T., Xiang, Y. T., Xiao, L., Hu, C. Q., Chiu, H. F. K., Psych., F. R. C., Ungvari, G. S., Correll, C. U., Lai, K. Y. C., Psych, M. R. C., Feng, L., Geng, Y., Phil, M., Feng, Y., & Wang, G. (2015). Measurement-based care versus standard care for major depression: a randomized controlled trial with blind raters. *The American Journal of Psychiatry*, 172(10), 1004–1013. doi:10.1176/appi.ajp.2015.14050652.

Henderson, A. A. (2013). Parenting skills as predictors of child and adolescent psychotherapy outcomes: Examining change in usual care settings (Publication No. 3613336) [Doctoral dissertation, Brigham Young University]. Proquest Dissertations & Theses Global.

Hewitt, P. L., Mikail, S. F., Dang, S. S., Kealy, D., & Flett, G. L. (2020). Dynamic-relational treatment of perfectionism: an illustrative case study. *Journal of Clinical Psychology*, 76(11), 2028–2040. doi:10.1002/jclp.23040.

Hill, C. E., Chui, H., & Baumann, E. (2013). Revisiting and re-envisioning the outcome problem in psychotherapy: an argument to include individualized and qualitative measurement. Psychotherapy, 50(1), 68–76. doi:10.1037/a0030571.

Hook, J. N., Davis, D., Owen, J., & DeBlaere, C. (2017). Cultural humility and the process of psychotherapy. In J. N. Hook, D. Davis, J. Owen, & C. DeBlaere, *Cultural humility: Engaging diverse identities in therapy* (pp. 91–112). American Psychological Association. doi:10.1037/0000037-005.

Horowitz, L. M., Alden, L. E., Wiggins, J. S., & Pincus, A. L. (2000). *IIP-64/IIP-32 professional manual.* Psychological Corporation.

Horvath, A. O. & Greenberg, L. S. (1989). Development and validation of the Working Alliance Inventory. *Journal of Counseling Psychology*, 36(2), 223–233. doi:10.1037/0022-0167.36.2.223.

Jacobson, N. S. & Truax, P. (1991). Clinical significance: A statistical approach to defining meaningful change in psychotherapy research. *Journal of Consulting and Clinical Psychology*, 59(1), 12–19. doi:10.1037/0022-006X.59.1.12.

Janis, R. A., Burlingame, G. M., Svien, H., Jensen, J., & Lundgreen, R. (2021). Group therapy for mood disorders: A meta-analysis. *Psychotherapy Research*, 31(3), 342–358. doi:10.1080/10503307.2020.1817603.

Johnson, J. E., Burlingame, G. M., Olsen, J. A., Davies, D. R., & Gleave, R. L. (2005). Group climate, cohesion, alliance, and empathy in group psychotherapy: Multilevel structural equation models. *Journal of Counseling Psychology*, 52(3), 310–321. doi:10.1037/0022-0167.52.3.310.

Krause, K. R. et al. (2021). International consensus on a standard set of outcome measures for child and youth anxiety, depression, obsessive-compulsive disorder, and post-traumatic stress disorder. *The Lancet Psychiatry*, 8(1), 76–86. doi:10.1016/S2215-0366(20)30356-30354.

Lambert, M. J. & Ogles, B. M. (2004). *The efficacy and effectiveness of psychotherapy.* In M. J. Lambert (Ed.), *Bergin and Garfield's handbook of psychotherapy and behavior change* (5th ed., pp. 139–193). Wiley.

Lambert, M. J., Kahler, M., Harmon, C., Burlingame, G., Shimokawa, K., & White, M. (2013). *Administration and scoring manual outcome questionnaire–45.* OQ Measures.

Lambert, M. J., Whipple, J. L., & Kleinstäuber, M. (2018). Collecting and delivering progress feedback: A meta-analysis of routine outcome monitoring. *Psychotherapy*, 55(4), 520–537. doi:10.1037/pst0000167.

Lewis, C. C., Boyd, M., Puspitasari, A., Navarro, E., Howard, J., Kassab, H., Hoffman, M., Scott, K., Lyon, A., Douglas, S., Simon, G., & Kroenke, K. (2019). Implementing measurement-based care in behavioral health: A review. *JAMA Psychiatry*, 76(3), 324–335. doi:10.1001/jamapsychiatry.2018.3329.

Lo Coco, G., Tasca, G. A., Hewitt, P. L., Mikail, S. F., & Kivlighan, D. M., Jr. (2019). Ruptures and repairs of group therapy alliance. An untold story in psychotherapy research. *Research in Psychotherapy*, 22(1), 58–70. doi:10.4081/ripppo.2019.352.

MacKenzie, K. R. (1981). Measurement of group climate. *International Journal of Group Psychotherapy*, 31(3), 287–295. doi:10.1080/00207284.1981.11491708.

MacNair-Semands, R. R. (2002). Predicting attendance and expectations for group therapy. *Group Dynamics: Theory, Research, and Practice*, 6(3), 219–228. doi:10.1037/1089-2699.6.3.219.

MacNair-Semands, R. R. (2014, August 7–10). Using an ethical framework to promote transformation in group. In MacNair-Semands, R. R. (Chair), Marmarosh, C. & Riva, M., *Ethical issues in working with individual and cultural differences in groups* [Symposium]. American Psychological Association 122nd Annual Convention, Washington, DC, United States.

McClendon, D. T. (2009). Relative sensitivity to change of psychotherapy outcome measures for children and adolescents: A comparison using parent- and self-report versions of the CBCL/6–18, BASC-2, and Y-OQ-2.01 (Publication No. 3362641) [Doctoral dissertation, Brigham Young University]. Proquest Dissertations & Theses Global.

McCrady, B. S. (2013). Health-care reform provides an opportunity for evidence-based alcohol treatment in the USA: The National Institute for Health and Clinical Excellence (NICE) guideline as a model. *Addiction*, 108(2), 231–232. doi:10.1111/j.1360-0443.2012.04052.x.

McFayden, T. C., Gatto, A. J., Dahiya, A. V., Antezana, L., Miyazaki, Y., & Cooper, L. D. (2021). Integrating measurement-based care into treatment for autism spectrum disorder: Insights from a community clinic. *Journal of Autism and Developmental Disorders*, 51(10), 3651–3661. doi:10.1007/s10803-020-04824-6.

Mellor-Clark, J., Cross, S., Macdonald, J., & Skjulsvik, T. (2016). Leading horses to water: Lessons from a decade of helping psychological therapy services use routine outcome measurement to improve practice. *Administration and Policy in Mental Health and Mental Health Services Research*, 43(3), 279–285. doi:10.1007/s10488-014-0587-8.

Muir, H. J., Coyne, A. E., Morrison, N. R., Boswell, J. F., & Constantino, M. J. (2019). Ethical implications of routine outcomes monitoring for patients, psychotherapists, and mental health care systems. *Psychotherapy*, 56(4), 459–469. doi:10.1037/pst0000246.

O'Keeffe, S., Martin, P., Target, M., & Midgley, N. (2019). 'I just stopped going': A mixed methods investigation into types of therapy dropout in adolescents with depression. *Frontiers in Psychology*, 10 (75), 1–14. doi:10.3389/fpsyg.2019.00075.

Packard, A. E., Warren, J. S., & Linford, L. B. (2020). Parent functioning and child psychotherapy outcomes: Predicting outcomes in usual care. *Journal of Clinical Psychology*, 77(1), 49–59. doi:10.1002/jclp.23032.

Porter, M. E. & Teisberg, E. O. (2006, May 2). *Redefining health care: creating value-based competition on results*. Harvard Business School Press. www.hbs.edu/ris/Publication%20Files/20060502%20NACDS%20-%20Final%2005012006%20for%20On%20Point_db5ede1d-3d06-41f0-85e3-c11658534a63.pdf.

Remedios, J. D. & Snyder, S. H. (2018). Intersectional oppression: Multiple stigmatized identities and perceptions of invisibility, discrimination, and stereotyping. *Journal of Social Issues*, 74(2), 265–281. doi:10.1111/josi.12268.

Ridley, C. R., Chih, D. W., & Olivera, R. J. (2000). Training in cultural schemas: An antidote to unintentional racism in clinical practice. *American Journal of Orthopsychiatry*, 70(1), 65–72. doi:10.1037/h0087771.

Rosen, B., Israeli, A., & Shortell, S. M. (Eds). (2012). Accountability and responsibility in health care: Issues in addressing an emerging global challenge (Vol. 1). World Scientific.

Salisbury, T. N. (2015). Predicting youth treatment failure: An investigation of clinical versus actuarial judgment (Publication No. 3643159) [Doctoral dissertation, Brigham Young University]. Proquest Dissertations & Theses Global.

Shimokawa, K., Lambert, M. J., & Smart, D. W. (2010). Enhancing treatment outcome of patients at risk of treatment failure: Meta-analytic and mega-analytic review of a psychotherapy quality assurance system. *Journal of Consulting and Clinical Psychology*, 78(3), 298–311. doi:10.1037/a0019247.

Singh, A. A., Merchant, N., Skudrzyk, B., & Ingene, D. (2012). Association for specialists in group work: Multicultural and social justice competence principles for group workers. *The Journal for Specialists in Group Work*, 37(4), 312–325. doi:10.1080/01933922.2012.721482.

Tam, H. E. & Ronan, K. (2017). The application of a feedback-informed approach in psychological service with youth: Systematic review and meta-analysis. *Clinical Psychology Review*, 55, 41–55. doi:10.1016/j.cpr.2017.04.005.

Tasca, G. A., Ritchie, K., Demidenko, N., Balfour, L., Krysanski, V., Weekes, K., Barber, A., Keating, L. & Bissada, H. (2013). Matching women with binge eating disorder to group treatment based on attachment anxiety: outcomes and moderating effects. *Psychotherapy Research*, 23(3), 301–314. doi:10.1080/10503307.2012.717309.

Tikkanen, R. & Abrams, M. K. (2020, January 30). U.S. health care from a global perspective, 2019: Higher spending, worse outcomes? The Commonwealth Fund. www.commonwealthfund.org/publications/issue-briefs/2020/jan/us-health-care-global-perspective-2019.

Trauer, T., Callaly, T., & Herrman, H. (2009). Attitudes of mental health staff to routine outcome measurement. *Journal of Mental Health*, 18(4), 288–297. doi:10.1080/09638230701879177.

Walfish, S., McAlister, B., O'Donnell, P., & Lambert, M. J. (2012). An investigation of self-assessment bias in mental health providers. *Psychological Reports*, 110(2), 639–644. doi:10.2466/02.07.17.PR0.110.2.639-644.

Wampold, B. E. & Imel, Z. E. (2015). *The great psychotherapy debate: The evidence for what makes psychotherapy work* (2nd ed.). Routledge/Taylor & Francis Group.

Warren, J. S., Nelson, P. L., Mondragon, S. A., Baldwin, S. A., & Burlingame, G. M. (2010). Youth psychotherapy change trajectories and outcomes in usual care: Community mental health versus managed care settings. *Journal of Consulting and Clinical Psychology*, 78(2), 144–155. doi:10.1037/a0018544.

Whittingham, M. (2017). *Attachment and interpersonal theory and group therapy: Two sides of the same coin.* International Journal of Group Psychotherapy, 67(2), 276–279. doi:10.1080/00207284.2016.1260463.

Whittingham, M. (2018). *Innovations in group assessment: how focused brief group therapy integrates formal measures to enhance treatment preparation*, process, and outcomes. Psychotherapy, 55(2), 186–190. doi:10.1037/pst0000153.

Whittingham, M. & Arlo, C. (2019). *AGPA Agency Survey* [*Report*]. AGPA National Convention, New York, United States.

Whittingham, M., Mallow, P., Marmarosh, C., L., & Scherer, M. (2021). Group therapy utilization and reimbursement under third party payment compared to other therapies: Nationwide data from FAIR Health [Symposium]. APA National Convention. Virtual.

Whittington, J. W., Nolan, K., Lewis, N., & Torres, T. (2015). Pursuing the triple aim: the first 7 years. *The Milbank Quarterly*, 93(2), 263–300. doi:10.1111/1468-0009.12122.

Wright, C. V., Goodheart, C., Bard, D., Bobbitt, B. L., Butt, Z., Lysell, K., McKay, D., & Stephens, K. (2020). Promoting measurement-based care and quality measure development: The APA mental and behavioral health registry initiative. *Psychological Services*, 17(3), 262–270. doi:10.1037/ser0000347.

Yalom, I. D. & Leszcz, M. (2020). *The theory and practice of group psychotherapy*. Basic Books.

Youn, S. J., Kraus, D. R., & Castonguay, L. G. (2012). The treatment outcome package: Facilitating practice and clinically relevant research. *Psychotherapy*, 49(2), 115–122. doi:10.1037/a0027932.

2 Group Selection, Group Composition, and Pre-Group Preparation

Anthony S. Joyce and Cheri L. Marmarosh

This chapter addresses the "front-end" work of the group leaders to *select* and *prepare* prospective members for group therapy. This investment is essential to identify appropriate candidates and facilitate the client's commitment to and comfort in the group. Thoughtful selection and intentional preparation can increase the likelihood that the group will develop cohesion and a positive working climate (Yalom & Leszcz, 2020). Selection represents a clinical assessment: the leader seeks to determine whether a client and the group will *mutually benefit* from the client's inclusion. In describing how to evaluate a client for group membership, we consider using measures of factors found to predict group dropout, process, or outcome in empirical studies. Use of measures can assist in formulating goals for therapy, facilitating group commitment—the goal of preparation—and promoting a client-leader working alliance.

Selection features a clinical focus on the individual client, i.e., whether the client meets inclusion/exclusion criteria or has attributes that would be of value to the group. In contrast, pre-group preparation (PGP) considers the client's relationships with the leader and group, highlights tasks the member will be asked to undertake in group, and addresses any preconceptions that could impact the client's commitment and participation. Preparation aims to foster the client's best use of the treatment once selection has determined the client is appropriate for the group.

Throughout our presentation, the assumed treatment context is an outpatient, open-ended process group therapy focusing on interpersonal learning, psychological insight, and character change (Yalom & Leszcz, 2020). Clinicians forming process groups have typically aimed for *heterogeneity* in terms of client personality and problem presentation and *homogeneity* in terms of "ego strength," i.e., resources and capacities (e.g., psychological mindedness). Readers should be mindful of variations associated with their specific approach (e.g., theoretical orientation, treatment duration, group focus, population, presumed mechanisms of change) and consider adaptations to the selection principles presented. For example, ego strength may be a central selection criterion for a process group involving frank feedback but less critical in a CBT group where there may be lower risk of psychological injury.

Following a discussion of general issues, the first subsection considers augmenting selection through the use of four measures of client readiness, expectations, and ego strength. The full set is recommended for leaders' selection activity but tailoring to clinical needs is possible. For example, the Group Therapy Questionnaire (MacNair-Semands, 2002) provides for a qualitative understanding of the client, including their cultural context, while the Group Readiness Questionnaire (Baker et al., 2013) allows for efficiency in its quantitative scoring of the client on readiness factors. Leaders could use one or the other, depending on objectives; on the other hand, employing both could allow for a convergent view of the client's suitability for group. We suggest many potentially useful measures in the chapter but assume that choice of one instrument or a battery will be based on their clinical utility

DOI: 10.4324/9781003255482-2

balanced against considerations of "assessment fatigue." To be clear, though, we are advocating for *more* investment in the selection process by administering and interpreting one or more relevant measures.

The next subsection suggests *alternative* measures for assessing type and intensity of symptoms, capacity for therapy process (alexithymia), and a problem deficit (reactance), to evaluate client *compatibility* for group. These represent useful adjuncts to evaluations of readiness for group by highlighting client strengths and weaknesses. In this and subsequent sections, measures are presented as *options* for leaders to consider for clinical use.

We next consider group *composition* as a more directed approach to selection activity—the focus being less on the individual client and more on the resulting "character" of the group-as-a-whole (Rutan et al., 2019). A critical dimension of composition involves the members' identities and sociocultural experiences; in the first subsection addressing composition we focus on two measures that can be helpful in achieving balanced representation in the group. A second subsection presents *transdiagnostic* measures that can provide information in line with the leaders' *theory of change*, deepening clinical understanding and allowing for *predictions* of in-group behavior and process. These mainly address personality traits that often have centrality to the interpersonal process approach, theory, or intervention style of the leaders. We highlight evidence that these factors can impact group development and functioning. We also address the pragmatics of group composition. Our central premise is that investing time to consider composition can deepen leaders' understanding of clients. From that understanding, group process and interventions can be predicted on the basis of a *measurement-based care* approach (Resnick et al., 2020), a form of *evidence-based* therapy.

The second half of the chapter considers methods of preparing selected clients to join and flourish in the group. Preparation can involve cognitive learning or education, vicarious or observational learning, behavioral practice, or some combination of all three, encompassing passive, active, or interactive elements. We specifically address goals of preparation, including a) establishing a member-leader working alliance, b) reducing client anxiety, addressing expectations for group, and correcting misconceptions, c) providing information on the norms and frame of group therapy (e.g., member and therapist roles, group contracts and process, and confidentiality), and d) developing consensus on group goals and objectives. We also consider how to address cultural factors during preparation, a critical update to the CORE-R (Burlingame et al., 2006).

Group Selection: Guidelines

In their review of this area, Yalom and Leszcz (2020) cogently define a central guiding principle: selection aims to ensure that the client does not *fail* as a member of the group. Failure can mean the client encounters problems with participation because of a *mismatch* with other members or the group, or eventually becomes a group dropout. Dropping out is invariably demoralizing for the client and also likely to negatively impact the remaining members, so selection to *prevent* failures is critical (Yalom & Leszcz, 2020). Thus, selection represents a clinical evaluation to determine *if the client is unable to engage in primary group tasks*, i.e., to examine interpersonal patterns, offer self-disclosures, and give and receive feedback. Group failures can arise, owing to logistical, intellectual, psychological, or interpersonal reasons. Logistical problems (e.g., work or travel issues, finances) and intellectual deficits are readily determined and would preclude group entry. Our focus is on interpersonal (both deficits and dynamics) and psychological factors (e.g., social inhibition) that determine selection decisions.

In addition to preventing failures, selection also aims to identify clients *most likely to benefit* from group, given presenting problems, clinical issues, and personal strengths. The range of suitability for certain client characteristics may be quite narrow. Take for example the capacity for assertiveness: too little and the client may feel "left behind" by the group process, too much and the client's behavior can border on aggressiveness and might be disruptive to that same process. Similarly, certain characteristics can be a counterweight to concerns regarding admittance, e.g., a capacity for self-reflection might provide balance against issues of anger dyscontrol and allow for group entry. Selection decisions often involve a *risk/benefit* analysis.

Principles guiding selection are relativistic. It is likely impossible to establish an "ideal" group based on "cherry-picking" clients from an available pool because many variables add to the complexity of selection decisions. These encompass the presentation of other prospective or active members (e.g., the presence of personality disorder), the characteristics of the group (e.g., newly implemented versus maturely functioning), leader qualities (e.g., degree of directiveness, experience), and the interactions involving these variables. Deliberate efforts to compose a new group or add to an existing group should judiciously focus on only a few dimensions so that the process can remain feasible and manageable. This is the perspective we adopt in the later discussion of composition. Selection becomes critical when the aim is to start a new group or fill vacancies (owing to therapeutic terminations, instrumental departures, or group dropouts) in existing groups. Appropriate selection obviously depends on having a pool of referrals available. The AGPA's clinical practice guidelines (Bernard et al., 2008) offer useful suggestions for establishing and maintaining referral sources, in both private practice and healthcare settings.

The selection process should consistently maintain a dual focus on *mutual benefit*. In sum, selection represents a thoughtful clinical assessment of *fit* between the prospective member and the group. This process can be augmented by employing relevant empirical measures.

Inclusion and Exclusion Criteria: General Issues

Selection decisions can frequently be made readily, that is, a client will be promptly *deselected* because of one or more exclusionary features (e.g., logistical issues, intellectual deficits). Meeting a *single* exclusion criterion is often sufficient for a decision against admittance. In contrast, applying inclusion criteria often means the client must meet a more complex "profile" to gain admittance. A two-stage screening process is helpful: first, rule out the presence of any characteristics that would immediately preclude admittance; second, conduct a more detailed assessment to determine the client's suitability and potential value to the group. Selection decisions about fit are less equivocal if the client's pathology is more profound and are more difficult if the client presents with a mix of features helpful *and* hindering in a group setting.

In some instances, a characteristic that justifies exclusion from one group can serve as an inclusion criterion for another (Yalom & Leszcz, 2020). For example, in a hospital outpatient service, clients presenting with schizoid or schizotypal personality issues were explicitly excluded from interpersonal process groups. One clinician made an intrepid decision to establish a homogenous group for clients on this spectrum, selecting on the basis of diagnosis. Over time, a capacity for effective work evolved in the group and members achieved outcomes that were unlikely had they been placed in the usual process group. Client characteristics can interact in selection decisions—strength on one characteristic (e.g., motivation) may outweigh concerns regarding other traits or issues (e.g., reactance); addressing these "trade-offs" allows for a *calculated* risk regarding admittance. The same characteristic might also demonstrate important variation across clients. For example, a treatment-naïve client with severe borderline personality disorder (BPD) may be unsuitable, but a client with BPD who has completed a course of DBT and can now tolerate interpersonal work can potentially be a valuable process group member. If the clinical context allows for sufficient preparatory attention to a client's issues, greater allowances might be made. Whittingham (2018) outlines pre-group interventions to "inoculate" clients against engaging in disruptive group behavior, e.g., focusing on a client's anger dyscontrol and facilitating more capacity for containment prior to group entry. Selection decisions often reflect a case-by-case consideration more than the application of explicit rules.

Exclusion Criteria. Many "rule of thumb" selection guidelines have been developed in line with the evolution of group practice (Yalom & Leszcz, 2020). Selection criteria are not absolute rules but instead guidelines regarding characteristics that are *relatively* important to include or exclude when adding to the group, i.e., each criterion must be viewed in light of other client variables and the purpose, maturity, and functioning of the group itself. Exclusion criteria identify whether the candidate's presence will disrupt or detract from the development of group cohesiveness, i.e., the client presents as divergent from or incompatible with other members or the group as a whole. Admittance to group is most often refused because of the client's clinical presentation; certain exclusion criteria represent obvious issues ruling out admittance, i.e., active substance abuse, brain damage, acute psychosis, sociopathy, hypochondriasis. Other "common sense" exclusion criteria may highlight issues calling for supportive or crisis-oriented interventions instead of a process group, e.g., acute crisis (marital issues, work or school termination, bereavement, or serious illness), profound depression with suicidal concerns, extreme social inhibition, or substance abuse that interferes with interpersonal and daily functioning (Yalom & Leszcz, 2020).

Regarding *presenting problems*, concerns are likely if the client:

- reports frequent interpersonal conflicts and consistent aggressiveness, defensiveness, agitation, or hostility in relationships;
- reports frequently engaging in self-defeating or self-destructive behaviors, including substance abuse, risky sexual behavior, or parasuicidal/suicidal gestures;
- reports somatic complaints or pain without linking psychological factors to these experiences, a form of externalization antithetical to an insight-oriented group process;
- demonstrates engaging in strong denial of clear issues; or
- shows an inability to adhere to "rules" such as a group contract (MacNair-Semands, 2002; Valbak, 2018; Yalom & Leszcz, 2020).

Client *capacities* may also be problematic. Questions of capacity often imply that the client would likely require a disproportionate degree of leader and group attention and support. For example, the individual may present as:

- intensely shy or avoidant and thus unprepared for group interaction;
- vague regarding issues of concern;
- failing to consider treatment appropriately seriously; or
- without any kind of network of friends or family to support group treatment.

Clinical issues specific to the particular client will often influence the group leader's decision about admittance. The client may report doubts about being able to feel comfortable or make open disclosures, or question the efficacy or value of the group approach. The leader may sense that the client would likely deviate from group norms or tasks (e.g., tendencies to be reactant or monopolize the discussion). A bias towards paranoid thinking, if sufficiently severe, could also impede the client's work and the level of trust in the group. Research has suggested that issues with low motivation, poor insight, angry hostility or provocativeness, and a reliance on denial and defensiveness predict poor group attendance or dropout

(MacNair-Semands, 2002; Yalom & Leszcz, 2020). An incompatibility with one or more group members (e.g., impatience with members who are hesitant, stereotyped views of BIPOC members), or the possibility that the client might jeopardize the safety of other members or the group (e.g., an antisocial or malignantly narcissistic client), could also represent grounds for exclusion. If the leader does refuse admittance, it is critical to convey the rationale for this decision and frame the exclusion as a therapeutic learning. Ethically, it is also incumbent on the leader to suggest or implement changes to the therapy plan and ensure that the client's needs are met in an alternative format.

Inclusion Criteria. Guidelines regarding inclusion can address presenting problem, capacities, and clinical issues associated with the client's *suitability* for group therapy. The principle here is to evaluate how well the client's presenting issues and their etiology mesh with the focus and mechanisms of change of the group treatment. With regard to *presenting problem*, the client:

- identifies difficulties in central relationships with family, partners, or friends;
- acknowledges that current relational issues are influenced by family of origin dynamics;
- reports feeling distress, including suicidal ideation, but shows a willingness to connect with others to examine these feelings and contract for safety, i.e., is *motivated* for treatment in general and for group specifically; and
- asserts that this motivation is not due to external influences or duress.

Meeting these criteria presumes a degree of client awareness. Not uncommonly, the client may *lack* self-awareness of interpersonal issues or present with character traits that are egosyntonic, i.e., not felt to represent problems. In these cases, it is important to identify other strengths valuable to group and devote some pre-group preparation to developing an interpersonal formulation of the client's issues (see Hewitt et al., 2018). In terms of *capacities*, the client:

- demonstrates some aptitude for psychological mindedness, self-observation, and frustration tolerance;
- can discuss the feelings associated with presenting problems to some degree and demonstrates insight or previous successful therapy experience;
- has one or more healthy relationships and demonstrates basic skills of interpersonal communication, reality testing, and empathy; and
- has sufficient medical/physical health to be able to participate fully in the group (Valbak, 2018; Yalom & Leszcz, 2020).

A common *clinical* issue occurs when the client has become overly dependent on an individual therapist and could benefit from the multiple transferences in group. Lastly, and pragmatically, the client should be able to commit to the meeting time and duration of the group.

In terms of an *ideal* prospective member, strengths would include a capacity and willingness to examine interpersonal patterns, to self-disclose, to engage in reflection on self and others, and to give and receive feedback, and with clear motivation to engage with other members (Yalom & Leszcz, 2020). More succinctly, Ogrodniczuk et al. (2003) found that three of the Big Five personality factors—extraversion, conscientiousness, and openness— were associated with positive outcomes in two forms of brief dynamic group therapy, while neuroticism (negative emotional reactivity) was linked to poor outcomes. Of course, many clients who do not meet the ideal can still benefit from group. Another simple principle: the *farther* the client is from the prototypic ideal, the more the leaders should invest in pre-group preparation. If a decision about admittance remains difficult, observing the client in a preparation session involving multiple prospective members (a "mini-group") might be considered as a "make or break" proposition.

The client's *motivation* is arguably the single most important criterion for selection (Yalom & Leszcz, 2020). The client's motivation for engagement in the group process can often compensate for risks associated with other issues, e.g., low psychological mindedness. The quality of the client's motivation can frequently "tip the scales" towards admittance in the context of a selection dilemma. For a process group, an obvious criterion for selection is the client's presentation of *recurrent difficulties in interpersonal relations*. Difficulties in the client's relationship with *self* can also be included. Even if the client's problem presentation is *not* expressed interpersonally, a link to relational conflicts or deficits can often be established during pre-group assessments. The range of interpersonal issues treatable in group is broad:

> "Loneliness, shyness and social withdrawal, inability to be intimate or to love, excessive competitiveness, aggressivity, abrasiveness, argumentativeness, suspiciousness, problems with authority, narcissism, an inability to share, to empathize, to accept criticism, a continuous need for admiration, feelings of unlovability, fears of assertiveness, obsequiousness, and dependency."
>
> (Yalom & Leszcz, 2020, p. 314)

More rarely, the client's issues might directly *inhibit* the development of relationships (e.g., a stultifying tendency to intellectualize) or reflect problems with self-regulation (e.g., reactance or impulsivity), but these can nonetheless represent suitable targets for group intervention. The client's acknowledgment of relational issues as fundamental, coupled with an understanding of the norms and process of group therapy achieved through preparation, can help promote the client's *expectancy* that engagement in group will prove beneficial. In turn, a positive expectancy can predict a beneficial outcome, so it is valuable to clarify the client's expectations about the group process and change as a third critical dimension of inclusion during the screening process.

Essential Measures for Group Selection: Readiness, Expectations, and Ego Strength

The group therapist's evaluation of the potential member can be augmented by making use of measures of client suitability. This usually occurs following an initial assessment (and often the source referral for group therapy), and thus constitutes a pre-group *screening*. The priority for screening is a clear evaluation of the client's *readiness* for group therapy. Marmarosh et al. (2013b) offer a synopsis of the critical elements of a screening interview using a model emphasizing interpersonal behavior and associated attachment style. Screenings can occupy one session with one or two leaders or can involve multiple meetings to determine suitability for the group (Whittingham, 2018). At the least, two sessions—an assessment session and a later meeting to review results with the client—would be well worth the effort. We describe four measures recommended as a battery for the leader's screening activity to illuminate client readiness, expectations, and ego strength.

Group Therapy Questionnaire (GTQ)

The GTQ (MacNair & Corazzini, 1994; MacNair-Semands, 2002) is retained from the CORE-R (Burlingame et al., 2006) because of its vital focus on information relevant to selection. The GTQ strikes a balance obtaining essential clinical data and information for a "deeper" formulation of the client's issues. A short form (and digital version) of the GTQ

Table 2.1 The Group Therapy Questionnaire-S

Item	Information
Name of instrument	**Group Therapy Questionnaire (GTQ-S)**
Authors	Rebecca R. MacNair-Semands & John G. Corazzini
Source	MacNair-Semands, R. R. (2019). The Group Therapy Questionnaire—Short Form. University of North Carolina, Charlotte, NC.
Translations	English
Brief description	The GTQ-S is a self-report instrument designed to assess pre-existing client variables affecting potential group behavior. The GTQ-S may be used to identify interpersonal difficulties in addition to other factors predictive of premature termination. It is often used during pre-group meetings to review clinical data related to potential group interactions.
Time requirements	Administration: 30 minutes or less Scoring: 10–15 minutes
Subscales and scoring	The GTQ-S comprises 25 items organized into 5 domains and features both Likert-type ratings and narrative inquiries. The domains include Counseling (Experiences and Expectations), Family (Relationship and Roles), Health/Mental Health (including items for suicidality and somatic symptoms), Interpersonal Problems (a 34-item checklist), and Therapy Considerations (Goals, Fears, Impediments). The measure can be scored manually; subscale scores represent sums and norms are provided in the manual. Quantitative subscale scores include expectations for group, substance abuse, somatic concerns, and factor scores for interpersonal problems (e.g., Dependency, Angry Hostility, Social Inhibition, and Low Ego Strength). Several items elicit narrative responses and can be used for discussion of cultural identity issues or expectancies, and to increase client interest and involvement in treatment.
Psychometric properties	Three-week test-retest reliabilities were: Alcohol/drug issues, .93; Expectations about group, .77; Interpersonal Problem scale (sum of factor scores), .89; Somatic concerns, .60.
Norms	The GTQ-S manual includes norms for the subscales, including interpersonal factor scores, based on samples of college students.
Administration types	Paper & pencil or digital versions.
Sensitivity to change	Several variables derived from the GTQ-S have demonstrated ability to predict poor attendance or premature termination, including hostility, alcohol/drug problems, somatic complaints, and social inhibition.
Analytics	Quantitative scores can be compared to norms in the manual; variables predictive of premature termination are critical in this regard. Narrative responses can provide indications of problems to address in pre-group meetings.
Benchmarking	NA
Sample references	MacNair, R. R., & Corazzini, J. (1994). Client factors influencing group therapy dropout. *Psychotherapy, 31*, 352–361. https://dx.doi.org/10.1037/h0090226 MacNair-Semands, R. R. (2002). Predicting attendance and expectations for group therapy. *Group Dynamics: Theory, Research, and Practice, 6*, 219–228. https://dx.doi.org/10.1037/1089-2699.6.3.219
Website resources	www.routledge.com/Core-Principles-of-Group-Psychotherapy-An-Integrated-Theory-Research/Kaklauskas-Greene/p/book/9780367203092 (using the button labeled *Support Materials* and choosing the folder entitled *Pre-group 1–10*).
How to obtain/Cost	The GTQ-S and manual are available for download at no cost at the website link above.

has been developed (MacNair-Semands, 2019). The GTQ-S offers a structured assessment of the client's personal and family history, goals, and interpersonal problems, and assesses factors found to predict group dropout (e.g., substance use, social inhibition). Usefully, the GTQ-S provides a framework for a problem formulation that could become the focus of a PGP interview.

The GTQ-S comprises 25 items organized into five domains, featuring both Likert-type ratings and narrative inquiries. The domains include Counseling (Experiences and Expectations), Family (Relationships and Roles), Health/Mental Health (including suicidality and somatic symptoms), Interpersonal Problems (a 34-item checklist), and Therapy Considerations (Goals, Fears, Impediments). A family genogram in the original GTQ was excluded but prompts have been added to the GTQ-S to address aspects of identity, covering racial, cultural, gender, sexuality, and other elements, a critical development of the measure. Narrative inquiries address the client's comfort with self-disclosure, capacity to examine relational patterns, and ability to be reflective on self and others. Ratings of interpersonal problems can be compiled to score four factors identified as critical in studies of group dropout: Angry Hostility, Dependency, Social Inhibition, and Low Ego Strength. High factor scores would represent areas of concern regarding group admittance. The GTQ-S takes less than 30 minutes to complete. The GTQ-S instrument and manuals can be downloaded at no cost from: www.routledge.com/Core-Principles-of-Group-Psychotherap y-An-Integrated-Theory-Research/Kaklauskas-Greene/p/book/9780367203092 (using the button labeled *Support Materials* and choosing the folder entitled *Pre-group 1–10*).

The GTQ source article (MacNair & Corazzini, 1994) describes analyses to predict premature termination from group therapy. Subscales serving as predictor variables included hostility, substance use, somatic issues, and social withdrawal. A discriminant analysis correctly classified over three-quarters of the sample as dropouts or continuers. In later work, MacNair-Semands (2002) reported that Angry Hostility and Social Inhibition emerged as significant predictors of poor attendance. Clients with previous therapy experience were found to report more positive expectations for group. Clients who reported substance use or somatic issues had fewer positive expectations which in turn predicted premature termination. Other systematic applications of the GTQ in the clinical setting are reported by Söchting et al. (2018) and Whittingham (2018).

Group Readiness Questionnaire (GRQ)

The GRQ (Baker et al., 2013) offers a quick, focused assessment of group readiness *factors*. The GRQ is an evolution of the Group Selection Questionnaire (Burlingame et al., 2011) and represents the state of the art of questionnaire development and validation—the psychometric quality and brevity of the GRQ commend its use for evaluating risk and predicting success in a clinical context. The self-report focuses on qualities of *appropriateness* for group therapy; regardless of the client's presenting problem and relational issues, a *minimum* level of interpersonal skill is required for group interaction. The GRQ assesses the client's positive and negative interpersonal characteristics and expectations regarding outcome of group therapy. Positive interpersonal characteristics have been found to predict remaining in treatment (Connelly et al., 1986) and benefit (Ogrodniczuk et al., 2002). Negative interpersonal characteristics, reflecting aggressiveness or behaviors that highlight the client's *deviancy* relative to other members, can interfere with group process and contribute to attrition (Yalom & Leszcz, 2020). The client may have unclear or distorted expectations about how group treatment unfolds and whether benefit may be possible, critical issues to address in PGP. In contrast, clients who expect the group to be helpful tend to achieve

Table 2.2 The Group Readiness Questionnaire

Item	Information
Name of instrument	*Group Readiness Questionnaire (GRQ)*
Authors	Elizabeth Baker, Gary M. Burlingame, Jonathan C. Cox, Mark E. Beecher, & Robert L. Gleave
Source	Baker, E., Burlingame, G. M., Cox, J. C., Beecher, M. E., & Gleave, R. L. (2013). The Group Readiness Questionnaire: A convergent validity analysis. *Group Dynamics: Theory, Research, and Practice, 17*(4), 299–314. https://dx.doi.org/10.1037/a0034477
Translations	English and Czech. Translations are available through www.oqmeasures.com.
Brief description	The GRQ is a brief assessment of qualities of *appropriateness* for group therapy, including positive and negative interpersonal characteristics and expectations regarding benefit from group. The GRQ comprises 19 items rated on a 5-point (1–5) Likert-type scale and was designed to provide therapists with an accurate screen of clients' fit for group therapy.
Time requirements	Administration: 5 minutes. Scoring: 5 minutes.
Subscales and scoring	Scores for a replicated three-factor structure are calculated by simple summation: Expectancy (3 items), Participation (positive interpersonal characteristics; 13 items), and Demeanor (negative characteristics; 3 items). A total score can also be calculated. Higher scores indicate *less* readiness and a greater need for attention during pre-group preparation.
Psychometric properties	In terms of predictive validity, GRQ subscales have demonstrated significant correlations with measures of group process, time in treatment (retention), and symptom change (outcome). Convergent validity has been demonstrated with subscales of the GTQ.
Norms	Norms can be found in Baker et al. (2013) and in the GRQ Manual. These are aggregate versions of sample values undifferentiated as to gender or ethnicity.
Administration types	Paper & pencil and digital versions.
Sensitivity to change	NA
Analytics	Based on multiple respondent samples, cut-off values for Expectancy, Participation, and the total score have been presented in the Manual, indicating when greater attention during pre-group preparation sessions is warranted.
Benchmarking	Earlier studies with versions of the GRQ involved community, outpatient, and inpatient samples; Baker et al. (2013) and the Manual offer discussion of sample differences.
Sample references	Burlingame, G. M., Cox, J. C., Davies, D. R., Layne, C. M., & Gleave, R. (2011). The Group Selection Questionnaire: Further refinements in group member selection. *Group Dynamics: Theory, Research, and Practice, 15*, 60–74. https://dx.doi.org/10.1037/a0020220 Krogel, J., Beecher, M., Presnell, J., Burlingame, G. & Simonsen. (2009). The Group Selection Questionnaire: A qualitative analysis of extreme scores. *International Journal of Group Psychotherapy, 59*(4), 529–542. https://dx.doi.org/10.1037/ijgp.2009.59.4.529
Website resources	The GRQ is available as part of an instrument bundle (also including the Group Climate Questionnaire – Short Form and the Group Questionnaire, both useful in tracking group process) at www.oqmeasures.com.
How to obtain/Cost	Contact sales@oqmeasures.com to request a quote; pricing depends on type of license needed. Further information is available at info@OQMeasures.com.

positive outcomes (Abouguendia et al., 2004). The GRQ is an efficient means of evaluating readiness in terms of the client's positive/negative characteristics and expectancies.

The GRQ comprises 19 Likert-type items (ratings of 1–5) requiring less than 5 minutes to complete. Given this brevity, the manual defines the GRQ as a screening tool to identify clients *most likely to require attention in PGP*. Scores for three factors can be calculated by simple summation: Expectancy (3 items), Participation (positive interpersonal characteristics; 13 items), and Demeanor (negative characteristics; 3 items). Expectancy and Participation are reverse scored; higher scores indicate *less* readiness and greater need for attention during PGP. The factors have been shown to have good concurrent validity, e.g., correlations with measures of group process and symptom change. Because of inconsistency across samples, the three items of the Demeanor factor are now presented as "critical indices" of unassertive or aggressive interpersonal behavior. A total GRQ score can also be calculated. In a convergent validity study of a college counseling sample, Baker et al. (2013) found that the GRQ total score was significantly correlated with the overall interpersonal problems score from the GTQ, suggesting the former can serve as an index of global problem severity. The manual (available for purchase from www.oqmeasures.com) describes the GRQ's development and provides norms, an item-level interpretive guide, and suggestions for addressing high factor or total scores during PGP.

Target Objectives

The Target Objectives procedure constitutes a method more than a singular measure, aimed at capturing *individualized* therapy goals based on the *client's* description of their own problems. The procedure was described in the seminal work of Battle et al. (1966) and has been employed in psychotherapy research since. The client is asked to list three goals or objectives they want to achieve in therapy. The leader helps the client define these goals in terms of specific, concrete behaviors (e.g., to be more open with my feelings during interactions), ideally in the interpersonal domain. The client then provides three ratings for each objective: *severity of distress* during the past month, *importance*, and *expected improvement* as a result of therapy. The leader can rate the same dimensions to derive parallel measures, or use expanded rating scales to address duration, frequency, intensity, pervasiveness, and disruptiveness. At the end of treatment, the client again rates each objective on distress, importance, and *observed* improvement. Benefit is represented by a pre-post difference score for severity of distress. Expected improvement reflects the client's outcome *expectancy*; extreme scores would be of concern (reflecting pessimism or idealization regarding therapy). Expected and observed improvement ratings can be contrasted as an indication of client satisfaction. Instructions and rating forms are found in Appendix I. An Excel scoring template is available for download on the publisher website. Studies of time-limited group therapy (Piper et al., 2001, 2007) showed the procedure could be consistently implemented across assessors (reliability estimates >.95). The objectives' *idiographic* nature means the ratings are highly sensitive to change over the course of treatment. This goal attainment method was used in a replication study of interpersonal relatedness variables as predictors of group outcome (Joyce et al., 2010) and an examination of the joint prediction afforded by psychological mindedness and group process variables (Kealy, Piper, Ogrodniczuk, et al., 2018).

Mental Functioning: M Axis Ratings from the Psychodiagnostic Chart

Ego strength is problematic to define clearly because it serves as an umbrella term for a number of mental functions, all of which are critical to evaluate in a clinical assessment. The group leader looks to select members who are homogeneous for ego strength, i.e., all

Table 2.3 The Target Objectives Procedure

Item	Information
Name of instrument	*Target Objectives*
Authors	Carolyn C. Battle, Stanley D. Imber, Rudolph Hoehn-Saric, Anthony R. Stone, Earl R. Nash, & Jerome D. Frank
Source	Battle, C. C., Imber, S. D., Hoehn-Saric, R., Stone, A. R., Nash, E. R., & Frank, J. D. (1966). Target complaints as criteria of improvement. *American Journal of Psychotherapy, 20,* 184–192. https://dx.doi.org/10.1176/appi.psychotherapy.1966.20.1.184
Translations	The Target Objectives procedure can be easily adapted for use in any language.
Brief description	The Target Objectives procedure (also referred to in the literature as Target Goals or Target Complaints) is an individualized measure of expectations for psychotherapy outcome based on a patient's description of the problems and difficulties for which they have sought treatment. As an idiographic measure, the procedure has inherent psychometric limitations but is recommended because of its direct relevance to individual patient experience, strong face validity, and sensitivity to change.
Time requirements	Administration: 15–30 minutes. Scoring: 10 minutes.
Subscales and scoring	There is no published manual outlining standardized procedures or normative data; most applications follow the guidelines in the seminal work by Battle et al. (1966). During pre-group screening, the client is asked to list, in their own words, three goals or objectives they most want to achieve in therapy. The effort is made to help the client define these objectives in concrete behavioral terms. Using both a 5- or 11-point Likert scale, clients then rate each objective according to: a) the severity of distress during the previous month (1 = slight severity, 5 = extreme severity); b) the importance of the objective to the client (1 = slight importance, 5 = extreme importance); and c) their expectation for improvement as a result of treatment (1 = extreme worsening, 6 = no change, 11 = extreme improvement). The group leader can also rate each target objective along the same dimensions. At the end of treatment, client and therapist can rate each objective according to: a) the severity of distress during the previous month; b) the importance of the objective to the client; and c) the degree of observed improvement/level of change since therapy began. (The leader can also engage in an alternative scoring option providing additional information, by rating each objective on the five dimensions of duration, frequency, intensity, pervasiveness, and disruptiveness.) Scoring consists of either summing or averaging the pre- and post-therapy ratings for each target objective. Change over treatment is typically expressed as a difference score.
Psychometric properties	The Target Objectives procedure has substantial face validity—the objectives jointly formulated by the client and leader are central to the client's treatment. Research use (e.g., Piper et al., 2007) has demonstrated that the procedure can be applied consistently across different raters. Concurrent validity studies suggest the client and therapist improvement ratings tap a broad factor of change and have been reported to correlate highly with standardized measures of outcome ($r = .71$). Battle et al. (1966) highlighted "reliable results" based on their observation that the majority of patients did not change the content or severity rating of their target objectives following an intensive psychiatric interview.
Norms	NA
Administration types	Paper & pencil.

Item	Information
Name of instrument	*Target Objectives*
Sensitivity to change	Studies by Piper et al. (2001, 2007) demonstrate that the Target Objectives procedure is highly sensitive to change as a function of treatment.
Analytics	Summed or averaged pre-therapy ratings of expected improvement reflect the client's outcome *expectancy* for treatment. Very low or high expectancy scores would be of concern: low scores suggest that the client may be pessimistic about therapy or not committed to change, while high scores suggest an overly idealized view of what therapy can do.
Benchmarking	NA
Sample references	Joyce, A. S., Ogrodniczuk, J. S., Piper, W. E., & Sheptycki, A. R. (2010). Interpersonal predictors of outcome following short-term group therapy for complicated grief: A replication. *Clinical Psychology and Psychotherapy, 17*, 122–135. https://dx.doi.org/10.1002/cpp.686 Kealy, D., Piper, W. E., Ogrodniczuk, J. S., Joyce, A. S., & Weideman, R. (2018). Individual goal achievement in group psychotherapy: The roles of psychological mindedness and group process in interpretive and supportive therapy for complicated grief. *Clinical Psychology and Psychotherapy*, 1–11. https://dx.doi.org/10.1002/cpp.2346 Piper, W. E., McCallum, M., Joyce, A. S., & Ogrodniczuk, J. S. (2001). Patient personality and time-limited group psychotherapy for complicated grief. *International Journal of Group Psychotherapy, 51*, 525–552. https://dx.doi.org/10.1521/ijgp.51.4.525.51307 Piper, W. E., Ogrodniczuk, J. S., Joyce, A. S., Weideman, R., & Rosie, J. S. (2007). Group composition and group therapy for complicated grief. *Journal of Consulting and Clinical Psychology, 75*, 116–125. https://dx.doi.org/10.1037/0022-006X.75.1.116
Website resources	Target Objectives procedure instructions and an Excel scoring program are available for free download from AGPA (www.agpa.org).
How to obtain/ Cost	Public domain.

members can reasonably be viewed as able to meet group demands for engagement, interaction, containment, and change. The M Axis is one of five assessment domains of the Psychodiagnostic Chart-2 (PDC) (Gordon & Bornstein, 2015, 2018). In turn, the PDC represents a clinical tool operationalizing the assessment approach of the Psychodynamic Diagnostic Manual (PDM) (Lingiardi et al., 2015) as an alternative to symptom-oriented diagnostic systems like the DSM-5 or ICD-10. We recommend the M Axis as a way to systematically evaluate ego strength but also encourage the reader to become acquainted with the full PDC and the latest edition of the PDM.

The M Axis offers a framework to evaluate the client on the 12 mental functions listed in Table 2.1. Based on encounters with the client (encompassing referral information, self-report data, clinical interview, and therapist responses), 5-point ratings of strength or impairment for each function are made and then aggregated into a global score for level of ego strength. The procedure can identify clients who may require additional preparation prior to group admittance. The PDC demonstrates good internal consistency and test-retest stability, with strong interrater reliability (Gordon & Bornstein, 2018; Gordon & Stoffey, 2014).

Clinical Vignette Part One

Dr. Abel Brown, a psychologist identifying as a White gay male, and Francis Ford, a psychiatric nurse identifying as a Black heterosexual female, had discussed starting an interpersonal process

Table 2.4 The 12 Mental Functions of the PDM-2 M Axis

Cognitive and affective processes	
1.	Capacity for regulation, attention, and learning (*attend to and process internal and external information, regulate focus, learn from experience*)
2.	Capacity for affective range, communication, and understanding (*ability to experience, express, and comprehend the full range of affects in a way that is appropriate*)
3.	Capacity for mentalization and reflective functioning (*to infer and reflect on own and others' mental states, and to use ideas to experience, describe, and express internal life*)
Identity and relationships	
4.	Capacity for differentiation and integration (*ability to construct and maintain a differentiated, realistic, coherent, and complex representation of self and other people*)
5.	Capacity for relationships and intimacy (*depth, range, and stability of the person's interpersonal relationships, ability to engage in pleasurable sexual fantasies and activities, and the ability to blend sexuality with emotional intimacy*)
6.	Self-esteem regulation and quality of internal experience (*level of confidence and self-regard*)
Defense and coping	
7.	Impulse control and regulation (*ability to modulate impulses and express them in adaptive, culture-appropriate ways*)
8.	Defensive functioning (*ability to modulate anxiety resulting from internal conflict, external challenge, or threat to the self without excessive distortion in self-perception and reality testing*)
9.	Adaptation, resiliency, and strength (*ability to cope effectively with uncertainty, loss, stress, and challenge with individual strengths, such as empathy and sensitivity to other peoples' needs and feelings, the ability to recognize alternative viewpoints, or to be appropriately assertive when necessary*)
Self-awareness and self-direction	
10.	Self-observing capacities, psychological mindedness (*motivated to introspect and observe own internal life mindfully and realistically, and use this information effectively*)
11.	Capacity to construct and use internal standards and ideals (*capacity to formulate internal values and ideals and to make mindful decisions based on a set of coherent, internally consistent underlying moral principles*)
12.	Meaning and purpose (*ability to construct a personal narrative that gives cohesion and meaning to personal choices, and a sense of directedness, purpose, and spirituality to grasp the broader implications of one's attitudes, beliefs, and behaviors*)

Adapted from Gordon & Bornstein (2017).

Note. PDM-2 = Psychodynamic Diagnostic Manual-Second Edition.

group together. They expressed this interest during staff meetings at the outpatient clinic. In short order, a dozen potential group members of diverse diagnosis and background were referred from the caseloads of busy colleagues. Abel and Francis agreed to each conduct pre-group screening interviews with six clients. They also assumed a measurement-based care perspective and asked each client to complete the GTQ-S in the waiting area prior to their screening interview. Abel and Francis met a week later to compile interview impressions and GTQ-S responses for eleven clients—one client could not attend her session with Francis because of a family crisis. For eight of the eleven clients, clinical impressions from the interview and GTQ-S data aligned well—all eight looked to be appropriate, strong candidates for the group. For three of the eight, the GTQ-S flagged issues that Francis and Abel agreed to explore

Table 2.5 The M Axis of the PDC-2

Item	Information
Name of instrument	*M Axis of the Psychodiagnostic Chart-2*
Authors	Robert M. Gordon & Robert F. Bornstein
Source	Gordon, R. M., & Bornstein, R. F. (2018). Construct validity of the Psychodiagnostic Chart: A transdiagnostic measure of personality organization, personality syndromes, mental functioning, and symptomatology. *Psychoanalytic Psychology, 35,* 280–288. https://dx.doi.org/0000-0003-1990-8644
Translations	In preparation.
Brief description	The M Axis is one of five assessment domains of the Psychodiagnostic Chart-2 (the others reflecting personality organization, personality syndromes, symptom patterns, and cultural/contextual considerations). In turn, the PDC-2 is a clinical tool operationalizing the assessment approach of the Psychodynamic Diagnostic Manual (PDM). The M Axis offers a framework to evaluate the client's standing on twelve critical mental functions. Based on sources of client data (e.g., referral information, self-report data, clinical interview, therapist responses), ratings of strength versus impairment are made for each function and then aggregated into an overall score for level of "ego strength."
Time requirements	The actual M Axis ratings may require less than 10 minutes but collection and review of clinical data can require considerable time and effort.
Subscales and scoring	The 12 mental functions are subsumed into four main domains: cognitive and affective processes; identity and relationships; defense and coping; and self-awareness and self-direction. The client's strengths and limitations are considered for each of the functions using a series of 5-point ratings. After being rated individually, the 12 M Axis mental function ratings are summarized to derive an overall severity score which can then be categorized into one of seven levels of functioning (ranging from healthy/optimal to major/severe deficits).
Psychometric properties	Test-retest reliabilities for the original version of the M Axis rating items (9 items versus 12 in the PDC-2) ranged between .77- .89. Consistency between raters was demonstrated for the version of the M Axis from the PDC-2, with a mean interrater correlation of .85 (coefficients ranging between .82- .92), demonstrating the relative ease of use of the rating items.
Norms	NA
Administration types	A digital version of the PDC-2 is available for download.
Sensitivity to change	NA
Analytics	The M Axis can be employed on its own to evaluate the client's ego strength, or as part of a more comprehensive clinical assessment of personality structure/function and client context using the PDC-2.
Benchmarking	NA
Sample references	Gordon, R. M., & Stoffey, R. W. (2014). Operationalizing the psychodynamic diagnostic manual: A preliminary study of the psychodiagnostic chart. *Bulletin of the Menninger Clinic, 78,* 1–15. https://dx.doi.org/10.1521/bumc.2014.78.1.1
Website resources	Gordon, R. M., & Bornstein, R. F. (2015). *The Psychodiagnostic Chart-2 v. 8.1 (PDC-2).* Retrieved from: www.researchgate.net/publication/292592861_Digital_Psychodiagnostic_Chart-2_PDC-2_v81.
How to obtain/Cost	The PDC-2, with the digital version of the M Axis rating, is available for free download at the address listed above.

further during PGP sessions. Lamar, a heterosexual Black male, reported a history of family violence and the expectation that the group should provide him with a "cure" within six months. Marlena, a heterosexual Latin-American female, alluded to difficulties with certain anniversaries in her life when she would be plagued with suicidal thoughts. Jacob, a transgender White male, expressed fears of being humiliated by a judgmental group. Abel and Francis resolved to engage therapeutically on the specific issue with each client during PGP. To cap the assessment process with these eight members, Francis and Abel used M Axis ratings to quantify clients' ego functioning, based on the referral, their interview experience, and the GTQ-S. Their ratings indicated that all eight appeared to have the capacity to respond well to the demands of the group. The M Axis ratings and the GTQ-S Ego Strength score showed good concordance. Two outliers on both measures indicated that additional support for those clients might be needed at times during treatment.

Lori, identifying as a heterosexual White female, had cancelled her group screen with Francis, arrived at the clinic with only minutes left to her rescheduled session. Francis realized that a quick assessment might help her decide if another rescheduling would be useful or if her impression of Lori's life as chaotic was a red flag regarding selection. Francis asked Lori if she would complete the GRQ and have a quick debrief meeting about the results; Lori was relieved that she remained a prospective member and agreed. In short order, Francis saw that Lori's scores for Participation and Expectancy were low, reflecting readiness for group therapy. Francis also noted that Lori's responses on the Demeanor items suggested issues with anger control. Francis decided to have Lori back for a full screening interview and completion of the GTQ-S. Subsequently, the interview and GTQ-S data confirmed Lori's suitability for the group.

Of the dozen referrals, four clients provided GTQ-S responses that Francis and Abel found concerning. One client reported estrangement from family, a paucity of supportive friendships, and little motivation to leave his apartment to socialize. The clinicians felt a life skills support group was more in line with the client's treatment needs. A second client had struck Abel as resistant to a therapeutic focus; this was confirmed by a high Angry Hostility score on the GTQ-S. He and Francis agreed to return the client to the referring therapist for more individual work. The GTQ-S data for the remaining two clients strongly reflected somatic concerns; the pair were referred to an affiliated team of psychiatrists, psychologists, and internal medicine specialists.

Francis and Abel decided to combine preparation with implementation of the Target Objectives procedure for each confirmed group member. Two preparation sessions were held with four members each; the formulation and ratings of objectives for each member were central to establishing a base of understanding, a good foundation for the launch of the group.

Assessment Alternatives: Diagnostic and Client Capacity Measures

Selection should provide for a thorough understanding of the client and a confident decision regarding group admission. A measurement-based care approach can also benefit from a reliable evaluation of symptoms and psychological capacities. The three measures introduced below offer an adjunct perspective to the assessment of readiness and consider the *interface* between the client and the group. All demonstrate good psychometrics and utility for informing treatment.

The Brief Symptom Inventory (BSI-53)

Knowledge of the client's symptoms is critical to clinical understanding and evaluating change. The Brief Symptom Inventory-53 is an evolution of the venerable Symptom

Table 2.6 The Brief Symptom Inventory

Item	Information
Name of instrument	*Brief Symptom Inventory (BSI-53)*
Authors	Leonard R. Derogatis
Source	Derogatis, L. R. (1993). *BSI: Administration, scoring, and procedures manual for the Brief Symptom Inventory* (3rd ed.). Minneapolis, MN: National Computer Systems.
Translations	The BSI has been translated into over two dozen languages.
Brief description	The Brief Symptom Inventory comprises 53 items and represents the short form of the well-known Symptom Checklist-90-Revised. The checklist is a self-report of symptoms associated with psychological distress/disorders. Ratings of symptom intensity are assigned using a 5-point (0–4) rating scale. The instrument provides scores for nine symptom dimensions and three global indices.
Time requirements	Administration: 10 minutes. Scoring: 10 minutes.
Subscales and scoring	Symptom domains include Somatization, Obsessive-Compulsive, Interpersonal Sensitivity, Depression, Anxiety, Hostility, Phobic Anxiety, Paranoid Ideation, and Psychoticism. Global scales include the Global Severity Index (GSI), Positive Symptom Distress Index, and Positive Symptom Total. The GSI is frequently used as a general severity and outcome measure; the index reflects both the number and intensity of symptoms.
Psychometric properties	Internal consistency, based on a sample of 719 outpatients, ranged from.71-.85 for the nine symptom scales. Two-week test-retest reliabilities, based on a sample of 60 nonpatients, ranged from.68-.91; the GSI demonstrated excellent stability (r =.90). The manual also summarizes studies addressing the BSI's validity, highlighting its sensitivity to manifestations of psychological distress and the impact of interventions designed to ameliorate it.
Norms	Norms are provided in the manual for a) psychiatric outpatients, b) community nonpatients, c) psychiatric inpatients, and d) community adolescents. Values are also gender-keyed but restricted to a binary definition.
Administration types	Paper & pencil or digital, depending on format purchased (see below).
Sensitivity to change	The manual summarizes studies demonstrating the sensitivity of the BSI, both in identification of 'caseness' and changes as a function of treatment.
Analytics	A value > 63 for the T-scores of the GSI or any two primary symptom scales is indicative of a psychiatric diagnosis.
Benchmarking	The manual offers information regarding the symptom profile of patients with anxiety, depressive, and somatoform disorders; stress conditions; suicidality; alcohol and substance abuse conditions; sexual victimization; and medical conditions.
Sample references	Derogatis, L. R. (2017). Symptom Checklist-90-Revised, Brief Symptom Inventory, and BSI-18. In M. E. Maruish (Ed.), *Handbook of psychological assessment in primary care settings* (p. 599–629). New York, NY: Routledge. Derogatis, L. R., & Melisaratos, N. (1983). The Brief Symptom Inventory: An introductory report. *Psychological Medicine, 13*, 585–605. https://dx.doi.org/10.1017/S0033291700048017
Website resources	An online version of the SCL-90-R is mentioned in Derogatis (2017) but there is no comment regarding the same for the BSI-53.
How to obtain/Cost	The BSI-53 is available for purchase from www.pearsonassessments.com with options ranging from single administrations at $6.40 to instrument kits starting at $74.20.

Checklist-90-R (Derogatis, 1993, 2017). This self-report comprises 53 Likert-type items, rated on a 0–4 scale of intensity, measuring symptom distress in nine primary domains (Somatization, Obsessive-Compulsive, Interpersonal Sensitivity, Depression, Anxiety, Hostility, Phobic Anxiety, Paranoid Ideation, and Psychoticism). Three global scales (Global Severity Index, Positive Symptom Distress Index, and Positive Symptom Total) offer summary measures; the GSI reflects both the *number* and *intensity* of symptoms and is often used as a general severity and outcome measure. Regarding selection for group therapy, high scores on the Somatization, Interpersonal Sensitivity, Hostility, and Paranoid Ideation scales would be of concern.

Gender (binary only) norms for the BSI-53 are available for psychiatric in- and outpatients, community non-patients, and community adolescents (Derogatis, 1993). For each subscale, raw scores are converted to T-scores, allowing for normative comparisons but also for evaluations *within* individual profiles (e.g., is the client's level of Depression higher than the level of Anxiety?). A T-score equal to or greater than 63 for the GSI or any two symptom scales is indicative of a psychiatric diagnosis. Reliability and validity of the BSI-53 is strong—there are literally hundreds of studies demonstrating the measure's predictive validity and sensitivity to change (Derogatis, 1993, 2017). The BSI-53 is available for purchase at www.pearsonassessments.com.

The Toronto Alexithymia Scale (TAS-20)

Moving from assessing the phenomenology of the client's symptoms, this measure addresses issues with an important *capacity* that has implications for the therapy process; it can be useful in selection and also in efforts at composition (see below). This capacity is elusive to define but generally involves a person's ability to think in terms of psychological constructs reflecting internal mental contents—beliefs, desires, intentions, emotions, etc. The TAS-20 assesses a *deficit* in the capacity to identify and articulate feelings.

Alexithymia ("no words for feelings" in Latin) refers to deficits in the cognitive processing and regulation of emotion, reflected by a limited capacity to symbolize and elaborate upon emotional experience (Taylor & Bagby, 2004). The alexithymic individual has difficulty differentiating and communicating feelings and tends to engage in "externally oriented" thinking, i.e., a focus on the concrete details of events. Alexithymic individuals have also been described as having an impoverished fantasy life, an impaired capacity for empathy, a propensity for impulsivity and use of primitive defenses, and a tendency to somatize emotions (Taylor & Bagby, 2004).

Alexithymia can be measured with the 20-item self-report TAS-20 (Bagby et al., 1994a, 1994b). In addition to a total score (with cutoffs), the TAS-20 provides scores for three reliable factors: Difficulty Identifying Feelings (and distinguishing feelings from bodily sensations), Difficulty Communicating Feelings, and Externally Oriented Thinking. Items are rated on a 5-point Likert scale. The TAS-20 has demonstrated strong internal consistency and test-retest reliability over a three-week period, with good convergent and divergent validity (Bagby et al., 1994a, 1994b). The TAS-20 scores of clinical samples proved to be significantly higher than those of nonclinical samples (Bagby et al., 1994b). Joyce et al. (2013) identified correlates of alexithymia for outpatients in an intensive, group-oriented partial hospital program, reporting associations with attachment avoidance, suppression of emotions, use of immature defenses, and severity of borderline personality disorder. The source articles offer essential information on the TAS-20 and scoring; a more detailed package is available for download from Dr. M. Bagby (rmichael.bagby@utoronto.ca) or through www.gtaylorpsychiatry.org.

Given that most therapies require self-reflection, interest in internal experience, and access to feelings, alexithymia has been reported to have an adverse effect on therapy

Table 2.7 The Toronto Alexithymia Scale

Item	Information
Name of instrument	*Toronto Alexithymia Scale (TAS-20)*
Authors	R. Michael Bagby, James D. A. Parker, & Graeme J. Taylor
Source	Bagby, R. M., Parker, J. D. A., & Taylor, G. J. (1994a). The twenty-item Toronto Alexithymia Scale—I. Item selection and cross-validation of the factor structure. *Journal of Psychosomatic Research, 38*, 23–32. doi: 10.1016/0022–3999(94)90005–1 Bagby, R. M., Taylor, G. J., & Parker, J. D. A. (1994b). The twenty-item Toronto Alexithymia Scale—II. Convergent, discriminant, and concurrent validity. *Journal of Psychosomatic Research, 38*, 33–40. https://dx.doi.org/10.1016/0022–3999(94)90006-x
Translations	In addition to the original English, the TAS has been translated into 18 languages.
Brief description	The TAS is a 20-item self-report addressing traits of the alexithymia construct. The items are rated on a 5-point scale ranging from 1 (strongly disagree) to 5 (strongly agree).
Time requirements	Administration: 10–15 minutes. Scoring: 10–15 minutes.
Subscales and scoring	In addition to a total score, the TAS-20 yields scores for three reliable and valid factor scales: Difficulty Identifying Feelings, Difficulty Communicating Feelings, and Externally Oriented Thinking. Higher scores indicate greater alexithymia.
Psychometric properties	The source article indicates that the TAS-20 demonstrated acceptable internal consistency, with Cronbach's alpha coefficients of .81 for the total score, and .78, .75, and .66 for the three factor scores, respectively. Similar values were obtained in a cross-validation sample of post-secondary students and with a sample of psychiatric patients. Test-retest reliability with an independent sample yielded a coefficient of .77, indicating good stability. Research using the TAS-20 demonstrates adequate levels of convergent and concurrent validity. The 3-factor structure is theoretically congruent with the alexithymia construct and has been found to be stable and replicable across clinical and non-clinical populations.
Norms	In the original validation study, men demonstrated significantly higher TAS-20 total scores than women. These differences were not apparent in the cross-validation sample or with the sample of psychiatric patients. However, the gender difference has emerged in other research studies using the TAS-20.
Administration types	Paper & pencil or formatted on a device.
Sensitivity to change	The TAS-20 has been employed as an individual difference and outcome measure in a range of studies (see the website below for examples) and has proven to be sensitive to change during active treatment.
Analytics	The alexithymic status of an individual can be categorized based on the use of cut-offs for the TAS-20 total score: Scores less than or equal to 51 reflect *non-alexithymia*, scores of 52–60 reflect *possible alexithymia*, and scores of 61 or greater reflect *full alexithymia*.
Benchmarking	The source articles provide score values for non-clinical and clinical samples. The research base for the TAS-20 provides additional examples of comparisons by respondent characteristics or settings.
Sample references	Taylor, G. J., & Bagby, R. M. (2004). New trends in alexithymia research. *Psychotherapy and Psychosomatics, 73*, 68–77. https://dx.doi.org/10.1159/000075537
How to obtain/ Cost	The source articles provide the essential information on the TAS-20 and its scoring. A package with more detailed information can be obtained from Dr. M. Bagby for a copyright fee of US$40.00 (go to www.gtaylorpsychiatry.org/tas.htm for more information).

outcome. Ogrodniczuk et al. (2005) found that alexithymia was associated with less improvement on two of three outcome factors in a trial of two forms of brief group therapy. These effects on outcome were mediated by the group therapist's *negative* response to the alexithymic client. Selection would aim for a minority proportion of alexithymic clients in the group. The idea is that the non-alexithymic majority can "carry" one or two alexithymic clients towards therapeutic benefit.

The literature suggests that improvements in alexithymia can be seen over time in group therapy (Kleinberg, 1996) as the client becomes more adept at dealing with emotion.

The inverse of alexithymia is represented by a capacity for reflective function, or mentalization, defined as the ability to understand and interpret one's own and others' behavior as an expression of *mental states* such as feelings, thoughts, fantasies, beliefs, and desires (Fonagy et al., 2002). RF signifies an appreciation of the motive nature of mental states not only in relation to others (as in empathy) but also in relation to the self (Katznelson, 2014). Clients with differing capacity to mentalize will also vary in their ability to engage in the therapy process, i.e., RF can be a *moderator* of therapy outcome (Gullestad et al., 2012). It is also likely that RF can *change* as a function of therapy and improved RF may be related to improved psychological function more generally (Allen et al., 2008). A promising self-report measure of RF has been developed by Fonagy et al. (2016). An 8-item version of the RFQ (as well as more elaborate 46- and 54-item versions) and scoring programs are available for free download at www.ucl.ac.uk. However, the website notes that downloads are for research and that the measure is "not yet suited for clinical purposes." With further validation, the RFQ will certainly represent a useful index for group selection; it is mentioned here for the reader to explore further.

Therapeutic Reactance Scale (TRS)

Group therapy offers members opportunities for personal examination and expression. For some members, however, group can represent a threat to autonomy: the norms may be perceived as restrictive and the emotional pull of interaction may be felt as intrusive. The motivation to respond with opposition to perceived threats to personal freedom has been defined as *reactance* (Brehm & Brehm, 1981). Reactance is an outgrowth of adaptive strivings for autonomy. Highly reactant individuals are "likely to be skeptical of others' intentions, competitive, intolerant and distrustful, secretive, and detached" (Seeman et al., 2005, p. 95). Studies indicate that reactance may be associated with separation-individuation issues (e.g., Siebel & Dowd, 2001). In a group setting, reactance may be activated by more directive leader interventions or peer pressures (Kealy, Joyce, Ogrodniczuk, et al., 2018). The latter team found that reactance was directly associated with reduced attendance and premature termination from an intensive group program. Reactance was also related to views of the group as excessively dependent on the therapists and as mired in tension and conflict. The authors suggest that the reactant client's capacity to reflect on mental states can become compromised when their sense of personal freedom is challenged.

The potential for reactance can be assessed using the TRS (Dowd et al., 1991). This 28-item self-report provides two subscale scores: Behavioral Reactance reflects tendencies to act in ways that oppose encouraged behaviors ("If I'm told what to do, I often do the opposite") while Verbal Reactance refers to an inclination to argue against and resist persuasion ("I feel it is important to stand up for what I believe than to be silent"). Items are rated on a scale ranging from *strongly disagree* (1) to *strongly agree* (4). The two subscales have shown good internal consistency (Dowd et al., 1991); values can be summed to provide an overall reactance score (see Seibel & Dowd, 2001). High TRS scores would indicate that the client may require more intensive preparation or even a course of individual therapy prior to group. Only a small proportion of the group's membership should demonstrate any degree of reactance, allowing the majority to offer a buffer against extreme displays of opposition. High scores on Behavioral Reactance would be of more concern given the potential for disruptiveness in group. The leader should keep in mind that reactant clients may actually want to address their reactivity in treatment. A thoughtful use of the TRS to limit the reactance potential in the group can facilitate this possibility.

Table 2.8 The Therapeutic Reactance Scale

Item	Information
Name of instrument	*Therapeutic Reactance Scale (TRS)*
Authors	E. Thomas Dowd, Christopher R. Milne, & Steven L. Wise.
Source	Dowd, E. T., Milne, C. R., & Wise, S. L. (1991). The therapeutic reactance scale: A measure of psychological reactance. *Journal of Counseling and Development, 69,* 541–545. https://dx.doi.org/10.1002/j.1556-6676.1991.tb02638.x
Translations	English.
Brief description	The TRS is a 28-item self-report of the tendency to respond in an oppositional manner to perceived threats to personal freedom. Items are rated on a 4-point scale ranging from *strongly disagree* (1) to *strongly agree* (4).
Time requirements	Administration: 10–15 minutes. Scoring: 10–15 minutes.
Subscales and scoring	Two subscale scores can be derived: Behavioral Reactance reflects tendencies to act in ways that oppose encouraged behaviors while Verbal Reactance reflects an inclination to argue against and resist persuasion. Scores can also be summed to provide an overall reactance score.
Psychometric properties	Item selection and factor analytic work to develop the TRS was rigorous. Internal consistency estimates were strong (.81 for Behavioral and .75 for Verbal Reactance, with the Total Score demonstrating a coefficient of .84). Test-retest reliabilities by subscale were consistently around .60, suggesting that reactance can reflect both trait and state elements. The two forms of reactance demonstrated a relatively low correlation ($r = .37$), suggesting they are relatively discrete constructs.
Norms	The source article provides descriptive statistics for TRS total scores from two samples (N=211, 150) of college students.
Administration types	Paper & pencil or formatted on a device.
Sensitivity to change	The TRS has largely been employed as an individual difference measure, to predict possible clinical implications.
Analytics	NA
Benchmarking	NA
Sample references	Brehm, S. S., & Brehm, J. W. (1981). *Psychological reactance: A theory of freedom and control.* New York, NY: Wiley Press. Dowd, E. T., & Wallbrown, F. (1993). Motivational components of client reactance. *Journal of Counseling & Development, 71,* 533–538. https://dx.doi.org/10.1002.j.1556-6676.1993.tb02237.x Kealy, D., Joyce, A. S., Ogrodniczuk, J. S., Ehrenthal, J. C., & Weber, R. (2018). Reactance and engagement in integrative group psychotherapy for personality dysfunction, *Journal of Psychotherapy Integration, 28,* 462–474. https://dx.doi.org/10.1037/int0000129
How to obtain/Cost	Available in the source article.

Group Composition: Aims and Pragmatics

Composition Aims. Beyond selecting clients likely to contribute to and benefit from the group, leaders can tackle *actively composing the group* as a foundation for greater cohesiveness. *Composition* refers to efforts to implement a "blend and balance" of personal characteristics among the clients making up the group (Kealy et al., 2016; Rutan et al., 2014). A thoughtful use of standardized measures to "plant the seeds" for cohesion can increase the *likelihood* of the group starting well and developing quickly. Below, we suggest reliable, validated measures that can be used in efforts to influence group composition. (A number already introduced— the TAS-20 or TRS—could be used in this manner.) It must be said that there is no "cookbook" for crafting an intended group composition—the activity is much more like educated guessing ("group composition is still a soft science" according to Yalom & Leszcz, 2020, p. 330). We suggest making use of measures that mesh with the leaders' group approach and employing the data to compose a particular "case mix" for the group. Other methods of composing groups should be acknowledged, e.g., Yalom and Leszcz (2020) describe implementing one-time "trial" group experiences, then composing ongoing groups based on observations of clients "in action."

Kealy et al. (2016) note that composition addresses the relative homogeneity or heterogeneity of group members' characteristics. These can range from demographic or clinical variables (gender, ethnicity, presenting problem) to measures of personality traits or capacities. In the case of the prototype process group, the measures described below can be used to aim for maximal heterogeneity in clients' areas of conflict and interpersonal style, while attending to homogeneity on indices of ego strength (e.g., M Axis ratings). As noted, choice of measures should be based on conceptual relevance to the intervention approach. Composition objectives (e.g., a diversity of IIP profiles) will likely mirror objectives of the group approach (e.g., clarifying problematic interpersonal patterns). A main objective is to aim for a balance of similarity and divergence on measures of interpersonal "style;" client variation can be critical to the emergence of cohesion.

Groups with more *focused* aims (commonly briefer in duration) typically call for greater homogeneity among members, e.g., groups for complicated grief may also target the interpersonal dependency associated with the syndrome (Piper et al., 2007). In contrast, longer-term process groups may require a *balance* of characteristics (e.g., a restricted proportion of clients scoring highly on a measure of perfectionism) or a *diversity* of scores on a particular dimension (e.g., attachment style). For example, use of the IIP can capture variations in interpersonal dominance among clients; the data might then be used to "cap" or offset the number who are highly dominant or submissive, or "over-balance" the composition towards friendly (versus hostile) dominance. Members determined to have liabilities regarding group admittance (e.g., volatility) *can* engage and improve if the group's make-up offers the requisite "holding" to support the client's therapeutic process. The group could be composed with this in mind. Piper et al. (2007) found that brief groups having a greater *proportion* of members with more mature interpersonal functioning (higher "quality of object relations") demonstrated greater benefit for their members overall, regardless of each *individual* member's QOR level. Thus, the presence of members with high QOR influenced the group sufficiently to also benefit those members with less mature relational functioning.

Composition Pragmatics. The group leader has fewer "degrees of freedom" when selecting members for an ongoing group, given the existing composition. In this case, a measure can be used in a targeted way to identify clients within a desired range on the characteristic. A more extensive composition process is feasible for a *new* group when assessment can be implemented with a pool of candidates. Having a conceptual basis for any composition undertaking is a must. This requires specifying some element of theory, group approach, or

technical strategy that is likely to interact with the client attribute and developing a rationale for linking the client variable to greater cohesion and more optimal group functioning.
Some guiding questions: What client variable (or combination of variables) is likely to be
critical in the group's development and why? The leader should attend to conceptual
overlap between measures; for example, a number of the suggested instruments address
interpersonal domains so a choice of a single measure should rely on the leaders' clinical
theory and group approach. Information needs should also be balanced against clients'
"assessment fatigue" when designing a brief battery for evaluation. Further, it should be
determined how the selected variable(s) will be represented in the group composition. Is the
aim to establish a *balance* of the characteristic across members, a certain *proportion* with the
characteristic, to admit or decline clients based on critical score *cutoffs*, or to *predict* or *identify*
potentially problematic group members? The purpose of the exercise—choosing one or
more measures, collecting assessments from a pool of clients, "crunching" the numbers and
composing the group based on the data—is to supplement selection efforts and help *formulate predictions* of interpersonal and group behavior, ultimately facilitating greater group
cohesion. We selected measures for composition based on likely clinical utility and/or
informative richness of interpretation. We believe the applied use of any of these measures
in a "clinically oriented research evaluation" process (the original words behind the acro-
nym CORE) has a considerable potential to enhance the clinician's work.

Questions of Composition: Ethnic Identity and Experiences of Discrimination

We start by considering the cultural dimension from the perspective of composition.
Attending to the influence of culture is always relevant in clinical work but is critically
important in the new millennium. Chen et al. (2008, p.1264) state:

> "Culture is often defined as a network of domain-specific knowledge structures shared
> by members of a visible or invisible sociocultural group. It is internalized into each
> individual's self-concept and functions as a set of templates that guide and govern
> interpersonal expectations, perceptions, and interpretations across social situations."

The authors further note that a group is a social microcosm, with members having diverse
cultural values and expectations. Greater cultural diversity "expands the multiple perspectives that are already available in the group but also limits within-group communication,
presenting an increased risk for misunderstanding and conflict" (p. 1264). Clarity about the
cultural diversity represented by the members is accordingly quite useful to the leader and
can bear on composition of a new group or when adding to an existing group (Ribeiro,
2020).

An understanding of identities—our clients' and our own—is a key by-product of the
selection and preparation process. It is important to have clarity about identities that provide some with *privilege* related to race, gender, sexual orientation, religion, ability, or
socioeconomic status, and about identities associated with experiences of *marginalization*, and
how these issues will be addressed in the group. Ribeiro (2020) outlines how group leaders
can be sensitive to intersecting identities and how this may influence group selection. The
GTQ-S described above addresses these issues by asking clients about aspects of their
identities they would want to share, or find challenging to examine, in the group.

Our discussion is framed in terms of the racial-cultural dimension—we specifically focus
on measures of ethnic identity and experiences of discrimination. This is not to discount the
importance of attending to other aspects of diversity such as gender and sexual orientation,

immigration status, or disability—the intersectionality of identities is a critical focus during PGP sessions. Our rationale here is that ethnocultural background can influence the expression of attachment behavior and relationships more generally, e.g., the perspectives associated with being raised in an individualistic versus collectivistic culture (see Marmarosh et al., 2013b). We suggest evaluating the ethnic identity of prospective members, and their experiences of discrimination, to estimate the likelihood the composed group will be both robust and supportive of discussions addressing privilege, racism, and cultural under-standing (Ribeiro, 2020). In contrast to the transdiagnostic measures suggested for compo-sition in the next section, where scores determine composition decisions, we propose using the two measures below to gain clarity about the cultural context of the members, followed by reflection on treatment strategy or possible modifications of approach. We also assume that a heterogenous group composition on cultural dimensions is preferred to facilitate giving voice to marginalized individuals alongside those who comprise the majority. Adhering to this principle does however go against findings that treatments engaging a *specific* cultural group have proven more effective than those offered to clients from a range of cultural backgrounds (see Smith et al., 2011). For a process group and in a wider context of a vigorous social justice movement, aiming for cultural and ethnic diversity of membership represents an aspirational goal. The racial/ethnic composition of the group will in turn determine the multicultural sensitivity demanded of the group therapist (Chen et al., 2008).

Using this lens, the composition aim is to delve into each member's ethnic identity and experiences of discrimination to better predict how interactions around racial differences might unfold, i.e., practising *cultural humility* (Hook et al., 2013) to facilitate *cultural sensitivity* in leader and members alike (Kaklauskas & Nettles, 2019). For example, the assessment may highlight how members differ in managing conflict based on background: Western-influenced members may endorse emotional expression, confrontation, and working through, while Eastern-influenced members may prioritize maintaining respectful transac-tions and emotional self-control. A group reflecting this cultural composition might require incorporation of a more inclusive rationale for interventions (see Chang-Caffaro & Caffaro, 2018). This would contrast with implementing more extensive *cultural adaptations* of group approaches for specific populations, e.g., using the language (and world view) of a defined ethnic group (Bernal & Sáez-Santiago, 2006; Chen et al., 2008).

An individual's ethnic identity development can influence their perceptions and experi-ence of a group that does not share the same minority status. As Kivlighan et al. (2019) point out, engaging in explicit conversations about race is critical for positive ethnic identity development among BIPOC individuals. Prospective minority group members with a strong ethnic identity will be well prepared to engage in explicit conversations about race in a mixed-race context. In contrast, prospective members from the White majority may experience distress and show defensiveness when challenged about a "racialized frame of reference" (DiAngelo, 2011) and demonstrate "White fragility" (Kivlighan et al., 2019).

The Multigroup Ethnic Identity Measure (MEIM)

Ethnic identity is a key constituent of self-concept and reflects the individual's assertion of membership in a social group together with a valued emotional attachment to that membership (Phinney, 1992). Cultures are unique in terms of history, traditions, and values but a sense of "belonging" to one's group is a common experience that transcends ethnic differences. The MEIM (Phinney, 1992) is a self-report questionnaire addressing common elements of ethnic identity—self-identification as an ethnic group member, sense of belonging, and positive atti-tudes toward one's group—and is appropriate for use with all clients. Ethnic identity achievement is viewed as a continuous variable, ranging from a lack of interest and commitment to endorsement of both exploration and invested identification.

The MEIM was developed over iterations with multiple diverse samples of high school and college students and demonstrates good internal consistency. Fourteen items assess the

Table 2.9 The Multigroup Ethnic Identity Measure

Item	Information
Name of instrument	*The Multigroup Ethnic Identity Measure (MEIM)*
Authors	Jean S. Phinney
Source	Phinney, J. S. (1992). The Multigroup Ethnic Identity Measure: A new scale for use with diverse groups. *Journal of Adolescent Research*, 7, 156–176. https://dx.doi.org/10.1177/074355489272003
Translations	English.
Brief description	The MEIM is a 14-item self-report instrument measuring the common elements of ethnic identity, and thus appropriate to all clients. These elements include self-identification as an ethnic group member, a sense of belonging, and positive attitudes towards one's group. Items are rated on a 4-point Likert scale to indicate agreement.
Time requirements	Administration: 10 minutes. Scoring: 10 minutes.
Subscales and scoring	The MEIM allows for the calculation of three scores: positive attitudes and a sense of belonging (5 items); ethnic identity achievement, including both exploration and resolution of identity issues (7 items); and ethnic behaviors and practices (2 items). Scoring involves reversing negatively worded item ratings, summation, and calculation of mean values; scores range between 1 (low ethnic identity) to 4 (high). Additional items address attitudes towards other ethnic groups.
Psychometric properties	The MEIM was validated on two samples, high school students ($N = 417$) and college students ($N = 136$), each reflecting representative diversity. Internal consistency estimates demonstrated good reliability for the overall scale (.81 and .90, respectively), and the subscales of Affirmation/Belonging (.75 and .86, respectively) and Ethnic Identity (.69 and .80, respectively).
Norms	Descriptive statistics are provided in the source article for the high school and college student samples; the latter demonstrated a significantly higher Ethnic Identity score and stronger correlations between MEIM subscales, as expected developmentally.
Administration types	Paper & pencil or formatted on a device.
Sensitivity to change	NA
Analytics	NA
Benchmarking	The source article indicates that minority high school respondents (Asian, Black, Hispanic, and ethnically mixed) had significantly higher Ethnic Identity scores than White high school respondents but did not differ significantly among themselves. For the minorities, Ethnic Identity was significantly related to self-esteem in both samples; this was not the case for White respondents.
How to obtain/Cost	The MEIM items and scoring instructions are available in the source article.

three common elements: positive attitudes and sense of belonging (5 items); ethnic identity achievement, including both exploration and resolution of identity issues (7 items); and ethnic behaviors and practices (2 items). Items are rated on a 4-point Likert scale to indicate agreement. Scoring involves reversing the ratings for negatively worded items, summation, and calculating mean values. Importantly for composing a therapy group, six items assess attitudes towards other ethnic groups, useful for identifying "red flags" regarding potential group interactions. The MEIM and scoring procedure are found in the source article (Phinney, 1992). Scores for the three elements loaded on a single factor, supporting the measure's conceptualization. Ethnic identity scores for minorities (Black, Asian, Hispanic) reflected more strength than scores for White respondents; higher correlations between ethnic identity and self-esteem were observed for minority groups than for Whites. Low scores on the MEIM reflect ethnic identity diffusion and high scores a strongly held and valued ethnic identity. The stronger the client's ethnic identity, the more likely positive feelings about their ethnic group will be maintained in the face of stereotypes or charged conversations about race. A weaker ethnic identity may flag vulnerability to stereotyping or marginalization in the group process. Use of the MEIM can support composition of a diverse membership and help ensure that clients are grounded in their ethnic identity as preparation for reflection on experiences of cultural conflict, racism, and discrimination.

Perception of Ethnic Discrimination Questionnaire (PEDQ)

Experiences with discrimination may result in the development of mistrust and avoidance among minority group members in the majority culture. These experiences can arise from interactions with individuals or at the systemic level. Prospective members from minorities, then, may feel particularly wary of other members or the group, with expectations of hostility or rejection in the group. If the group's composition reflects the majority (White) group, the structure is vulnerable to recapitulating dominant-minority power dynamics (Marmarosh et al., 2013b), an effect that could be exacerbated by inclusion of minority members with experiences of discrimination. It is critical to understand the impact of racism and discrimination to adequately address the potential for stereotyping (Kaklauskas & Nettles, 2019) and recapitulation of injustice between members who hold privilege and those who do not (Chang-Caffaro & Caffaro, 2018).

Ethnicity-related stress refers to the perception of events and situations as having threat value because of one's membership in a particular ethnic group (Contrada et al., 2001). Relative to other measures (e.g., the Perceived Racism Scale; McNeilly et al., 1996) which are designed specifically for African American respondents, the PEDQ is appropriate for use with all ethnic groups. A brief community version of the PEDQ was developed by Brondolo et al. (2005) and is available for download at https://attcnetwork.org/sites/defa ult/files/2020-12/2-PEDQ-CV-B.pdf.

The Brief PEDQ-Community Version consists of 17 items and measures five reliable factors. Lifetime Exposure, represented by the mean of all items, assesses exposure to race-based discrimination over the client's life. Exclusion/Rejection assesses experiences where the respondent has felt isolated, excluded, or ignored because of race/ethnicity. Stigmatization/ Devaluation reflects experiences of being treated in a demeaning or stigmatizing manner. Discrimination at Work/School assesses unfair treatment in environments important to the client. Finally, Threat/Aggression reflects the degree to which the respondent felt that they (or their property) were threatened or harmed because of their race or ethnicity. Strong internal consistency (.7 or above) of the factors was reported (Brondolo et al., 2005). Blacks and Latinos reported greater discrimination; factor scores of minority

Table 2.10 The Perception of Ethnic Discrimination Questionnaire

Item	Information
Name of instrument	*Perception of Ethnic Discrimination Questionnaire (PEDQ)*
Authors	Elizabeth Brondolo, Kim P. Kelly, Vonetta Coakley, Tamar Gordon, Shola Thompson, Erika Levy, Andrea Cassells, Jonathan N. Tobin, Monica Sweeney, & Richard J. Contrada
Source	Brondolo, E., Kelly, K. P., Coakley, V., Gordon, T., Thompson, S., Levy, E., Cassells, A., Tobin, J. N., Sweeney, M., & Contrada, R. J. (2005). The Perceived Ethnic Discrimination Questionnaire: Development and preliminary validation of a community version. *Journal of Applied Social Psychology, 35*, 335–365. https://dx.doi.org/10.1111/j.1559-1816.2005.tb02124.x
Translations	English.
Brief description	The PEDQ is a 17-item self-report questionnaire inquiring about the individual's experiences of ethnic discrimination, as a form of chronic or recurrent ethnicity-related stress. For the community version of the measure, items were revised to target the life experiences of community-dwelling adults (the original instrument targets experiences of college students). The PEDQ is appropriate for use with all ethnic groups, in contrast to other measures (e.g., the Perceived Racism Scale) designed specifically for African American respondents.
Time requirements	Administration: 10–15 minutes. Scoring: 10 minutes.
Subscales and scoring	The PEDQ assesses five reliable factors: Lifetime Exposure (the mean of all items captures exposure to race-based discrimination over the course of the client's life); Exclusion/Rejection; Stigmatization/Devaluation; Discrimination at Work/School; and Threat/Aggression.
Psychometric properties	The brief version of the PEDQ was validated with a sample of 340 individuals (128 college students and 212 members of the community drawn from primary care practices). The sample was characterized by large proportions of African American and Latino respondents. Internal consistency reliability of the Lifetime Exposure and other factors ranged between .69- .87. The community sample was found to report higher levels of lifetime exposure to threat and harassment than the student sample. The source article also provides evidence of the measure's construct and convergent-discriminant validity.
Norms	Normative score values are provided in the source article for two validation samples. The first sample ($N = 301$) offers descriptive statistics on the subscales for Black and Latino participants, and for American-versus foreign-born participants. Data from the second sample ($N = 340$) contrasts college student and community-dwelling participants.
Administration types	Paper & pencil or formatted on a device.
Sensitivity to change	NA
Analytics	NA
Benchmarking	In initial administrations of the PEDQ, Blacks and Latinos reported higher levels of discrimination; the scores of ethnic minority respondents were also more likely to correlate with appraisals of threat and measures of anxiety, cynicism, and hostile attributions.
Sample references	Contrada, R. J., Ashmore, R. D., Gary, M. L., Coups, E., Egeth, J. D., Sewell, A., Ewell, K., Goyal, T. M., Chasse, V. (2001). Measures of ethnicity-related stress: Psychometric properties, ethnic group differences, and associations with well-being. *Journal of Applied Social Psychology, 31*, 1775–1820. https://dx.doi.org/10.1111/j.1559-1816.2001.tb00205.x
How to obtain/Cost	The PEDQ is available for free download at: https://attcnetwork.org/sites/default/files/2020-12/2-PEDQ-CV-B.pdf.

respondents demonstrated correlations with threat appraisals and personality indices (anxiety, cynicism, and hostile attributions).

Minority ethnic group clients who report experiences of discrimination may be vulnerable to racially charged interactions in a diverse group. This vulnerability could manifest as reactivity, defensiveness, or withdrawal, and may be offset by a strong ethnic identity. A clear snapshot of members' ethnic identity and experiences of discrimination can highlight individual resilience and weakness and, ultimately, the group's capacity to address issues of cultural conflict.

Clinical Vignette Part Two

Francis also had clinical interests in maternal health and the mother-infant bond. She contacted social agencies to announce the start of a "skills and support" group for first-time and single mothers from the diverse community surrounding the hospital where the clinic was located. The "skills" focus was to encourage responsiveness and mentalizing by the young mothers, and "support" involved providing a safe place to network and share parenting experiences. Francis was excited about the prospect of the group after receiving several phone calls soon after posting her announcement. She was also struck by the diversity of the callers, noting that the group could potentially include White, Black, Hispanic, and South Asian identities. Mindful of recent racial tensions in the area, Francis felt it would be important to gauge the prospective members' ethnic identity and experiences of discrimination before launching the group to ensure she was aware of any potential issues beyond the focus on maternal functioning. Prior to her screening sessions with young mothers who had expressed interest, Francis asked them to complete the MEIM and PEDQ and then dedicated a portion of each hour to reviewing the responses. Francis was struck by the strong valuation of ethnic identity among the three Black, two East Indian, and, in particular, four South Asian mothers. During their screening sessions, two of the latter mothers each highlighted how the Covid-19 pandemic and related social issues had prompted a deliberate re-investment in their ethnic identity. Chu Ha and Daiyu also reported recent experiences of discrimination in the community stemming from fear and misinformation about the origins of the virus. Francis acknowledged the ongoing vigilance that Daiyu and Chu Ha were feeling as pandemic-related tensions continued as a "live" issue. Both mothers expressed some trepidation about their reception in the group. Francis solicited an agreement from Daiyu and Chu Ha to open up discussion about their recent experiences in the first session of the group.

Ten mothers attended the first session. Francis outlined the dual purpose of the group and educated the women about norms and group process. After introductions, including the names of each mother's children, Francis disclosed what Daiyu and Chu Ha had reported on the MEIM and PEDQ and encouraged an open discussion of their experiences. She was aware of steeling herself for the possibility of microaggressions or worse from any of the non-Asian mothers. Instead, she felt a wave of relief and encouragement when the members showed Daiyu and Chu Ha sympathy and support. Shristi and Janet, an East Indian and Black mother, respectively, disclosed their own experiences of discrimination and how they had coped with the impact on their well-being. The lively discussion indicated to Francis that addressing the issue directly and quickly had helped to facilitate cohesion and successfully launch the group.

Questions of Composition: Transdiagnostic Variables

Four measures were chosen to represent client variables relevant across a range of psychiatric conditions and the treatments for those conditions. Each transdiagnostic variable reflects an important element of the human experience: depression, attachment, inter-personal distress, or struggles to attain some form of "perfection." Each measure represents a rich research base and a literature worthy of study. Importantly, the measures offer a bridge between understanding of the client and the group leaders' *theory of change*. They thus represent potentially useful conceptual tools for composition and formulating predictions regarding group process.

Depressive Experiences Questionnaire (DEQ)

The DEQ was selected for multiple reasons. First, it is an exceptionally well-validated questionnaire with a solid evidence base for the predictive utility of the DEQ factor scores. Quality is also reflected in the theoretical underpinning provided by Blatt's (2008) "two-polarities" model of human psychological development, positing a reciprocal dialectic of processes associated with *self-definition* and *interpersonal relatedness*. Second, the measure offers a "high level" overview of personality, identifying the client's principal psychological concerns. Third, clinical research with the DEQ and refinement of the Dependency factor (into facets for maladaptive Neediness and healthier Relatedness) can suggest "red flags" regarding clients being considered for the group's composition.

According to Blatt (2008), healthy personality involves a progressive integration of self-definition with a capacity for interpersonal relatedness, i.e., developing a balance between achievement-related and affiliative needs. The dialectic between these developmental strands is interactive and recursive: more mature relatedness facilitates the establishment of a stable and positive sense of self which in turn facilitates greater relational growth (Blatt, 2008). Life crises, biological predispositions, and interactions between the two can result in over-investment in one developmental line to the detriment of the other, giving rise to use of compensatory or defensive responses, i.e., psychological disorders. The main application of the two-polarities model has been in research on major depression; notably, studies have not focused on *symptoms* but rather the *life experiences* that are central to depression (Blatt, 2004). Maladaptive expressions of self-definition and relatedness have been implicated in other disorders, e.g., PTSD (Cox et al., 2004) or eating disorder (Boone et al., 2014).

Two forms of depression have been identified in studies involving case reviews and DEQ data (Blatt, 2008). A primarily *self-critical* depression ("introjective" in Blatt's terminology) is characterized by feelings of failure, guilt, and unworthiness. The individual is harshly self-evaluative and concerned about being criticized or losing the approval of others. There are strivings for achievement and perfection, competitiveness, and frequent efforts at compensation to maintain an image of success and the approval of others. These clients can isolate themselves and relationships they do have are often fraught with ambivalence and anger. Individuals who are self-critical and struggle with feelings of guilt and worthlessness can frequently be at risk of suicide (Blatt, 2008). In contrast, a primarily *dependent* depression ("anaclitic") is marked by feelings of loneliness and hopelessness, often with fears of abandonment or being without sufficient love, nurturance, or protection. Separations and other forms of loss elicit anxiety and can precipitate a depressive episode; the individual will often employ denial of feelings or a frantic search for alternative sources of caring. Difficulties expressing anger, somatic concerns and manipulative suicide attempts are frequent expressions of "masked" depression of the anaclitic type (Blatt & Zuroff, 1992). Importantly, the two presentations demonstrate differential responses to treatment. The self-critical intro-jective client tends to have difficulty establishing a strong alliance, does poorly in time-limited formats, and shows more responsiveness to exploratory, insight-oriented interventions. The dependent anaclitic client is more receptive to the interpersonal and supportive dimensions of therapy (Blatt, 2008). Introjective clients change primarily in terms of their symptoms and cognitive functioning while anaclitic clients achieve interpersonal changes (Blatt & Zuroff, 1992). Clients presenting with a mix of self-critical and dependent issues face a higher likelihood of depression but may also be more responsive to long-term intensive dynamic treatments (Blatt, 2004).

The DEQ questionnaire comprises 66 7-point Likert-type rating items assessing feelings about the self and interpersonal relations relevant to depression, e.g., a distorted or depreciated sense of self and others, helplessness, difficulties with anger or self-blame and guilt, loss of autonomy, or distortions in family relations. Reliability and validity of the measure are strong (Blatt, 2004). Three stable factors—Self-Criticism, Dependency, and Efficacy—have been identified across independent samples (Zuroff et al., 1990). The Efficacy dimension reflects well-being, felt competence, and independence. The scoring program allows for derivation of *facets* of the Dependency factor (Blatt et al., 1995): the Neediness facet reflects feelings of helplessness, fears of separation and rejection, and concerns about loss of support, while the Relatedness facet reflects more adaptive concerns about disruption of a specific significant attachment. Extreme scores on either Self-Criticism or Dependency would flag issues for group admittance. These concerns could be mitigated by higher scores on the Efficacy factor or the Relatedness facet (Blatt, 2004). A high Neediness score would be a "red flag" regarding including the client in the group. For composition, a *balance* between members on the Self-Criticism and Dependency factors would allow for maximal heterogeneity of psychological concerns and sufficient interpersonal tension to provide opportunities for learning (Bernard et al., 2008). The DEQ and scoring programs can be downloaded from the home page of David Zuroff of the Department of Psychology, McGill University (www.psych.mcgill.ca).

Table 2.11 The Depressive Experiences Questionnaire

Item	Information
Name of instrument	*Depressive Experiences Questionnaire (DEQ)*
Authors	Sidney J. Blatt, Joseph P. D'Afflitti, & Donald M. Quinlan
Source	Blatt, S. J., D'Afflitti, J. P., & Quinlan, D. M. (1976). Experiences of depression in normal young adults. *Journal of Abnormal Psychology, 85,* 383–389. https://dx.doi.org/10.1037.0021-843X.85.4.383
Translations	Primarily English, but the DEQ has been translated into several languages, including Chinese, Portuguese, and Italian.
Brief description	The DEQ is a 66-item self-report questionnaire assessing feelings about the self and interpersonal relationships thought to be relevant to depression but not manifest symptoms of depression in themselves. Items are rated for agreement on a 7-point Likert-type scale, are oriented in both positive and negative directions, and tap into issues such as a distorted or depreciated sense of self and others, dependency, helplessness, egocentricity, fear of loss, ambivalence, difficulties with anger or self-blame and guilt, loss of autonomy, and distortions in family relations. Importantly, the DEQ assesses primarily stable personality characteristics rather than depressed mood or other state variables.
Time requirements	Administration: 30–45 minutes. Scoring: 15–30 minutes.

Item	Information
Name of instrument	*Depressive Experiences Questionnaire (DEQ)*

Subscales and scoring	Three highly stable factors—Dependency, Self-Criticism, and Efficacy—have been identified in several independent samples (both clinical and non-clinical). Dependency reflects concerns about abandonment, loneliness, or being without support ("anaclitic"). Self-Criticism reflects concerns about feelings of failure, guilt, and unworthiness ("introjective"). The Efficacy factor reflects optimism, well-being, and felt competence. Scoring programs are available for SPSS or SAS.
Psychometric properties	Internal consistency reliability for the three DEQ factors is strong (Blatt et al., 1982): .81 for Dependency, .80 for Self-Criticism, and .72 for Efficacy. Test-retest reliabilities at 5- and 13-week intervals were .89 and .81 for Dependency, .83 and .75 for Self-Criticism, and .75 and .72 for Efficacy, suggesting the DEQ factors have good stability. Considerable evidence supports the construct validity of the DEQ Dependency and Self-Criticism scales, particularly in terms of relationships with gold standard measures of depression.
Norms	Blatt et al. (1982) provide normative values for the DEQ factors for males and females within clinical and non-clinical samples. Research has often identified differences between males and females (the latter tend to score more highly on Dependency) but the factor structure of the DEQ is consistent across samples. See Blatt (2004) for details.
Administration types	Paper & pencil or formatted on a device.
Sensitivity to change	Blatt (2004) suggests that more research is needed on the DEQ as a change measure but notes evidence that the factor scales can predict later mental health status.
Analytics	The scoring program allows for derivation of two facets of the Dependency factor (Blatt et al., 1995), a less adaptive Neediness and a more adaptive Relatedness.
Benchmarking	Blatt (2004) summarizes studies addressing DEQ scores in clinical versus non-clinical samples, between male and female respondents, and over time in clinical treatment.
Sample references	Blatt, S. J. (2004). *Experiences of depression: Theoretical, clinical, and research perspectives.* Washington, DC: American Psychological Association Press. Blatt, S.J., Quinlan, D.M., Chevron, E. S., MacDonald, C., & Zuroff, D. (1982). Dependency and self-criticism: Psychological dimensions of depression. *Journal of Consulting and Clinical Psychology, 50,* 113–124. https://dx.doi.org/10.1037//0022.006x.50.1.113 Blatt, S. J., Zohar, A. H., Quinlan, D. M., Zuroff, D. C., & Mongrain, M. (1995). Subscales within the dependency factor of the Depressive Experiences Questionnaire. *Journal of Personality Assessment, 64,* 319–339. https://dx.doi.org/10.1207/s15327752jpa6402_11 Luyten, P., Sabbe, B., Blatt, S. J., Meganck, S., Jansen, B., De Grave, C., Maes, F., & Corveleyn, J. (2007). Dependency and self-criticism: Relationship with major depressive disorder, severity of depression, and clinical presentation. *Depression and Anxiety, 24,* 586–596. https://dx.doi.org/10.1002/da.20272
How to obtain/Cost	Information on obtaining the DEQ and scoring programs at no cost can be found on the home page of Dr. David Zuroff of McGill University (www.psych.mcgill.ca).

Experiences in Close Relationships Scale (ECR-12)

The client's attachment "style" can influence the quality of the working alliance (Bucci et al., 2016) and the outcome of individual therapy (Levy et al., 2011). The same is true in group therapy (Kirchmann et al., 2009; Lawson & Brossart, 2009; Tasca et al., 2013). The literature offers useful summaries of this linkage: A special issue of the *International Journal of Group Psychotherapy* (Volume 67, Issue 2, 2017) is a contemporary synthesis of the area. Marmarosh et al. (2013a) apply attachment theory to group practice. Tasca et al. (2021) meld attachment theory and a psychodynamic approach to group therapy, highlighting how theory can guide selection and intervention in group therapy.

Adult attachment style can be measured efficiently with the 12-item form of the Experiences in Close Relationships Scale (ECR-12), a short version of the original 36-item ECR Scale (Lafontaine et al., 2016; Tasca et al., 2018). The ECR (Brennan et al., 1998) was itself a synthesis of measures developed by various investigators and based on factor analyses of over 400 items from those measures. Two relatively orthogonal dimensions were identified by Brennan et al. (1998). Attachment *anxiety* reflects a fear of rejection or abandonment, with an excessive need of approval from others, and distress when an attachment figure is unavailable or unresponsive. Attachment *avoidance* reflects a fear of dependence and intimacy, an excessive need for self-reliance, and reluctance to self-disclose. People who score highly on these dimensions are assumed to have an *insecure* attachment orientation, with various orientations reflected by combinations of scores on the two dimensions. Low anxiety coupled with high avoidance reflects *dismissing* attachment. High anxiety together with low avoidance reflects *preoccupied* attachment. High scores on both dimensions reflects *fearful* attachment. Clients with low anxiety and avoidance can be viewed as having a *secure* attachment orientation.

The self-report ECR-12 asks respondents to rate agreement (on a 7-point scale) with 12 items descriptive of feelings in close relationships. There is good evidence for the reliability and predictive validity of the ECR-12 (Lafontaine et al., 2016; see Tasca et al., 2018 for items and scoring.) Anxiously attached clients do well in relational group treatments that focus on fostering emotional regulation and cohesion. In contrast, avoidant clients tend to be repelled by pressures to be more intimate or more cohesive as a group. Members with a preoccupied orientation may present as more needy and show poor compliance with treatment expectations or norms (Dozier, 1990). Clients presenting with dismissing attachment are problematic to engage in interpersonal work and, if in a minority position in the group, at risk of dropout. When composing a group, including clients with more secure attachment, or with relatively less attachment anxiety or avoidance, can be beneficial for those members with less relational capacity as well as for the group as a whole (Kivlighan et al., 2017; Marmarosh, 2014; Piper et al., 2007). If the group mix allows for work on attachment concerns with sufficient support and cohesion, the leaders can consider including clients with a more dismissing avoidant style.

Applications of attachment theory and research in the context of group therapy is currently a highly active area (see Marmarosh et al., 2013a). Research has moved beyond evaluating member attachment orientations to also consider the *therapist's* attachment style or the member and therapist attachments to the *group* (Markin & Marmarosh, 2010; Marmarosh, 2014; Smith et al., 1999). An expanded view of attachment in the group context shows great potential for understanding therapy process and offers the reader rich dividends with further exploration.

Table 2.12 The Experiences in Close Relationships Scale

Item	Information
Name of instrument	*Experiences in Close Relationships Scale (ECR-12)*
Authors	Marie-France Lafontaine, Audrey Brassard, Yvan Lussier, Pierre Valois, Philip R. Shaver, & Susan M. Johnson
Source	Lafontaine, M-F., Brassard, A., Lussier, Y., Valois, P., Shaver, P. R., & Johnson, S. M. (2016). Selecting the best items for a short-form of the Experiences in Close Relationships Questionnaire. *European Journal of Psychological Assessment, 32*, 140–154. https://dx.doi.org/10.1027/1015-5759/a000243
Translations	English and French versions are available. The original 36-item ECR (Brennan et al., 1998) has been translated into Chinese, French, Dutch, Hebrew, Italian, Japanese, and Spanish.
Brief description	The ECR-12 provides a brief and efficient assessment of attachment dimensions in significant relationships. The ECR-12 is a self-report that asks respondents to rate agreement (on a 7-point Likert-type scale) with 12 items descriptive of feelings in close relationships. The instrument provides scores for two relatively orthogonal dimensions of attachment Anxiety and Avoidance. The ECR-12 was developed using Item Response Theory analyses to examine the performance of items from the original ECR. Six items with the greatest discriminatory power for each of the two attachment dimensions were selected. Notably, the ECR-12 is not affected by any gender response bias, i.e., men and women were found to endorse the items in the same way, and the factor structure also demonstrated relative invariance across gender (the assessment of bias was limited to the binary distinction). ECR-12 items and scoring instructions are available in Tasca et al. (2018).
Time requirements	Administration: 10 minutes. Scoring: 10 minutes.
Subscales and scoring	Anxiety reflects a fear of rejection or abandonment, an excessive need for approval from others, and distress in the absence of an attachment figure. Avoidance reflects a fear of dependency or intimacy, an excessive need for self-reliance, and reluctance to self-disclose.
Psychometric properties	Scores on the ECR-12 were found to correlate highly with the corresponding subscale from the full ECR (all *r*s >.85). Test-retest reliabilities over the course of a full year were strong (see Lafontaine et al., 2016), indicating good stability. Internal consistency of each subscale showed little variation across independent samples and genders, with coefficients of.78-.87 for Anxiety and.74-.83 for Avoidance (see Lafontaine et al., 2016). Convergent validity was demonstrated by correlations with measures of psychological distress and relationship satisfaction. Tasca et al. (2018) also provide evidence for internal consistency, test-retest reliability, convergent validity, and concurrent validity, based on a sample of treatment-seeking patients with eating disorder. Notably, patients with higher levels of attachment Anxiety were more likely to complete treatment than those with lower levels.
Norms	Tasca et al. (2018) provide mean values on the ECR-12 factors for five distinct groups of eating disorder patients (restricting anorexia, anorexia with binging/purging, bulimia nervosa, binge-eating disorder, and eating disorder NOS).
Administration types	Paper & pencil or formatted on a device.
Sensitivity to change	NA

Item	Information
Name of instrument	*Experiences in Close Relationships Scale (ECR-12)*
Analytics	Various orientations are reflected by the combination of scores on the two dimensions. Low anxiety coupled with high avoidance reflects *dismissing* attachment. High anxiety together with low avoidance reflects *preoccupied* attachment. High scores on both dimensions reflects *fearful* attachment. Clients with low levels of anxiety and avoidance can be viewed as having a *secure* attachment orientation
Benchmarking	NA
Sample references	Brennan, K.A., Clark, C.L., & Shaver, P.R. (1998). Self-report measurement of adult attachment: An integrated overview. In J.A. Simpson & W.S. Rholes (Eds), *Attachment theory and close relationships* (pp. 46–76). New York: Guilford Press.
	Tasca, G. A., Brugnera, A., Baldwin, D., Carlucci, S., Compare, A., Balfour, L., Proulx, G., Gick, M., & Lafontaine, M-F. (2018). Reliability and validity of the Experiences in Close Relationships Scale-12: Attachment dimensions in a clinical sample with eating disorders. *International Journal of Eating Disorders, 51,* 18–27. https://dx.doi.org/10.1002/eat.22807
How to obtain/Cost	See Tasca et al. (2018) for ECR-12 items and directions for scoring.

The Inventory of Interpersonal Problems (IIP-32)

Apart from character orientation or attachment "style," interpersonal *problems* can be assessed with a short form of the original IIP-64 (Horowitz et al., 1988). The IIP-32 (Horowitz et al., 2000) is a self-report of interpersonal problems that either constitute difficulties in executing certain behaviors ("It is hard for me to …") or difficulties in exercising restraint ("I do … too much"). The instrument is based upon interpersonal theories of behavior (e.g., Kiesler, 1996) and consists of 8 subscales of 4 items each, rated on a 5-point (0–4) scale. Scores can be represented geometrically as a circumplex that depicts the client's relational pattern on two orthogonal axes (see Figure 2.1).

The vertical axis represents Dominance (from submissive to domineering) while the horizontal axis represents Warmth (from cold to overly nurturant). Each subscale represents an *octant* on the circumplex; a "spider plot" can graphically represent the client's IIP profile. Subscales assess problems related to: being manipulating, controlling, and/or too aggressive toward others (Domineering); being distrustful, suspicious, and self-centered (Vindictive); difficulty expressing affection and maintaining relationships (Cold); being too socially anxious or shy (Socially Inhibited); difficulty being assertive (Nonassertive); difficulty expressing anger and being exploitable (Overly Accommodating); being overly caring and permissive of others (Self-Sacrificing); and being intrusive, attention-seeking, and inappropriately open (Intrusive). Subscales are scored by calculating a mean for associated items, using raw scores or a T-score transformation. A total score of overall interpersonal distress can be derived. *Extreme* scores in any octant or for global distress would be of concern. Scores reflecting *hostile dominance* have been associated with problems in the therapy process (Horowitz et al., 2000). Note that a relabeling of descriptors would be recommended if IIP scores are used for feedback to clients.

The IIP-32 has strong psychometric properties and the circumplex structure has been confirmed across studies and populations; reviews of research and norms are offered in the IIP manual. Using the original IIP, Kivlighan and Angelone (1992) found that members who perceived themselves as dominant experienced the group climate as more avoiding and tense. Fjelstad et al. (2017) found that members scoring highly on the domineering and cold

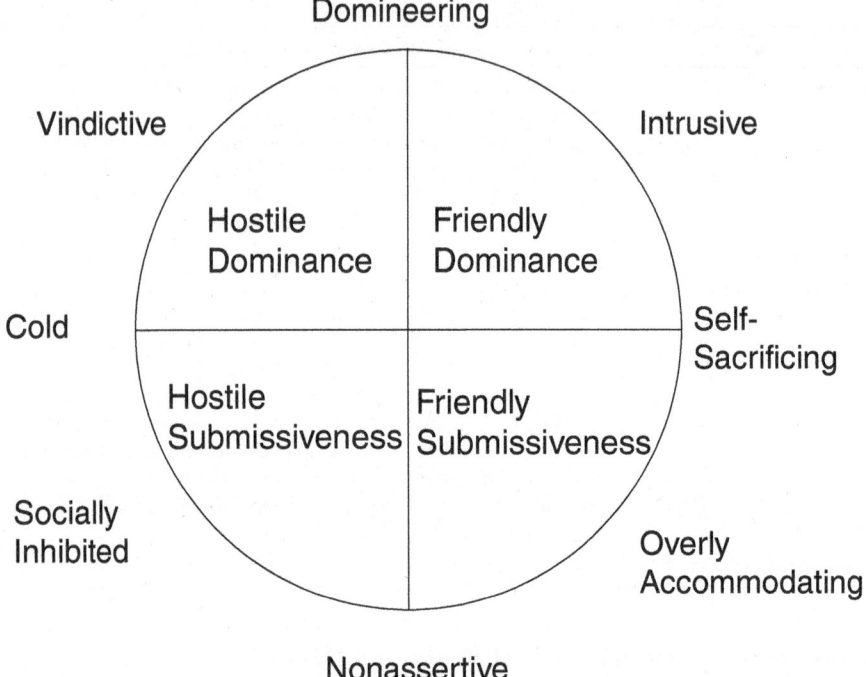

Figure 2.1 The Interpersonal Problems Circumplex
Source: Ruiz et al. (2004).

Table 2.13 The Inventory of Interpersonal Problems

Item	Information
Name of instrument	*Inventory of Interpersonal Problems (IIP-32)*
Authors	Leonard M. Horowitz, Saul E. Rosenberg, Barbara A. Baer, Gilbert Ureño, & Valerie S. Villaseñor.
Source	Horowitz, L. M., Rosenberg, S. E., Baer, B. A., Ureño, G., & Villaseñor, V. S. (1988). Inventory of Interpersonal Problems: Psychometric properties and clinical applications. *Journal of Consulting and Clinical Psychology, 56*, 885–892. https://dx.doi.org/10.1037/0022-006X.56.6.885 Horowitz, L. M., Aiden, L. E., Wiggins, J. S., & Pincus, A. L. (2000). *Inventory of Interpersonal Problems manual.* Odessa, FL: The Psychological Corporation.
Translations	English, Dutch, French, Korean, Slovenian, Danish, German, Norwegian, Swedish.
Brief description	The IIP-32 (Horowitz et al., 2000) is a short version of the original IIP (Horowitz et al., 1988) and offers a self-report of problems in interpersonal interactions that either constitute difficulties in executing certain behaviors ("It is hard for me to …") or difficulties in exercising restraint ("I do … too much"). The instrument follows in the tradition of interpersonal theories of human behavior (e.g., Kiesler, 1996). The IIP-32 consists of 8 subscales of 4 items each; items are rated for how well they describe the respondent on a 5-point (0 = Not at all to 4 = Extremely) Likert-type scale.
Time requirements	Administration: 10–15 minutes. Scoring: 15–20 minutes.

Item	Information
Name of instrument	*Inventory of Interpersonal Problems (IIP-32)*

Subscales and scoring	The 8 subscales each reflect a different dimension of interpersonal function: Domineering, Vindictive, Cold, Socially Inhibited, Non-assertive, Overly Accommodating, Self-Sacrificing, and Intrusive. The scores can be represented geometrically as a *circumplex* that depicts the client's relational pattern on two orthogonal axes—the vertical axis represents Dominance (from submissive to domineering) while the horizontal axis represents Warmth (from cold to overly nurturant). Each subscale is scored by calculating the mean rating of the four associated items, using raw scores or transforming the latter into T-scores. A total score reflecting overall interpersonal distress can also be calculated. Higher scores indicate greater interpersonal problems.
Psychometric properties	The IIP has strong psychometric properties and is one of the most frequently used measures in psychotherapy research. The circumplex structure has been confirmed in several studies and appears to be stable across different cultures. Horowitz et al. (2000) report strong test-retest reliability for the total score ($r = .78$) in their standardization sample, as well as strong correlations with the longer IIP ($rs = .88-.98$). Internal consistency coefficients ranged between .68- .87 across the 8 subscales; the total score demonstrated a high degree of internal reliability (alpha $= .93$).
Norms	The manual for the IIP-32 includes representative norms for clinical and non-clinical samples. The research literature provides data for specific subgroups (e.g., patients with personality disorders).
Administration types	Paper & pencil or formatted on a device.
Sensitivity to change	There is extensive evidence that the IIP is highly sensitive to the effects of treatment, underscoring its value as an outcome measure in psychotherapy research (e.g., Lorentzen & Høglend, 2004).
Analytics	*Ipsatized* versions of the IIP-32 subscale scores can also be calculated. These scores represent the individual's level of difficulty on each subscale after taking the individual's *overall level of interpersonal difficulty* into account. Ipsatized scores highlight those areas of the circumplex where the client demonstrates the greatest difficulty.
Benchmarking	The research literature is replete with examples of studies where the IIP was employed to differentiate groups, in both clinical and non-clinical settings. Entering search terms reflecting specific disorders or target areas for intervention will likely yield representative studies.
Sample references	Fjelstad, A., Høglend, P., & Lorentzen, S. (2017). Patterns of change in interpersonal problems during and after short-term and long-term psychodynamic group therapy: A randomized clinical trial. *Psychotherapy Research, 27*, 350–61. https://dx.doi.org/10.1080/10503307.2015.1102357 Kiesler, D. J. (1996). *Contemporary interpersonal theory and research: Personality, psychopathology, and psychotherapy*. New York, NY: Wiley. Kivlighan, D. M., & Angelone, E. O. (1992). Interpersonal problems: Variables influencing participants' perception of group climate. *Journal of Counseling Psychology, 39*, 468–472. https://dx.doi.org/10.1037/0022-0167.39.4.468 Lorentzen, S., & Høglend, P. (2004). Predictors of change during long-term analytic group psychotherapy. *Psychotherapy and Psychosomatics, 73*, 25–35. https://dx.doi.org/10.1159/000074437
How to obtain/Cost	The IIP (both short and full versions) is available for purchase at www.mindgarden.com. The manual is available for US$50.00; various purchase options for the instrument are available.

octants were more challenging to engage in group; they also determined that these clients could still make gains with appropriate PGP (see also Lorentzen & Høglend, 2004). Ogrodniczuk et al. (2009) reported that clients presenting with narcissistic issues were more likely to drop out of group prematurely; these clients also scored highly on the domineering, vindictive, and intrusive octants. Whittingham (2018) shows how the IIP can be used to generate a problem formulation, linking interpersonal distress to symptoms, attachment issues, and identity concerns. The IIP-32 instrument and manual (including norms) is available for purchase at www.mindgarden.com.

The Perfectionistic Self-Presentation Scale (PSPS)

Regardless of diagnosis or problem presentation, many clients struggle with issues of perfectionism. Perfectionism has been associated with a range of mental health issues, including chronic feelings of failure, guilt, procrastination and indecisiveness, shame, and low self-regard (Hewitt & Flett, 1991a). It is viewed as a core vulnerability and transdiagnostic personality factor in diverse client presentations (Hewitt et al., 2018). Perfectionistic concerns may be driven by various motivations, i.e., to elicit approval from others for presentation or performance or to conceal perceived inadequacies, but these invariably interfere with work success, relationship stability, or positive self-regard. Research has also documented how perfectionism can impede an effective therapy process and is negatively associated with treatment outcome (Blatt, 2004; Blatt et al., 1998; Miller et al., 2017). It can be critical to evaluate clients' perfectionism and ensure that the group composition allows for containment and confrontation of these issues.

Evaluation of perfectionism can be multidimensional and address a) the personality traits that underpin perfectionistic behavior (Hewitt & Flett, 1991a, b), b) the interpersonal expression of the client's perfectionism, and/or c) the intrapersonal representation of perfectionism as defined by the client's self-dialogue and self-regard (Hewitt et al., 2017). A comprehensive evaluation of these domains would be recommended if perfectionism represented the target for intervention, for example, when implementing the psychodynamic-interpersonal group approach described by Hewitt and colleagues (2015, 2018; Tasca et al., 2021). For composing a process group, a focus on the *interpersonal expression* of perfectionism is most pertinent. The development and validation of the PSPS is described by Hewitt et al. (2003). The measure consists of 27 items rated on a 7-point Likert scale. Three factor scores are provided: a) Perfectionistic Self-Promotion reflects the need to project oneself as perfect to others; b) Non-Display of Imperfection reflects fears of being seen publicly as behaving in a less than perfect manner; and c) Non-Disclosure of Imperfection reflects the tendency to avoid admission of shortcomings. The factors have demonstrated strong internal consistency, good test-retest reliability, and concurrent validity (e.g., expected correlations with the trait subscales of the Multidimensional Perfectionism Scale; Hewitt & Flett, 1991a, b). The PSPS, scoring guidelines, and norms are available online at Dr. Hewitt's website (https://hewittlab.psych.ubc.ca).

A high level of Perfectionistic Self-Promotion reflects a need to gain admiration but will likely come across as interpersonally aversive, i.e., self-centered and narcissistic. A sense of guardedness can also be central (Hewitt et al., 2003, p. 1311). A high score on the Non-Display factor implies that the client will wish to avoid scrutiny of their behavior and possible exposure of shortcomings. Similarly, a high score on the Non-Disclosure factor would imply the client may have difficulty with group pressures to examine personal faults or failures. Thus, high scores on the latter two factors would indicate the client may come across as distant and unengaging or need additional preparation. Composition would aim to achieve balance in the membership in order to counter and contain the self-presentation style of one or more clients.

Table 2.14 The Perfectionistic Self-Presentation Scale

Item	Information
Name of instrument	*The Perfectionistic Self-Presentation Scale (PSPS)*
Authors	Paul L. Hewitt, Gordon L. Flett, Simon B. Sherry, Marie Habke, Melanie Parkin, Raymond W. Lam, Bruce McMurtry, Evelyn Ediger, Paul Fairlie, & Murray B. Stein
Source	Hewitt, P. L., Flett, G. L., Sherry, S. B., Habke, M., Parkin, M., Lam, R. W., McMurtry, B., Ediger, E., Fairlie, P., & Stein, M. B. (2003). The interpersonal expression of perfection: Perfectionistic self-presentation and psychological distress. *Journal of Personality and Social Psychology, 84*, 1303–1325. https://dx.doi.org/10.1037/0022-3514.84.6.1303
Translations	English.
Brief description	The PSPS provides an assessment of both self-promoting and self-concealing elements of a maladaptive perfectionistic self-presentation style. The self-report measure consists of 27 items rated on a 7-point Likert scale (1 = *Disagree strongly* to 7 = *Agree strongly*).
Time requirements	Administration: 10 minutes. Scoring: 10 minutes.
Subscales and scoring	The PSPS provides scores for three reliable and valid factors: Perfectionistic Self-Promotion (the need to project oneself as perfect), Non-Display of Imperfection (fears of being seen publicly as behaving less than perfectly), and Non-Disclosure of Imperfection (the tendency to avoid admissions of shortcomings).
Psychometric properties	Validation of the PSPS was accomplished with seven samples of respondents (including university students, community members, psychiatric patients, or members of a depression self-help organization). The factor structure demonstrated high consistency across samples and gender. Internal consistency values range between .78 and .86 for the subscales, reflecting good reliability. Two samples were employed to evaluate test-retest reliability, at 3 weeks and at 4 months. The values for Perfectionistic Self-Promotion were .83 and .81; for Non-Display of Imperfection, .84 and .81; and for Non-Disclosure of Imperfection, .74 and .79. These figures demonstrate good stability of the factor scores. The source article also documents relationships between the PSPS factors and measures of defensiveness, poor self-regard, depression, and social anxiety.
Norms	Hewitt et al. (2003) provide descriptive statistics regarding the three PSPS subscales for student, community, and clinical samples.
Administration types	Paper & pencil or formatted on a device.
Sensitivity to change	The PSPS has not been evaluated as an outcome measure.
Analytics	NA
Benchmarking	NA
Sample references	Blatt, S. J., Zuroff, D. C., Bondi, C. M., Sanislow, C. A. III, Pilkonis, P. A. (1998). When and how perfectionism impedes the brief treatment of depression: Further analyses of the National Institute of Mental Health Treatment of Depression Collaborative Research Program. *Journal of Consulting and Clinical Psychology, 66*, 428–428. https://dx.doi.org/10.1037/0022-006X.66.2.423 Hewitt, P. L., Flett, G. L., & Mikhail, S. F. (2017). *Perfectionism: A relational approach to conceptualization, assessment, and treatment.* New York, NY: Guilford Publications. Hewitt, P. L., Mikail, S. F., Flett, G. L., & Dang, S. S. (2018). Specific formulation feedback in dynamic-relational group psychotherapy of perfectionism. *Psychotherapy, 55*, 179–185. https://dx.doi.org/10.1037/pst0000137
How to obtain/Cost	The PSPS, scoring instructions, and normative data are available for download at Dr. Hewitt's website (https://hewittlab.psych.ubc.ca).

Clinical Vignette Part Three

Dr. Ashley Morgan, a senior psychiatrist in the clinic and colleague of Abel and Francis, specialized in treatment of mood disorder. She believed the most effective group approach for depressed clients involved a balance of intervention strategies, emphasizing an interpretive development of insight on the one hand and support of "responsive relating" on the other. Ashley further believed that clients varied in ability to make use of these two strategies, i.e., some preferred building a narrative understanding while others responded more to relationship provisions in group. Ashley had a collection of regular clients in mind and raised the idea of continuing work in a process group with each of them, emphasizing that the multiple perspectives and sources of support would prove beneficial (regardless of the client's intervention preference). Nine clients indicating a willingness to shift therapy to a group format represented Ashley's selection "pool" for the group. Blatt's two-polarities model had helped Ashley appreciate distinctions between depressed clients; she was interested in what the DEQ might tell her about the clients being considered, over and above her clinical experience with each one. Aware of the pitfalls associated with perfectionism in treatment, Ashley also decided to use the PSPS to identify clients struggling with perfectionistic self-presentation issues. Each client completed the measures following an individual session; the combined 93 rating items required 45–60 minutes for each client.

Ashley found that the DEQ suggested a "mixed" profile for three of the nine clients, i.e., equivalent and moderate scores for Self-Criticism and Dependency. These clients also had moderate scores for Efficacy, reflecting some resilience. The remaining six clients demonstrated a differentiation in their primary psychological concerns, with three each scoring relatively highly for one of the two main factors. One client scored highly on Self-Criticism, highlighting a source of distress Ashley had not identified in the client's individual sessions. She decided further individual therapy was needed. With the rest, Ashley predicted that she could put more emphasis on interpretive understanding with those scoring highly on Self-Criticism, and engage in "responsive support" with those scoring highly on Dependency. Her expectations were tempered by review of the PSPS data. For the most part, the clients scored in the low to moderate range on the three PSPS factors. For two—both of whom had scored highly on DEQ Self- Criticism—the PSPS data indicated high levels on the Non-Display of Imperfection factor. Accordingly, in PGP sessions with these clients, Ashley explored concerns about criticism and emphasized the safe space offered by the group; both reported decreased anxiety about the group after the session. After the group's start, Ashley found that the members were operating at a "deeper" level of process than she had experienced in prior groups. She attributed this to the benefit of combining her therapy model with Blatt's theory and the data from the two measures.

Pre-Group Preparation

Preparation for group begins before a new member has their first group session, and it usually starts during the group screening after the referral to group is made. As described above, the leaders can invest time reviewing assessment measures as part of the screening process, and they can use these same data during PGP after a member is selected and agrees to join the group. Multiple studies point to the importance of providing new members with an accurate description of what they will experience in the group (MacNair & Corazzini, 1994; Markin & Marmarosh, 2010; Shechtman & Dvir, 2006). Pre-group orientation sessions are linked to better group attendance and may help prevent dropout (McNair-Semands, 2002; Yalom & Leszcz, 2020).

Bernard and colleagues (2008) emphasize the importance of reviewing group *objectives, processes,* and *roles* with incoming group members. Group leaders can incorporate preparation into the group intake process or they can schedule distinct preparation sessions for members prior to their entry into the group. The leaders decide how much preparation they will offer members. In hospital settings there may be less time to screen or prepare members for ongoing groups; in outpatient clinics there may be more time before the group starts while leaders are recruiting other members. Regardless of time constraints, we recommend having some basic preparation for group members, even if brief.

PGP can range in length from the one or two sessions of a screening interview to multiple individual or small group sessions while the leader assembles the remaining clients necessary to form the group. Yalom and Leszcz (2020) suggest meeting at least periodically with candidates, even by phone, to avoid possible dropout during the period of recruitment. Orientation sessions featuring preparation activities that parallel the tasks of the group appear to be particularly beneficial because they provide exposure to what the group process will involve (Bernard et al., 2008; Yalom & Leszcz, 2020). Preparation sessions can convey didactic material (information about how group therapy promotes change), encourage interpersonal feedback (engaging here-and-now interactions), or offer video presentations (observing process in another group).

Pre-Group Preparation

Key Objectives

In addition to providing information and education, three key objectives in PGP are the formation of the working alliance with the group leaders, promoting a sense of universality, and facilitating group cohesion between members (Yalom & Leszcz, 2020). In addition, the leaders aim to reduce initial anxiety and address myths or misconceptions about beginning the group. The leaders provide education about group to facilitate informed consent, and they seek consensus between the leaders and incoming members regarding group goals (Bernard et al., 2008; Burlingame et al., 2002; Rutan et al., 2014).

Fostering the Alliance with the Leaders

The alliance comprises multiple elements: a shared sense that the group leader values the member, a leader-member agreement on the tasks of therapy, and a shared vision of the goals for the group (Horvath, 2001). Developing a healthy working alliance is a key component of a successful group; researchers have found that a strong alliance is significantly related to the quality of therapy process and outcome (Alldredge et al., 2021). Not only have reviews found a strong relationship between alliance and treatment benefit (Martin et al., 2000), but they have shown that PGP is critical in the initial development of the alliance and the subsequent emergence of group cohesion (Rutan, 2021). Yalom and Leszcz (2020) observe that the first step to creating strong alliances amongst the members is to promote a shared mutual affiliation with the group leader. Burlingame et al. (2002) recommend that the leader utilize the emerging alliance from the PGP session(s) with individual group members to facilitate subsequent development of group cohesion and inter-member alliances.

Clinical Vignette Part Four

During a preparation session co-led by Francis and Abel, the leaders relied on active listening, empathy, and curiosity to help the five candidates explore the reasons they were considering group treatment. The leaders also relied on data from the measures they had previously administered to the clients. At the outset of the preparation session, the leaders express curiosity regarding how members experience the session and focus on listening to them before intervening. Lamar, the one Black man in the group, shares a painful history of emotional abuse in childhood and difficulties trusting people as an adult. Lamar discloses experiences of avoiding intimacy as an adult and shares his hope that group would help address his relationship issues. The leaders empathize with the pain of Lamar's early experiences and help him clarify a pattern of fleeing relationships out of fear of being hurt. The leaders note that these disclosures were consistent with Lamar's feedback on the GTQ-S and ECR-12 and encourage Lamar's expression of these issues in the group as important to his treatment. Francis and Abel help Lamar see how group could be helpful in addressing this avoidance and the fears of conflict and abuse that motivate his impulse to flee. They also raise how difficult it may be for Lamar, as a Black man, to express anger and to feel understood. Jacob, a White transgender male, reaches out to Lamar and describes similar experiences of being devalued. Abel raises the systemic issues that Black people face and notes that this can also be the experience of people who are transgender or endorse other identities. Lamar describes his experiences of discrimination and agrees that he worries about how others will see him in groups, especially those with White majorities. Lamar appears to direct his comments primarily to Francis, a Black woman, and she highlights the challenge of trusting people of a different race, particularly in a White majority context. Francis also notes how Jacob was able to show empathy regarding Lamar's experiences of discrimination even though the men come from different racial backgrounds. Together, the group discuss strategies for addressing the likely emergence of racial differences, fear, anger, and conflict in the upcoming group. The leaders' empathy and goal-setting helps the members gain trust in the leaders, establishes a client-leader alliance, and plants the seeds for group cohesion.

Fostering Universality during Preparation

When members come together in the group for the first time, it is common for them to share personal details that they may never have shared before. Members may open up about their mental health concerns, experiences of loss, health issues, or painful feelings. Often, they experience *universality*, the sense of not being alone in their wretchedness (Yalom & Leszcz, 2020). This experience of *being with others who understand* helps reduce feelings of loneliness, shame, and alienation. Group leaders can foster universality during PGP by letting members know that they will not be alone in the group and that other members will likely share some of the same struggles.

Clinical Vignette Part Five

During a PGP session, the leaders noted that Marlena had scored highly for Social Inhibition and indicated concerns of being rejected by the group members on the GTQ-S. When asked about this concern, Marlena says that she often feels that people will not like her and worries about others criticizing her. She immigrated to the United States from Mexico as a child and often feels different and judged by others. She notes that her accent bothers her and that she will often stay quiet so she can "fit in." Francis and Abel empathize with this struggle and invite other members to share if they have similar feelings. Jacob responds immediately, sharing his childhood feelings of being different. He speaks openly about his gender identity and how being transgender impacted his family and friends. He also expresses worry that he will be rejected by the group. Lamar, a Black male, shares his experiences of being a "unicorn" in an all-white school. He discloses fears of coming to the group and not being wanted, based on being the only minority group member. After contributions by different members in the session, Francis asks Marlena how she was feeling. Marlena sighed and said she had not been expecting to have other people in the group understand her. She expresses relief hearing that other members have also struggled with trusting people and groups and says she feels comfortable talking with others she would be joining in the group.

Fostering Group Cohesion

Theorists have highlighted the importance of group cohesion for years (Yalom & Leszcz, 2020), arguing it is one of the most valuable factors in group work. Forsyth (2021) describes cohesion as a feeling of unity or collaboration. Cohesive groups reflect attraction to the group, foster emotional connection, and offer support and structure. Cohesion has been referred to as the "glue" that keeps the members in the group; in a cohesive therapy group, members can disagree or express conflict yet continue to feel a sense of belonging (Forsyth, 2021). A group struggling with cohesion often feels less safe and more avoidant of genuine disclosures. Members are more at risk of dropping out of groups that lack cohesion. Researchers have found that cohesion positively correlates with increased member self-esteem, reduced symptoms, and higher rates of goal attainment (e.g., Tschuschke & Dies, 1994). The greater the cohesion in the group the more members attend sessions (Ogrodniczuk et al., 2006), stay in the group, endure conflict, and empathize with one another (Alonso, 2011). A meta-analysis examining the cohesion-outcome relationship across 40 studies indicated that cohesion significantly predicted outcome in both in- and outpatient settings (Burlingame et al., 2019).

Johnson et al. (2005) found that empathy by leaders and/or members was related to positive relationships in the therapy group. Researchers have also shown that leaders who promote interpersonal interaction and prioritize the cultivation of cohesion facilitate a greater bond among members (Burlingame et al., 2019). One of the most *inhibiting* leadership factors is a leader's inability to tolerate emotional reactions in the group (Mikulincer & Shaver, 2016). A leader's inability to express or accept caring, address conflict, or engage in exploration of members' avoidant behaviors (e.g., lateness, missed sessions) will negatively influence the development of cohesion (Yalom & Leszcz, 2020). Smokowski et al. (1999) found that dropout from group increased when members experienced leaders as not adequately supporting or protecting them. Leaders may inhibit members from expressing negative feelings towards other members or the leader, preventing the group from confronting and repairing conflict (Marmarosh & Van Horn, 2011). This avoidance of honest dialogue can prompt some members to withdraw or drop out.

During PGP, the group leader can establish the foundations of cohesion by reviewing policies regarding attendance, addressing confidentiality and boundaries, sharing regarding upcoming breaks in treatment (e.g., owing to commitments or vacations), discussing the group process and behaviors that ensure safety and privacy, and attending to how the leader will address difficult conversations in the group. Making therapeutic use of encounters occurring during preparation can reinforce the leader's efforts and help set the parameters for safety within the group. Knowing what to expect and sharing a commitment, the members can have trust in the group and be more open to taking risks.

Clinical Vignette Part Six

The group leaders met with incoming members in a virtual preparation session to "prime" the members for the group. The leaders had reviewed individual client responses on the

GTQ-S and were aware of the different member's goals and fears about group. The leaders started by reviewing the group treatment, explaining how many members would be starting, and providing information about time and format of the sessions. The leaders reviewed the therapy agreement explaining the limits of confidentiality for online treatment and the group contract (see handouts below). The leaders addressed the process of group and the importance of respecting privacy, attending sessions, and letting the group know about planned absences. The leaders discussed commitment to the group and being transparent about any decisions to leave the group. When the session was opened up for questions, members asked about group being a second-rate treatment and the leaders were able to address this myth by providing information supporting the efficacy of group therapy (see handouts). The preparation session also involved watching a short video depicting group process. By the close of the session, the members reported feeling less anxious, expressed confidence about the treatment, and disclosed insight about how group might address their issues. There was less anxiety about the process and enthusiasm for the group's start in a few weeks.

Addressing Diversity During PGP Sessions

Considering how to address cultural factors during preparation represents an important update to the CORE-R. This perspective encompasses the domains of intersecting identities and client experiences of discrimination and oppression. Although joining a group tends to be anxiety-inducing for most members (Bernard et al, 2008; Yalom & Leszcz, 2020), this anxiety tends to manifest uniquely for clients with experiences of oppression, abuse, neglect, and trauma. Aided by use of measures like the PEDQ (see discussion of composition above), the leader can get a sense of how experiences of racism, sexism, xenophobia, homophobia, or other forms of discrimination have impacted prospective members before preparing them for joining group. Ribeiro (2020) argues that during PGP, the leader is encouraged to bring up race, class, gender, and any intersecting identities within the group and to explore how these identities may influence the group process. Leaders are encouraged to share preferred pronouns during preparation and let members know that group is a place where all will be valued regardless of their identities.

It is also helpful to prepare members for possible microaggressions in the group, and to explore how members may react when these occur (Lefforge et al., 2020; Miles et al., 2021). Microaggressions are defined as subtle forms of discrimination, often unintentional and unconscious, that send negative and denigrating messages to a person or group based on an identity that has historically been marginalized (Sue et al., 2007). The emergence of microaggressions can influence the climate of the group (Lefforge et al., 2020; Miles et al., 2021). A common microaggression in group is when members assume everyone has the same sexual orientation without considering that some are gay or bisexual; another is when a leader continues to use an incorrect pronoun to address members who are transgender (Rutan, 2021). Despite a lack of intention to be hurtful, these comments can cause ruptures to the alliances in the group (Miles et al., 2021). An alliance rupture can reflect a subtle tension in a group or it can be a more pervasive conflict between members, leaders, or the entire group (Lo Coco et al., 2021). Ruptures are unavoidable. Many members come to group to work on their ability to address conflict, be genuine, and find ways of repairing relational struggles; ruptures thus reflect therapeutic opportunities if leaders can facilitate a process of clarification and resolution. During PGP, leaders can help members develop readiness for ruptures by asking them how they are likely to respond to a microaggression and how they would like the group leader to address these during sessions. It is the leaders' job to help members with privilege to listen without being defensive and to help the group be open to conversations about diverse identities (Debiak, 2007). It is also the leaders' job to support marginalized members in confronting these ruptures and to safeguard them from feeling overburdened in the group (Lefforge et al., 2020).

Clinical Vignette Part Seven

During a PGP session, Marlena, a cisgender Latin-American female, asked about the identities of group members. Abel, the White male co-leader, described the diverse identities in the group, noting that there were only two other BIPOC members out of a membership of seven. Marlena quickly asked about the gender of these members and appeared anxious when the leader said that both were men. The leader noticed the anxiety and recalled the experiences of discrimination Marlena had reported on the PEDQ. The leader asked more about these and Marlena described her fear that she would be the only woman of color in the group. When Abel asked her to continue, Marlena shared painful examples of being the only woman of color in her graduate class, at work, and in her professional groups. She gave multiple examples of being alone and frustrated when people said things that were offensive. Marlena said she had learned to be silent and accommodating, despite feeling angry, hurt, and alone. She said that one of her goals identified during pre-group screening was to be able to talk more openly about her true feelings and said that having other women of color in the group would help her feel able to take more risks. Marlena looked directly at Francis, the Black co-leader; in response, Francis smiled and praised Marlena's capacity to take a risk in the group by expressing her true feelings. Abel shared his desire to support her, and they explored ways they could work together to address her fears and to challenge any microaggressions that might occur in the group. Abel also explored how his being a White leader might influence the members' safety and ability to feel understood in the group. He asked the members, "If I were to say something in the group that offended you, would my being a White man make it hard to tell me what you think or feel, to confront me?" Marlena initially avoided the question, but after other group members spoke up, she said, "I think it would. I would not want to offend you. I would worry that you would get angry, and then I would want to leave the group." Francis explored how Marlena had pulled back and empathized with her anxiety; together they discussed the impact of race on being able to express anger directly, especially to a White authority figure. Jacob spoke up to say that he had felt offended in the group when Abel said there were two male members, pointing out that he identified as transgender and employed the pronoun "they." Abel welcomed the feedback and expressed appreciation for Jacob's correction. Jacob said that he was "used to people misunderstanding" their gender identity and, like Marlena, would often avoid informing other people of this. Dr. Brown said that he valued the honesty of these disclosures and acknowledged the anger that arose from being misunderstood. He expressed that he would try to understand the group members to the best of his ability and would be open to owning his privilege as a White leader and how that affected the group members. Abel added that he would not be angry if they revealed negative feelings about microaggressions he might express in the group. The PGP session helped the members consider how anger may feel dangerous and how race and gender identity issues can affect the safety in groups. The session opened the door for the clients to feel understood regarding how identity factors could hinder their ability to be open and honest in the group. Importantly, the leaders helped the members begin a challenging conversation about race, sexual identity, gender, and power that did not lead to feeling attacked or more frustrated, isolated, or misunderstood. The members had already started to do the work of group therapy.

Inoculating Group Members During Preparation

Preparation aims to reduce anxiety about group by helping members identify the interpersonal struggles that interfere with their relationships and would serve as a focus for work in group. In the Focused Brief Group Therapy model, Whittingham (2018) argues that the leader can help prepare members by "inoculating" them for the interpersonal challenges they are likely to experience in the group. For example, if a member struggles with being passive aggressive in his relationships, the leader can help the member imagine this passivity emerging in the group and discuss ways the leader and member can prepare for that. Whittingham relies on the IIP-32 (see above) to help prepare members, but many of the screening tools described earlier can be used.

In a similar approach, leaders can rely on attachment theory and the ECR-12 (see above) to help prepare a member for the group (Marmarosh et al., 2013a). For example, new members with higher levels of attachment anxiety on the ECR-12 may be more likely to seek reassurance and feedback from members and leaders (Marmarosh et al., 2013a, b; Mikulincer & Shaver, 2016; Tasca et al., 2006). They may become anxious and/or frustrated with the silences in group and have worries about being rejected. The leader may help the member prepare for the interpersonal interactions that generally occur during the first few group sessions and encourage direct expressions of their fears to fellow members. Members with more avoidance on the ECR-12 often shut down or withdraw, which may inhibit the necessary interactions that can facilitate change over time (Marmarosh et al., 2013b; Tasca et al., 2021). Leaders can best prepare more avoidant group members by helping them imagine how they would respond to transactions in the group situation (Marmarosh et al., 2013b). Helping the members prepare for these transactions can increase their insight and motivation to try something different in group, such as talking about their desire to withdraw when they feel too much pressure to be close (Tasca et al., 2006).

Clinical Vignette Part Eight

Jacob, a Black male transgender client, was referred to group to address struggles in intimate relationships. Jacob had completed the ECR-12 and the leaders determined that he was extremely fearful of being rejected and often pulled away in relationships to prevent potential disappointment. Francis and Abel also reviewed the GTQ-S and noted that Jacob reported fears of being rejected in the group and described how he "felt very far away" from other family members. Abel asked Jacob about this depiction and his fears of being rejected in the group. Jacob shared prior experiences of being shamed in his family and bullied in school for gender non-conformity. The leader explored Jacob's fears of what might transpire in the group and, with him, formulated a plan for addressing the withdrawal that would likely occur in the group based on years of avoiding relationships. The leaders also considered the use of endorsed pronouns, sharing the gender identities of members in the group they knew about. Finally, the leaders intentionally recruited another transgender client to establish a subgroup that could provide support and enhance universality.

Checklist of Procedural Issues to Address During Preparation

Preparing selected clients for entry into group definitely requires an educational focus in addition to an emphasis on establishing a working alliance and fostering a sense of universality and cohesiveness. The leaders' "to-do" list would include the following:

- Review myths about group therapy (e.g., group is a cheap and diluted therapy)
- Provide coherent explanation about group therapy and its processes
- Review goals for each member and objectives of the group
- Explore expectations of the member for group attendance and confidentiality
- Discuss common group problems (group versus individual goals, tardiness, absence of adequate airtime, irregular attendance)
- Discuss common individual problems (fear of rejection, self-disclosure, loss of individuality, repeating social failures, being left behind, avoidance of conflict)
- Explain the time, place, length, breaks, and duration of the therapy
- Review organizational and administrative issues (e.g., fee collection, online format)

Handouts for Pre-Group Preparation

Handouts to use during PGP are designed to facilitate effective groups. A selected set is provided with this chapter (see Handouts in Appendix II). These vary in purpose. Some are used to orient a member to the group process while others include contracts used to outline and formalize a commitment to the group. The handouts can benefit client understanding of the group process and group norms in a concrete manner, helping to create a healthy group climate.

It is recommended that group leaders review the handouts and choose those that best match the type of group, client mix, setting, theoretical approach, and norms of their practice or clinic/agency. Handouts may be adapted to fit the agency or practice as needed. For example, group leaders in an inpatient setting may not need to focus on the norms around attendance if group is a required part of the patient's program. The confidentiality contract, however, may be useful for explaining to patients the commitment to each other's privacy expected for the group experience within the hospital milieu. In one setting, the handout offering examples of how to present the concept of group treatment may be beneficial for therapists in training looking to offer group for new clients they meet on intake, while in another setting the written descriptions of group may better fit the agency procedures. Recently, there has been an increase in online group tele-therapy (Weinberg, 2020) and it is important to have revised handouts that address the needs of members in online group treatment. A brief description of each handout follows.

Presenting Group Therapy to New Members

A list of examples used to educate potential group referrals about the benefits of group is provided. These examples include reasons why group therapy may be the treatment of choice for selected clients and how direct feedback about interpersonal style can be helpful in a group setting. Effectiveness of group therapy, how group works, and common myths about group therapy are discussed. This handout describes how incoming members may get the most out of their group experience and avoid common obstacles to success in group treatment. The handout clarifies norms and expectations regarding confidentiality, attendance, socializing with other members, contact between group sessions, and alcohol and drug use.

Group Therapy Contract/Agreement and Policies

This handout was designed for the group member. It can be used as an informal contract between the leader and group member.

Group Confidentiality Agreement

An agreement on the confidentiality expectations of the group treatment can be formalized if required by the organization or institution.

Online Group Therapy Agreement

Telehealth services, more widespread as a function of the Covid-19 pandemic, remain novel. A clear specification of rights and responsibilities when using technology for therapeutic purposes is a prudent strategy.

Conclusion

Group screening and preparation are critical aspects of group practice, and we have only scratched the surface of how to best assess potential members, determine fit with the group, and prepare each member for group treatment. This chapter focused on the most critical aspects of group selection, composition, and preparation based on contemporary theory, evidence-based assessments, and recommendations grounded in years of research. The chapter should not replace formal course work, training in group therapy, or supervision of group practice. Group interventions are often complex, and one chapter cannot fully address the many ways group therapists select candidates, consider composition, and prepare members for group treatment.

In addition, this chapter focused on interpersonal process groups as the prototype, but there are many approaches that recommend specific protocols for the selection and preparation of members. For example, Dialectical Behavioral Group Therapy recommends specific activities for PGP that are different from dynamic interpersonal group therapy. Groups led in different settings may require different processes. Counseling center groups, private practice groups, inpatient groups, groups in forensic settings, and groups in medical settings may all incorporate different criteria for admission, different requirements for composition, and different processes for preparing new members.

Despite these limitations, the chapter does introduce important elements that were not emphasized in the past, such as considering members' experiences of discrimination and attending to intersecting identities within a group (Ribeiro, 2020). Systemic issues can play out in group, and leaders must be ready to prepare members to address challenging conversations about racism, sexism, homophobia, ableism, discrimination, and privilege. In addition, Covid-19 has changed the way we engage with clients. More than ever, we are using online group formats, and this will certainly influence how we select and prepare members for virtual treatment. We included updated confidentiality forms and recommendations for leaders considering how to prepare members for an online format. Ongoing group research will help us gain a better sense of members who may not be good candidates for online groups but would be excellent candidates for a face-to-face group. Acknowledging a need for additional research in this domain, we do know that when leaders make deliberate efforts to select and prepare members for group therapy, members are more engaged, less likely to drop out, and more likely to benefit from the group.

References

Abouguendia, M., Joyce, A. S., Piper, W. E., & Ogrodniczuk, J. S. (2004). Alliance as a mediator of expectancy effects in short-term group psychotherapy. *Group Dynamics: Theory, Research, and Practice*, 8, 3–12. doi:10.1037/1089-2699.8.1.3.

Alldredge, C. T., Burlingame, G. M., Yang, C., & Rosendahl, J. (2021). Alliance in group therapy: A meta-analysis. *Group Dynamics: Theory, Research, and Practice*, 25, 13–28. doi:10.1037/gdn0000135.

Allen, J. G., Fonagy, P., & Bateman, A. W. (2008). *Mentalizing in clinical practice*. Washington, DC: American Psychiatric Publishing.

Alonso, J. T. (2011). Cohesion's relationship to outcome in group psychotherapy: A meta-analytic review of empirical research (Doctoral dissertation). Brigham Young University, Provo, UT.

Bagby, R. M., Parker, J. D. A., & Taylor, G. J. (1994a). The twenty-item Toronto Alexithymia Scale—I. Item selection and cross-validation of the factor structure. *Journal of Psychosomatic Research*, 38, 23–32. doi:10.1016/0022-3999(94)90005-1.

Bagby, R. M., Taylor, G. J., & Parker, J. D. A. (1994b). The twenty-item Toronto Alexithymia Scale—II. Convergent, discriminant, and concurrent validity. *Journal of Psychosomatic Research*, 38, 33–40. doi:10.1016/0022-3999(94)90006-x.

Baker, E., Burlingame, G. M., Cox, J. C., Beecher, M. E., & Gleave, R. L. (2013). The Group Readiness Questionnaire: A convergent validity analysis. *Group Dynamics: Theory, Research, and Practice*, 17, 299–314. doi:10.1037/a0034477.

Battle, C. C., Imber, S. D., Hoehn-Saric, R., Stone, A. R., Nash, E. R., & Frank, J. D. (1966). Target complaints as criteria of improvement. *American Journal of Psychotherapy*, 20, 184–192. doi:10.1176/appi.psychotherapy.1966.20.1.184.

Bernal, G. & Sáez-Santiago, E. (2006). Culturally centered psychosocial interventions. *Journal of Community Psychology*, 34, 121–132. doi:10.1002/jcop.20096.

Bernard, H., Burlingame, G., Flores, P., Greene, L., Joyce, A., Kobos, J. C., Leszcz, M., MacNair-Semands, R. R., Piper, W. E., Slocum McEneaney, A. M., and Feirman, D. (2008). Clinical practice guidelines for group psychotherapy. *International Journal of Group Psychotherapy*, 58, 455–542. doi:10.1521/ijgp.2008.58.4.455.

Blatt, S. J. (2004). *Experiences of depression: Theoretical, clinical, and research perspectives*. Washington, DC: American Psychological Association Press.

Blatt, S. J. (2008). *Polarities of experience: Relatedness and self-definition in personality development, psychopathology, and the therapeutic process*. Washington, DC: American Psychological Association Press.

Blatt, S. J., Zohar, A. H., Quinlan, D. M., Zuroff, D. C., & Mongrain, M. (1995). Subscales within the dependency factor of the Depressive Experiences Questionnaire. *Journal of Personality Assessment*, 64, 319–339. doi:10.1207/s15327752jpa6402_11.

Blatt, S. J. & Zuroff, D. C. (1992). Interpersonal relatedness and self-definition: Two prototypes for depression. *Clinical Psychology Review*, 12, 527–562. doi:10.1016/0272-7358%2892%2990070-O.

Blatt, S. J., Zuroff, D. C., Bondi, C. M., Sanislow, C. A. III, Pilkonis, P. A. (1998). When and how perfectionism impedes the brief treatment of depression: Further analyses of the National Institute of Mental Health Treatment of Depression Collaborative Research Program. *Journal of Consulting and Clinical Psychology*, 66, 428–428. doi:10.1037/0022-006X.66.2.423.

Boone, L., Claes, L., & Luyten, P. (2014). Too strict or too loose? Perfectionism and impulsivity: The relation with eating disorder symptoms using a person-centered approach. *Eating Behaviors*, 15, 17–23. doi:10.1016/j.eatbeh.2013.10.013.

Brehm, S. S. & Brehm, J. W. (1981). *Psychological reactance: A theory of freedom and control*. New York, NY: Wiley Press.

Brennan, K. A., Clark, C. L., & Shaver, P. R. (1998). Self-report measurement of adult attachment: An integrated overview. In J. A. Simpson & W. S. Rholes (Eds), *Attachment theory and close relationships* (pp. 46–76). New York: Guilford Press.

Brondolo, E., Kelly, K. P., Coakley, V., Gordon, T., Thompson, S., Levy, E., Cassells, A., Tobin, J. N., Sweeney, M., & Contrada, R. J. (2005). The Perceived Ethnic Discrimination Questionnaire: Development and preliminary validation of a community version. *Journal of Applied Social Psychology*, 35, 335–365. doi:10.1111/j.1559-1816.2005.tb02124.x.

Bucci, S., Seymour-Hyde, A., Harris, A., & Berry, K. (2016). Client and therapist attachment styles and working alliance. *Clinical Psychology & Psychotherapy*, 23, 155–165. doi:10.1002/cpp.1944.

Burlingame, G. M., McClendon, D. T., & Yang, C. (2019). Cohesion in group therapy. In J. C. Norcross & M. J. Lambert (Eds), *Psychotherapy relationships that work: Evidence-based therapist contributions, Vol. 1* (3rd ed.; pp. 205–244). New York, NY: Oxford University Press.

Burlingame, G. M., Cox, J. C., Davies, D. R., Layne, C. M., & Gleave, R. (2011). The Group Selection Questionnaire: Further refinements in group member selection. *Group Dynamics: Theory, Research, and Practice*, 15, 60–74. doi:10.1037/a0020220.

Burlingame, G. M., Fuhriman, A., & Johnson, J. (2002). Cohesion in group psychotherapy. In J. C. Norcross (Ed.), *Psychotherapy relationships that work: Therapist contributions and responsiveness to patients* (pp. 71–88). New York: Oxford University Press.

Burlingame, G. M., Strauss, B., Joyce, A., MacNair-Semands, R., MacKenzie, K. R., Ogrodniczuk, J., & Taylor, S. (2006). *CORE Battery—Revised: An assessment tool kit for promoting optimal group selection, process and outcome.* New York, NY: American Group Psychotherapy Association.

Chang-Caffaro, S. & Caffaro, J. (2018). Differences that make a difference: Diversity and the process group leader. *International Journal of Group Psychotherapy*, 68, 483–497. doi:10.1080/00207284.2018.1469958.

Chen, E. C., Kakkad, D., & Balzano, J. (2008). Multicultural competency and evidence-based practice in group therapy. *Journal of Clinical Psychology*, 64, 1261–1278. doi:10.1002/jclp.20533.

Connelly, J. L., Piper, W. E., de Carufel, F. L., & Debbane, E. G. (1986). Premature termination in group psychotherapy: Pretherapy and early therapy predictors. *International Journal of Group Psychotherapy*, 36, 145–152.

Contrada, R. J., Ashmore, R. D., Gary, M. L., Coups, E., Egeth, J. D., Sewell, A., Ewell, K., Goyal, T. M., and Chasse, V. (2001). Measures of ethnicity-related stress: Psychometric properties, ethnic group differences, and associations with well-being. *Journal of Applied Social Psychology*, 31, 1775–1820. doi:10.1111/j.1559-1816.2001.tb00205.x.

Cox, B. J., MacPherson, P. S. R., Enns, M. W., & McWilliams, L. A. (2004). Neuroticism and self-criticism associated with posttraumatic stress disorder in a nationally representative sample. *Behavior Research and Therapy*, 42, 105–114. doi:10.1016/S0005-7967(03)00105-0.

Debiak, D. (2007). Attending to diversity in group psychotherapy: An ethical imperative. *International Journal of Group Psychotherapy*, 57, 1–12. doi:10.1521/ijgp.2007.57.1.1.

Derogatis, L. R. (1993). *BSI: Administration, scoring, and procedures manual for the Brief Symptom Inventory* (3rd ed.). Minneapolis, MN: National Computer Systems.

Derogatis, L. R. (2017). Symptom Checklist-90-Revised, Brief Symptom Inventory, and BSI-18. In M. E. Maruish (Ed.), *Handbook of psychological assessment in primary care settings* (pp. 599–629). New York, NY: Routledge.

DiAngelo, R. (2011). White fragility. *International Journal of Critical Pedagogy*, 3, 54–70.

Dowd, E. T., Milne, C. R., & Wise, S. L. (1991). The therapeutic reactance scale: A measure of psychological reactance. *Journal of Counseling and Development*, 69, 541–545. doi:10.1002/j.1556-6676.1991.tb02638.x.

Dozier, M. (1990). Attachment organization and treatment use for adults with serious psychopathological disorders. *Development and Psychopathology*, 2, 47–60. doi:10.1017/S0954579400000584.

Fjelstad, A., Høglend, P., & Lorentzen, S. (2017). Patterns of change in interpersonal problems during and after short-term and long-term psychodynamic group therapy: A randomized clinical trial. *Psychotherapy Research*, 27, 350–361. doi:10.1080/10503307.2015.1102357.

Fonagy, P., Gergely, G., Jurist, E., & Target, M. (2002). *Affect regulation, mentalization, and the development of the self.* New York, NY: Other Press.

Fonagy, P., Luyten, P., Moulton-Perkins, A., Lee, Y.-W., Warren, F., Howard, S., Ghinal, R., Fearon, P., & Lowyck, B. (2016). Development and validation of a self-report measure of mentalizing: The Reflective Functioning Questionnaire. *PloS ONE*, 11, e0158678. doi:10.1371/journal.pone.0158678.

Forsyth, D. R. (2021). Recent advances in the study of group cohesion. *Group Dynamics: Theory, Research, and Practice*, 25, 213–228. doi:10.1037/gdn0000163.

Gordon, R. M. & Bornstein, R. F. (2015). *The Psychodiagnostic Chart-2 v. 8.1 (PDC-2)*. Retrieved from www.researchgate.net/publication/292592861_Digital_Psychodiagnostic_Chart-2_PDC-2_v81.

Gordon, R. M. & Bornstein, R. F. (2018). Construct validity of the Psychodiagnostic Chart: A trans-diagnostic measure of personality organization, personality syndromes, mental functioning, and symptomatology. *Psychoanalytic Psychology*, 35, 280–288. doi:0000-0003-1990-8644.

Gordon, R. M. & Stoffey, R. W. (2014). Operationalizing the psychodynamic diagnostic manual: A preliminary study of the psychodiagnostic chart. *Bulletin of the Menninger Clinic*, 78, 1–15. doi:10.1521/bumc.2014.78.1.1.

Gullestad, F. S., Johansen, M. S., Høglend, P., Karterud, S., & Wilberg, T. (2012). Mentalization as a moderator of treatment effects: Findings from a randomized clinical trial for personality disorders. *Psychotherapy Research*, 23, 674–689. doi:10.1080/10503307.2012.684103.

Hewitt, P. L. & Flett, G. L. (1991a). Perfectionism in the self and social contexts: Conceptualization, assessment, and association with psychopathology. *Journal of Personality and Social Psychology*, 60, 456–470. doi:10.1037/0022-3514.60.3.456.

Hewitt, P. L. & Flett, G. L. (1991b). The Multidimensional Perfectionism Scale: Reliability, validity, and psychometric properties in psychiatric samples. *Psychological Assessment: A Journal of Consulting and Clinical Psychology*, 3, 464–468. doi:10.1037/1040-3590.3.3.464.

Hewitt, P. L., Flett, G. L., & Mikhail, S. F. (2017). *Perfectionism: A relational approach to conceptualization, assessment, and treatment.* New York, NY: Guilford Publications.

Hewitt, P. L., Flett, G. L., Sherry, S. B., Habke, M., Parkin, M., Lam, R. W., McMurtry, B., Ediger, E., Fairlie, P., & Stein, M. B. (2003). The interpersonal expression of perfection: Perfectionistic self-presentation and psychological distress. *Journal of Personality and Social Psychology*, 84, 1303–1325. doi:10.1037/0022-3514.84.6.1303.

Hewitt, P. L., Mikail, S. F., Flett, G. L., & Dang, S. S. (2018). Specific formulation feedback in dynamic-relational group psychotherapy of perfectionism. *Psychotherapy*, 55, 179–185. doi:10.1037/pst0000137.

Hewitt, P. L., Mikhail, S. F., Flett, G. L., Tasca, G. A., Flynn, C. A., Deng, X., Kaldas, J., & Chen, C. (2015). Psychodynamic/interpersonal group psychotherapy for perfectionism: Evaluating the effectiveness of a short-term treatment. *Psychotherapy*, 52, 205–217. doi:10.1037/pst0000016.

Hook, J. N., Davis, D. E., Owen, J., Worthington, E. L., & Utsey, S. O. (2013). Cultural humility: Measuring openness to culturally diverse clients. *Journal of Counseling Psychology*, 60, 353–366. doi:10.1037/a0032595.

Horowitz, L. M., Aiden, L. E., Wiggins, J. S., & Pincus, A. L. (2000). *Inventory of Interpersonal Problems manual.* Odessa, FL: The Psychological Corporation.

Horowitz, L. M., Rosenberg, S. E., Baer, B. A., Ureño, G., & Villaseñor, V. S. (1988). Inventory of Interpersonal Problems: Psychometric properties and clinical applications. *Journal of Consulting and Clinical Psychology*, 56, 885–892. doi:10.1037/0022-006X.56.6.885.

Horvath, A. O. (2001). The alliance. *Psychotherapy: Theory, Research, Practice, Training*, 38, 365–372. doi:10.1037/0033-3204.38.4.365.

Johnson, J. E., Burlingame, G. M., Olsen, J. A., Davies, D. R., & Gleave, R. L. (2005). Group climate, cohesion, alliance, and empathy in group psychotherapy: Multilevel structural equation models. *Journal of Counseling Psychology*, 52, 310–321. doi:10.1037/0022-0167.52.3.310.

Joyce, A. S., Fujiwara, E., Cristall, M., Ruddy, C., & Ogrodniczuk, J. S. (2013). Clinical correlates of alexithymia among patients with personality disorder. *Psychotherapy Research*, 23, 690–704. doi:10.1080/10503307.2013.803628.

Joyce, A. S., Ogrodniczuk, J. S., Piper, W. E., & Sheptycki, A. R. (2010). Interpersonal predictors of outcome following short-term group therapy for complicated grief: A replication. *Clinical Psychology and Psychotherapy*, 17, 122–135. doi:10.1002/cpp.686.

Kaklauskas, F. J. & Nettles, R. (2019). Towards multicultural and diversity proficiency as a group psychotherapist. In F. J. Kaklauskas & L. R. Greene (Eds), *Core principles of group psychotherapy: An integrated theory, research, and practice training manual* (pp. 25–45). New York, NY: Routledge. doi:10.4324/9780429260803.

Katznelson, H. (2014). Reflective functioning: A review. *Clinical Psychology Review*, 34, 107–117. doi:10.1016/j.cpr.2013.12.003.

Kealy, D., Joyce, A. S., Ogrodniczuk, J. S., Ehrenthal, J. C., & Weber, R. (2018). Reactance and engagement in integrative group psychotherapy for personality dysfunction, *Journal of Psychotherapy Integration*, 28, 462–474. doi:10.1037/int0000129.

Kealy, D., Ogrodniczuk, J. S., Piper, W. E., & Sierra-Hernandez, C. A. (2016). When it is not a good fit: Clinical errors in patient selection and group composition in group psychotherapy. *Psychotherapy*, 53, 308–313. doi:10.1037/pst0000069.

Kealy, D., Piper, W. E., Ogrodniczuk, J. S., Joyce, A. S., & Weideman, R. (2018). Individual goal achievement in group psychotherapy: The roles of psychological mindedness and group process in interpretive and supportive therapy for complicated grief. *Clinical Psychology and Psychotherapy*, 1–11. doi:10.1002/cpp.2346.

Kiesler, D. J. (1996). *Contemporary interpersonal theory and research: Personality, psychopathology, and psychotherapy*. New York, NY: Wiley.

Kirchmann, H., Mestel, R., Schreiber-Willnow, K., Mattke, D., Seidler, K. P., Daudert, E., Nickel, R., Papenhausen, R., Eckert, J., & Strauss, B. (2009). Associations among attachment characteristics, patients' assessment of therapeutic factors, and treatment outcome following inpatient psychodynamic group psychotherapy. *Psychotherapy Research*, 19, 234–248. doi:10.1080/10503300902798367.

Kivlighan, D. M. & Angelone, E. O. (1992). Interpersonal problems: Variables influencing participants' perception of group climate. *Journal of Counseling Psychology*, 39, 468–472. doi:10.1037/0022-0167.39.4.468.

Kivlighan, D. M., Lo Coco, G., Gullo, S., Pazzagli, C., & Mazzeschi, C. (2017). Attachment anxiety and attachment avoidance: Members' attachment fit with their group and group relationships. *International Journal of Group Psychotherapy*, 67, 223–239. doi:10.1080/00207284.2016.1260464.

Kivlighan, D. M. III, Drinane, J. M., Tao, K. W., Owen, J., & Ming Liu, W. (2019). Detrimental effect of fragile groups: Examining the role of cultural comfort for group therapy members of color. *Journal of Counseling Psychology*, 66, 763–770. doi:10.1037/cou0000352.

Kleinberg, J. L. (1996). Working with the alexithymic patient in groups. *Psychoanalysis and Psychotherapy*, 13, 76–85.

Lafontaine, M-F., Brassard, A., Lussier, Y., Valois, P., Shaver, P. R., & Johnson, S. M. (2016). Selecting the best items for a short-form of the Experiences in Close Relationships Questionnaire. *European Journal of Psychological Assessment*, 32, 140–154. doi:10.1027/1015-5759/a000243.

Lawson, D. M. & Brossart, D. F. (2009). Attachment, interpersonal problems, and treatment outcome in group therapy for intimate partner violence. *Psychology of Men & Masculinity*, 10, 288–301. doi:10.1037/a0017043.

Lefforge, N. L., Mclaughlin, S., Goates-Jones, M., & Mejia, C. (2020). A training model for addressing microaggressions in group psychotherapy. *International Journal of Group Psychotherapy*, 70, 1–28. doi:10.1080/00207284.2019.1680989.

Levy, K. N., Ellison, W. D., Scott, L. N., & Bernecker, S. L. (2011). Attachment style. In J. C. Norcross (Ed.), *Psychotherapy relationships that work: Evidence-based responsiveness* (pp. 378–401). New York, NY: Oxford University Press. doi:10.1093/acprof.oso/9780199737208.003.0019.

Lingiardi, V., McWilliams, N., Bornstein, R. F., Gazzillo, F., & Gordon, R. M. (2015). The Psychodynamic Diagnostic Manual Version 2 (PDM-2): Assessing patients for improved clinical practice and research. *Psychoanalytic Psychology*, 32, 94–115. doi:10.1037/a0038546.

Lo Coco, G., Tasca, G. A., Hewitt, P. L., Mikail, S. F., & Kivlighan, J. D. M. (2019). Ruptures and repairs of group therapy alliance. An untold story in psychotherapy research. *Research in Psychotherapy: Psychopathology, Process and Outcome*, 22, 58–70. doi:10.4081/ripppo.2019.352.

Lorentzen, S. & Høglend, P. (2004). Predictors of change during long-term analytic group psychotherapy. *Psychotherapy and Psychosomatics*, 73, 25–35. doi:10.1159/000074437.

MacNair, R. R. & Corazzini, J. (1994). Client factors influencing group therapy dropout. *Psychotherapy*, 31, 352–361. doi:10.1037/h0090226.

MacNair-Semands, R. R. (2002). Predicting attendance and expectations for group therapy. *Group Dynamics: Theory, Research, and Practice*, 6, 219–228. doi:10.1037/1089-2699.6.3.219.

MacNair-Semands, R. R. (2019). *The Group Therapy Questionnaire—Short Form*. University of North Carolina, Charlotte, NC.

Markin, R. D. & Marmarosh, C. L. (2010). Application of adult attachment theory to group member transference and the group therapy process. *Psychotherapy*, 47, 111–121. doi:10.1037/a0018840.

Marmarosh, C. L. (2014). Empirical research on attachment in group psychotherapy: Moving the field forward. *Psychotherapy*, 51, 88–92. doi:10.1037/a0032523.

Marmarosh, C. L., Markin, R. D., & Spiegel, E. B. (2013a). *Attachment in group psychotherapy*. Washington, DC: American Psychological Association Press.

Marmarosh, C. L., Markin, R. D., & Spiegel, E. B. (2013b). Assembling the group: Screening, placing, and preparing group members. In C. L. Marmarosh, R. D. Markin, & E. B. Spiegel (Eds), *Attachment in group psychotherapy* (pp. 67–95). Washington, DC: American Psychological Association Press. doi:10.1037/14186-005.

Marmarosh, C. L. & Van Horn, S. M. (2011). Cohesion in counseling and psychotherapy groups. In R. K. Conyne (Ed.), *The Oxford handbook of group counseling* (pp. 137–163). New York, NY: Oxford University Press. doi:10.1093/oxfordhb/9780195394450.013.0009.

Martin, D. J., Garske, J. P., & Davis, M. K. (2000). Relation of the therapeutic alliance with outcome and other variables: A meta-analytic review. *Journal of Consulting and Clinical Psychology*, 68, 438–450. doi:10.1037/0022-006X.68.3.438.

McNeilly, M. D., Anderson, N. B., Armstead, C. A., Clark, R., Corbett, M., Robinson, E. L., Pieper, C. F., & Lepisto, E. M. (1996). The Perceived Racism Scale: A multidimensional assessment of the experience of White racism among African Americans. *Ethnicity & Disease*, 6, 154–166. doi:10.1037/t70724-000.

Mikulincer, M. & Shaver, P. R. (2016). *Attachment in adulthood: Structure, dynamics, and change* (2nd ed.). New York, NY: Guilford Press.

Miles, J. R., Anders, C., Kivlighan, D. M. III, & Belcher Platt, A. A. (2021). Cultural ruptures: Addressing microaggressions in group therapy. *Group Dynamics: Theory, Research, and Practice*, 25, 74–88. doi:10.1037/gdn0000149.

Miller, R., Hilsenroth, M. J., & Hewitt, P. L. (2017). Perfectionism and therapeutic alliance: A review of the clinical research. *Research in Psychotherapy: Psychopathology, Process and Outcome*, 20, 19–29.

Ogrodniczuk, J. S., Piper, W. E., & Joyce, A. S. (2005). The negative effect of alexithymia on the outcome of group therapy for complicated grief: What role might the therapist play? *Comprehensive Psychiatry*, 46, 206–213. doi:10.1016/j.comppsych.2004.08.005.

Ogrodniczuk, J. S., Piper, W. E., & Joyce, A. S. (2006). Treatment compliance among patients with personality disorders receiving group psychotherapy: What are the roles of interpersonal distress and cohesion? *Psychiatry: Interpersonal and Biological Processes*, 69, 249–261. doi:10.1521/psyc.2006.69.3.249.

Ogrodniczuk, J. S., Piper, W. E., Joyce, A. S., McCallum, M., & Rosie, J. S. (2003). NEO-Five Factor personality traits as predictors of response to two forms of group psychotherapy. *International Journal of Group Psychotherapy*, 53, 417–442. doi:10.1521/ijgp.53.4.417.42832.

Ogrodniczuk, J. S., Piper, W. E., Joyce, A. S., Steinberg, P. I., & Duggal, S. (2009). Interpersonal problems associated with narcissism among psychiatric outpatients. *Journal of Psychiatric Research*, 43, 837–842. doi:10.1016/j.jpsychires.2008.12.005.

Ogrodniczuk, J. S., Piper, W. E., McCallum, M., Joyce, A. S., & Rosie, J. S. (2002). Interpersonal predictors of group therapy outcome for complicated grief. *International Journal of Group Psychotherapy*, 52, 511–535. doi:10.1521/ijgp.52.4.511.45520.

Phinney, J. S. (1992). The Multigroup Ethnic Identity Measure: A new scale for use with diverse groups. *Journal of Adolescent Research*, 7, 156–176. doi:10.1177/074355489272003.

Piper, W. E., McCallum, M., Joyce, A. S., & Ogrodniczuk, J. S. (2001). Patient personality and time-limited group psychotherapy for complicated grief. *International Journal of Group Psychotherapy*, 51, 525–552. doi:10.1521/ijgp.51.4.525.51307.

Piper, W. E., Ogrodniczuk, J. S., Joyce, A. S., Weideman, R., & Rosie, J. S. (2007). Group composition and group therapy for complicated grief. *Journal of Consulting and Clinical Psychology*, 75, 116–125. doi:10.1037/0022-006X.75.1.116.

Resnick, S. G., Oehlert, M. E., Hoff, R. A., & Kearney, L. K. (2020). Measurement-based care and psychological assessment: Using measurement to enhance psychological treatment. *Psychological Services*, 17, 233–237. doi:10.1037/ser0000491.

Ribeiro, M. (2020). *Examining Social Identities and Diversity Issues in Group Therapy: Knocking at the Boundaries.* New York, NY: Routledge.

Ruiz, M. A., Pincus, A. L., Borkovec, T. D., Echemendia, R. J., Castonguay, L. G., & Ragusa, S. A. (2004). Validity of the Inventory of Interpersonal Problems for predicting treatment outcome: An investigation with the Pennsylvania Practice Research Network. *Journal of Personality Assessment*, 83, 213–222. doi:10.1027/s15327752jpa8303_05.

Rutan, J. S. (2021). Rupture and repair: Using leader errors in psychodynamic group psychotherapy. *International Journal of Group Psychotherapy*, 71, 310–331. doi:101080/00207284.2020.1808471.

Rutan, J. S., Greene, L. R., & Kaklauskas, F. J. (2019). Preparing to begin a new group. In F. J. Kaklauskas, & L. R. Greene (Eds), *Core principles of group psychotherapy: An integrated theory, research, and practice training manual* (pp. 89–99). New York, NY: Routledge. doi:10.4324/9780429260803.

Rutan, J. S., Stone, W. N., & Shay, J. J. (2014). *Psychodynamic group psychotherapy*. New York, NY: Guilford Press Publications.

Shechtman, Z. & Dvir, V. (2006). Attachment style as a predictor of behavior in group counseling with preadolescents. *Group Dynamics: Theory, Research, and Practice*, 10, 29–42. doi:10.1037/1089-2699.10.1.29.

Seeman, E. A., Buboltz, W. C., Thomas, A., Soper, B., & Wilkinson, L. (2005). Normal personality variables and their relationship to psychological reactance. *Individual Differences Research*, 3, 88–98. doi:10.1037.t09859-000.

Seibel, C. A. & Dowd, E. T. (2001). Personality characteristics associated with psychological reactance. *Journal of Clinical Psychology*, 57, 963–969. doi:10.1002/jclp.1062.

Smith, E. R., Murphy, J., & Coats, S. (1999). Attachment to groups: Theory and management. *Journal of Personality and Social Psychology*, 77, 94–110. doi:10.1037/0022-3414.77.1.94.

Smith, T. B., Domenech Rodríguez, M. M., & Bernal, G. (2011). Culture. In J. C. Norcross (Ed.), *Psychotherapy relationships that work: Evidence-based responsiveness* (pp. 317–335). New York, NY: Oxford University Press. doi:10.1093/acprof:oso/9780199737208.001.0001.

Smokowski, P. R., Rose, S., Todar, K., & Reardon, K. (1999). Postgroup-casualty status, group events, and leader behavior: An early look into the dynamics of damaging group experiences. *Research on Social Work Practice*, 9, 555–574. doi:10.1177/10497315990090050.

Söchting, I., Lau, M., & Ogrodniczuk, J. (2018). Predicting compliance in group CBT using the Group Therapy Questionnaire. *International Journal of Group Psychotherapy*, 68, 184–194. doi:10.1080/00207284.2017.1371569.

Sue, D. W., Capodilupo, C. M., Torino, G. C., Bucceri, J. M., Holder, A., Nadal, K. L., & Esquilin, M. (2007). Racial microaggressions in everyday life: Implications for clinical practice. *American Psychologist*, 62, 271–286. doi:10.1037/0003-066X.62.4.271.

Tasca, G. A., Brugnera, A., Baldwin, D., Carlucci, S., Compare, A., Balfour, L., Proulx, G., Gick, M., & Lafontaine, M.-F. (2018). Reliability and validity of the Experiences in Close Relationships Scale-12: Attachment dimensions in a clinical sample with eating disorders. *International Journal of Eating Disorders*, 51, 18–27. doi:10.1002/eat.22807.

Tasca, G. A., Mikhail, S. F., & Hewitt, P. L. (2021). *Group psychodynamic-interpersonal psychotherapy: An evidence-based transdiagnostic approach*. Washington, DC: American Psychological Association Press.

Tasca, G. A., Ritchie, K., Conrad, G., Balfour, L., Gayton, J., Lybanon, V., & Bissada, H. (2006). Attachment scales predict outcome in a randomized controlled trial of two group therapies for binge eating disorder: An aptitude by treatment interaction. *Psychotherapy Research*, 16, 106–121. doi:10.1080/105033005000909.

Tasca, G. A., Ritchie, K., Demidenko, N., Balfour, L., Krysanski, V., Weekes, K., Barber, A., Keating, L., & Bissada, H. (2013). Matching women with binge eating disorder to group treatment based on attachment anxiety: Outcomes and moderating effects. *Psychotherapy Research*, 23, 301–314. doi:10.1080.10503307.2012.717309.

Taylor, G. J. & Bagby, R. M. (2004). New trends in alexithymia research. *Psychotherapy and Psychosomatics*, 73, 68–77. doi:10.1159/000075537.

Tschuschke, V. & Dies, R. R. (1994). Intensive analysis of therapeutic factors and outcome in long–term inpatient groups. *International Journal of Group Psychotherapy*, 44, 185–208.

Valbak, K. (2018). Preparing for group analytic psychotherapy: Meeting the new patient. *Group Analysis*, 51, 159–174. doi:10.1177/0533316418764385.

Weinberg, H. (2020). Online group psychotherapy: Challenges and possibilities during COVID-19— A practice review. *Group Dynamics: Theory, Research, and Practice*, 24, 201. doi:10.1037/gdn0000140.

Whittingham, M. (2018). Group assessment: How Focused Brief Group Therapy integrates formal measures to enhance treatment preparation, process, and outcomes. *Psychotherapy*, 55, 186–190. doi:10.1037/pst0000153.

Yalom, I. and Leszcz, M. (2020). *The Theory and Practice of Group Psychotherapy* (6th ed.). New York: Basic Books.

Zuroff, D. C., Quinlan, D. M., & Blatt, S. J. (1990). Psychometric properties of the Depressive Experiences Questionnaire in a college population. *Journal of Personality Assessment*, 55, 65–72. doi:10.1207/s15327752jpa5501&2_7.

3 Process Measures

Joseph R. Miles, Bernhard M. Strauss and Les R. Greene

In one of the more authoritative analyses on the topic of *group process*, Brown (2003) observed that, while the term is a core concept in understanding group life, there is no generally agreed upon definition. Because it is multidimensional, it is difficult to pin down in a concise and clinically informative manner. Burlingame et al. (2006), for example, equated group process with "whatever occurs in the group therapy session" (p. 43). Other conceptualizations have tried to more clearly specify and delineate the components of group process. For example, Brown (2003) proposed that process is the:

> "here-and-now experience in the group that describes how the group is functioning, the quality of the relationships between and among the members and with the leader, the emotional experiences and reactions of the group, and the group's strongest desires and fears."
>
> (p. 228)

These broad and abstract definitions, while accurate, may not be so helpful in guiding and focusing the group therapist's attention or helping the therapist think about what is going on, amidst the continuing bombardment of clinical material from seemingly all directions in the here-and-now of the group. Perhaps, as Pascual-Leone and Andreescu (2013) posited, a clinically relevant understanding of process can be acquired through the study of group process measures. In essence, these clinical researchers suggested that the clearest way to understand group process is through a positivist approach of mastering the extant operational definitions of process—that is, learning how group process has been formally assessed; the interrelationships among measures of process; and the relationships between group structure, process, and outcomes can help therapists develop hypotheses about what is happening in the group and what interventions would be useful.

A review of the empirical literature on group process measurement reveals that group process has been conceived of in multifarious ways: a) as single robust variables best exemplified by measures of cohesion (Burlingame, McClendon, & Alonso, 2011a, b; Burlingame, McClendon, & Yang, 2018) and as systems of integrated variables (Beck & Lewis, 2000); b) as self-report measures of members' experiences and rater observations of members' behaviors; and c) as overt interpersonal behaviors (such as arguing with the leader) but also as dimensions that must be inferred because they are hidden, unspoken, or out of awareness (such as emotions, cognitions, attitudes, emotional and defensive needs). Regarding covert or latent phenomena, group process also includes motivational and dynamic components as key elements. In thinking about group process, the group therapist needs to ask questions such as "What is the group trying to do at this moment, particularly in terms of the structuring and quality of the here-and-now relationships? What are the emotional needs of the group that are being enacted (e.g., finding a protector or guarantor for safety and security or looking for a target to blame)? What are the overt and covert agendas the group is trying to achieve in terms of official task achievement and

DOI: 10.4324/9781003255482-3

emotional needs and gratifications?" As we discuss below, thinking about the interior of the group—the quality of the interpersonal relationships, the emotional needs being enacted, the wishes and fears activated in the moment—is crucial work for the therapist and the group precisely because the amassing research provides compelling evidence for the significant link between process and outcome (cf. Burlingame & Strauss, 2021).

The primary aim of this chapter is to review and recommend psychometrically sound and clinically useful measures to monitor process variables in group sessions. We discuss why it is important for group practitioners to think about and assess process in an ongoing way, both at the individual member level and at the level of the group-as-a-whole. We also describe how group process must be understood in relation to group structure, on one hand, and outcome or goal attainment, on the other. We also include a discussion of issues related to culture and diversity in group psychotherapy, as there has been increased acknowledgement in group therapy research and practice that these factors significantly influence group process. We provide a description of selected process measures and a brief section on measures relevant to leadership and conclude with our summary and recommendations.

Throughout the chapter, we aim to illustrate the utility of the group process measures we discuss through an ongoing hypothetical case example. We offer vignettes of a psychotherapy group at a counseling center at a large, public, university in the US with a diverse student population. The group is interpersonal in orientation, fashioned after the model by Yalom and Leszcz (2020). One of the co-leaders is Stacy, a staff psychologist and a Black, cisgender, heterosexual woman. Mike, a pre-doctoral intern under Stacy's supervision, and a White, cisgender, gay man, is the other co-leader. The group has eight members, and includes women and men. Two of the members identify as People of Color and six as White. All group members have provided informed consent as a part of their group orientation to complete group process measures after every third session. Specifically, they all complete the Group Questionnaire (GQ), Therapeutic Factors Inventory (TFI-19), the Critical Incidents measure (CI), and the Multicultural Orientation Inventory – Group Version (MCO-G), all of which are described below. Stacy explained to Mike in an early supervision session that she values the collecting of group process data and, after considerable deliberation, chose these particular measures for several reasons in order to better understand where the group is with respect to group climate and cohesion; to get another perspective, beyond her clinical observations on what individual group members are experiencing in sessions, including adverse reactions that she had not seen directly in the group; and to learn how group members are feeling with regard to the group's *multicultural orientation* (i.e., the extent to which cultural issues are addressed, and the comfort the group has in talking about cultural issues).

Why is it Necessary for Practitioners to Know about Group Process Measures and Monitoring?

The *primary* rationale for employing process measures is to provide an alternative perspective on what is happening in the group, beyond the therapist's viewpoint. Group life is very complex and the observations and experiences of even the most seasoned group therapist may miss or overlook important emotional dynamics. Moreover, the therapist's own biases and emotional needs may distort perceptions and understandings of what is happening in the group and its individual members. Chapman et al. (2012), for example, found that group therapists underestimated the number of group patients experiencing deterioration in therapy and were not accurate in judging clients' experiences of the therapeutic alliance.

Of course, self-report measures completed by group members are also not foolproof. As suggested in Chapter 1, members' own emotional and defensive needs may lead to deviations—either exaggerations or minimizations—from their actual internal experiences. The point, then, is that routine monitoring is precisely useful through its comparison to the therapist's subjective take on what is going on. If the two perspectives are similar, then the therapist has more reason to trust their own understandings and interpretations. However, divergence in these two perspectives provides a kind of "red flag" warning for the therapist to stop and reconsider—through exploration within self and with the group—what is actually happening (cf. Miller et al., 2015). In the experience of those clinician-researchers who have implemented and integrated measures into clinical practice, Gleave et al. (2017) declared:

> "I find outcome and process measures extremely helpful as I lead my groups. Although I believe in and trust my intuition and feel fairly confident in interpreting the interactions and processes in my groups, it is clear to me that I cannot capture everything each person is thinking or feeling through my observations. I find clients' voices, provided through the measures, to be another way for them to let me know about their experience."
>
> (p. 155)

There are a number of other reasons for administering measures to explore group process. In an age of increasing accountability in clinical practice, the formal and systematic monitoring of group process (and outcomes) through measures like the Group Questionnaire (GQ) is an important component of being an evidence-based practitioner. Employing measures, routinely or on an ad hoc basis, defines practice-based evidence that offers an accountability beyond the therapist's subjective construal of what is happening and what has happened. Moreover, there is mounting evidence suggesting that providing feedback to group psychotherapy clients may actually improve outcomes (Burlingame, Whitcomb et al., 2018; Griner et al., 2018); Slone et al., 2015; Woodland et al., 2022). In addition, the use of process measures has been shown to be helpful in detecting and repairing alliance ruptures and misalliances (Burlingame, Alldredge et al., 2021; Burlingame, Whitcomb et al., 2018).

Of course, in considering the implementation of process measures into one's practice, the therapist needs to be mindful of resistances and barriers that need to be sensitively understood and resolved (Gleave et al., 2017). Overcoming patients' suspicions (Solstad et al., 2019; Solstad et al., 2021; Solstad et al., 2021) about the use of such measures is a primary challenge and efforts must be directed at developing a collaborative spirit between therapist and patients in using instruments. Yalom and Leszcz (2020) recommended engaging clients in the feedback process by helping them see its importance (suggesting that one might frame the assessment process as analogous to bloodwork a physician might do to assist in providing appropriate care). Similarly, the therapist must be open to exploring one's own resistances to and rationalizations for the use of measurement and monitoring, given the potential of receiving negative feedback about the group process or one's own effectiveness from patients (Miller et al., 2015).

Returning to our case example, Stacy explains to Mike in supervision that there are important potential benefits of considering group process theory and research, and of formally assessing group processes with validated measures. Because of this, she tells him, in addition to the counseling center's periodic outcome measures, she asks members of all her groups to complete a brief set of post-session evaluation measures, clearly explaining to the group members the intention of such measures, namely to provide her, her co-leader, and the group feedback about the session. Stacy tells Mike there may be negative aspects of the overall process that they discover through these measures that might have gone undetected by their clinical observations and that could ultimately and adversely affect outcome unless addressed in the group. Stacy explains that she discusses the feedback from the assessments in her meetings with her co-leader, but also brings the information gleaned from the assessments into sessions when she feels it would help the group by providing an opportunity for the group to reflect on how the group and its individual members are faring. Next, we introduce a model of group process that has helped guide how Stacy thinks about the "anatomy" and "physiology" of groups and why she collects and uses group process measures.

The Anatomy and Physiology of Groups

While the focus of this chapter is group process, this construct needs to be viewed in relation to other core concepts of group life, particularly social structure. Analogous to living organisms characterized by their distinct anatomical forms and physiological functions, groups as social systems can be uniquely defined and described by their structural and functional properties. And, as implied in Figure 3.1, which lists key structural and dynamics properties of groups that have been extensively studied (Burlingame et al., 2004; Burlingame et al., 2008), there are intricate and reciprocal dynamic relationships between structure and process. For example, as most experienced group therapists understand, imposing too much structure (e.g., keeping to a rigidly scripted agenda in a psychoeducational group) may suppress important processes (such as the expression of fears about the group) that could interfere with commitment to the learning task unless adequately explored and understood; on the other hand, too little structure may be an invitation for more developmentally primitive group processes such as scapegoating or fight-flight enactments).

We believe it is essential for group leaders, as well as researchers, to be knowledgeable about group form and process and to continuously explore what is happening in the group from both of these perspectives. Unfortunately, too much formal research on therapy groups fails to adequately describe and assess their structural and dynamic properties and thus leaves unaddressed how these properties influence therapeutic outcomes. We believe future progress in outcome research *must* include measures of well-known group properties to at least rule them in or out as potential contributors to therapeutic change. Such research would also positively impact clinical practice (see Burlingame et al. 2008, for more detailed description) by giving clinicians more knowledge about the anticipation of conflict, withdrawal of single members, or dropout.

As shown in Figure 3.1, structure can be considered both from the therapist's initial steps in establishing boundaries and defining format, that is, the *imposed* or "official" structure (e. g., selecting who is in, prescribing the rules and roles for the members, defining what the work is in the group, and establishing the when and where of the group), and from the

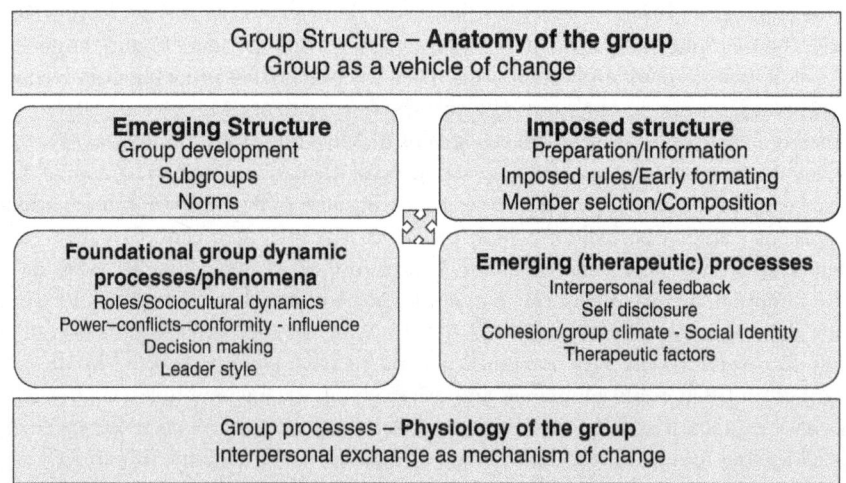

Figure 3.1 Interrelationships Between Group Structure and Group Process
Source: Burlingame et al. (2013).

emergent structure, referring to the kinds of unofficial and often covert social-emotional arrangements that arise in the group over time and that can powerfully shape behavior and relationships in the group. Emergent structure describes the "group personality" and refers to three component constructs: developmental patterns, subgroups, and norms.

Group Developmental Patterns

Many theories of group life posit that groups go through predictable arrangements or configurations of work investment and emotional dynamics over time. Greene and Kaklauskas (2020b) reviewed these patterns as: 1) progressive linear-models such as the stages of forming, storming, norming, performing, and adjourning posited by Tuckman and Jensen (1977); 2) life cycle models that posit early, middle, and late phases of group life analogous to human life development such as those constructed by MacKenzie (1997) and Wheelan (2005); and 3) pendular or recurring-cycle models such as Bion's (1961) model of the dynamic interplay between work and defense.

Results of studies aimed at detecting these proposed invariant developmental stages in group life have been mixed, at best, however, leading some to propose that models of group development be viewed heuristically and "not in too literal a manner" (Ogrodniczuk et al., 2021, p. 244). The best clinical wisdom to date is that putative group phases might not necessarily occur in every group and might not happen in a specific sequence. There are simply too many factors and unforeseen events that can affect the course of the group, including keeping it stuck in one phase or regressing to an earlier phase. Having a "chart of the voyage" (Yalom & Leszcz, 2020, p. 397) in mind, however, helps a group leader reflect on where the group is in terms of capacities for psychological work and coping with various emotional needs and tensions. Such an appraisal, along with reflections on where the group has been in the past, can serve to guide the therapist's interventions in order to move the group further towards achieving its goals. For example, assessing the group as stuck in a culture of conflict will require interventions aimed directly at this issue before other work can be accomplished.

Of the measures available for monitoring process, the Group Climate Questionnaire (GCQ) (MacKenzie, 1981, 1983) seems well suited for capturing phases of group development by comparing three clinically robust dimensions of Engagement (reflecting members' commitment to the work and to the group), Conflict (capturing perceived emotional tension), and Avoidance (fleeing from the work and the group). For example, a session characterized by low avoidance and conflict and high engagement can be thought of as typifying the performing stage of group life.

Returning to our hypothetical case example, after the third session, Mike notes to Stacy that the group seems to be going exceptionally well—everyone seems to like and care about each other and the group and there seems to be relatively little conflict. Stacy suggests that they look together at the GCQ data they have recently collected through their administration of the GQ. As Mike hypothesized, the data, overall, suggest a high level of engagement and low levels of conflict and avoidance in the group. Stacy is pleased with this portrait and hopes to reinforce the values and culture in the group that have led to it. She adds that they should continue to monitor the GCQ feedback to see if this pattern is sustained or whether less optimal patterns arise, owing to unforeseen circumstances or as the group approaches termination. She wants to look at the data in an aggregated manner to get a snapshot of the group as whole but also look at individual member contributions to see if they deviate from the collective picture (cf. Gold & Kivlighan, 2018).

Subgroups

Another component of emergent structure is the formation of subgroups. To reduce the complexity of group life, it is not infrequent that a member joins with select others to experience the gratification of bonding with some and to distance from others. Clinically important, Gantt and Agazarian (2017) distinguish between functional and dysfunctional subgroups, the former formed on the basis of similar beliefs, values, emotional needs, or "valencies" (cf. Stock & Thelen, 1958). As these theorists have suggested, functional subgroups can help the group discover differences in the apparently similar and discover similarities in the apparently different, all processed in a contained, safe manner. In contrast, dysfunctional subgroups serve defensive needs by externalizing undesirable and threatening aspects of self onto another subgroup and then keeping that other subgroup at arms distance, a polarizing, us-versus-them dynamic that disrupts group-as-a-whole harmony and cohesion (Greene & Kaklauskas, 2020a). While there have been comparatively few empirical studies of subgrouping, one promising line of investigation has been the construction and preliminary validation of the Functional Subgrouping Questionnaire-2, a brief self-report inventory tapping members' perceptions of subgroup formation from a systems-centered approach (O'Neill et al., 2013; Whitcomb et al., 2018).

Group Norms

Group norms define the implicit and explicit rules that regulate the members' and leaders' interpersonal behavior and characterize the uniqueness of a group identity by describing and prescribing how it is to be in the group. Some norms can be articulated by the therapist in the initial planning of the group and pre-group orientation sessions, but other norms come about through the process of the group over time as group members create rules, often covert, about how to be and relate in the group. Members often learn about these covert rules when they bump up against them and experience group pressures and reinforcements to conform to them. It is clinically important for the therapist to assess whether these emergent norms are consistent with therapeutic work or whether they primarily serve defensive needs and inhibit therapeutic growth and development (Greene, 2020). Empirically, it has been shown, for example, that in interpersonal therapy groups, members' self-disclosure, combined with constructive interpersonal exchange, task orientation on the side of the leader, and engagement within the entire group is predictive for productive group development, whereas hostility and aggression, withdrawal, or boundary violations are likely to have negative effects (Strauss, 2021).

In our hypothetical case example, after their sixth session Stacy notes to Mike that she thinks there might be some dysfunctional subgrouping occurring, along with some anti-therapeutic norms. Mike asks what gives her that feeling and she says she heard two of the group members discussing a coffee outing they had together outside of the group. She also started to notice that these members avoided conflict with one another and were not providing difficult feedback. Stacy recalls Yalom and Leszcz's (2020) warning that subgrouping may reflect a problem in group development, which can lead to the development of anti-therapeutic norms. She suggests they look at the group members' responses on the GQ to better understand the relationships and development of the group. In particular, she wants to see if the results of the process measures from these two members deviated from the rest of the group, a finding that could support her concern about dysfunctional subgrouping. She also suggests the CI might give them a nuanced sense of how individual members are experiencing these sessions and give them a clearer understanding of what she was perceiving as dysfunctional subgrouping.

Group Physiology

Foundational Group Processes

As displayed in Figure 3.1, there are a number of foundational group processes, considered universal in all kinds of groups and empirically studied from such diverse and disparate fields as social psychology, group dynamics, organizational psychology, and sports psychology. These universal group process concepts are considered to have relevance for the practice of group psychotherapy which requires not just technical expertise on the part of the leader but a deep understanding of the processes and dynamics that pervade the group therapy situation (Parks & Tasca, 2020). While beyond the scope of this volume to review these literatures, Burlingame et al. (2013) have encouraged group clinicians to become more acquainted with foundational group processes given that these basic and universal group processes—such as social psychological processes of conformity and social influence, inclusion and exclusion, principles of cooperation, power, and the management of conflict—occur in all kinds of groups, including therapy groups (Forsyth, 2010; Parks & Tasca, 2021). For example, the social psychological study of conflict development, escalation, and resolution in small groups (e.g., Lewicki et al., 2006) has been conceptually linked to and has implications for the relatively recent notions of rupture and repair in group therapy (Lo Coco et al., 2019). As Fuhriman and Burlingame (1994) stated some time ago, there is an enormous potential for improving our conceptual and empirical understanding of therapy groups in the theories and empirical literature on task groups from social and organizational psychological perspectives. The recent efforts of Parks and Tasca (2020) to foster synergies between group psychology and group therapy reflect one promising attempt to bridge gaps between separated worlds.

Emerging Processes

Therapeutic factors, perhaps the best known of emerging processes in therapeutic groups, refer to those processes, both intrapsychic and interpersonal, that promote therapeutic change: universality, altruism, instillation of hope, imparting information, corrective recapitulation of family experience, development of socializing techniques, imitative behavior, cohesion, existential factors, catharsis, interpersonal learning by input and output, and self-understanding (cf. Corsini & Rosenberg, 1955; Greene, Barlow, & Kaklauskas, 2020; Yalom & Leszcz, 2020).

In recent years, there have been empirical attempts to consolidate this listing and thus make it more useful as a guide for therapist interventions. Kivlighan and Holmes (2004), for example, developed a typology of four kinds of therapeutic groups based on clusters of salient therapeutic factors as perceived by group members: affective-insight groups (exemplified by psychodynamic therapy groups), affective support groups (such as trauma support groups), cognitive support groups (like 12-step support groups), and cognitive insight groups (such as cognitive behavioral therapy groups). Clinically this study underscores the importance of the therapist's exploring what processes the group members consider to be most therapeutically useful in their groups. Other recent attempts to detect higher-order dimensions within the list of therapeutic factors are based on studies with the TFI (Joyce et al., 2011; MacNair-Semands et al., 2010; Tasca et al., 2016), which are described below. Greene, Barlow, and Kasklauskas (2020) have reviewed specific concepts of therapeutic factors derived from attachment theory (e.g., empathic attunement, mentalization), interpersonal theory (e.g., creating corrective emotional experiences), and cognitive behavioral perspectives (e.g., group-based learning) that can help to clarify the question about what works in different small group treatments.

Sociocultural Dynamics: Culture and Diversity in Group Process

One additional important consideration related to group process that has received overdue attention in recent years is the role of culture and cultural differences in the group. Group members bring with them their diverse backgrounds, including their racial, ethnic, gender, sexual orientation, disability, national, and religious identifications among other dimensions of difference. From this perspective, all groups can be considered "multicultural" (Chen et al., 2003; Cone-Uemura & Bentley, 2018). Viewed as social microcosms, then, they have the potential to replicate oppressive societal dynamics (e.g., racism, classism, sexism) but also to provide corrective, affirming, and socially just experiences. To provide the latter, group psychotherapists must: 1) be aware of historical (and current) institutional bias in the field and its impact on the theory and practice of group psychotherapy; 2) examine their own identities, biases, and experiences with privilege and oppression and how they impact their group practice; 3) work toward developing multicultural competencies; and 4) cultivate a multicultural orientation (Cone-Uemura & Bentley, 2018; Kaklauskas & Nettles, 2020) in their clinical work. To be sure, developing multicultural competencies and a multicultural orientation are lifelong pursuits (see Cone-Uemura & Bentley, 2018; Kaklauskas & Nettles 2020 for more comprehensive discussions of cultural issues). Here we focus primarily on cultural issues as a part of group process, specifically the enactment of microaggressions and the fostering of a group multicultural orientation, both of which are discussed next.

Cultural Ruptures: Microaggressions in Group Psychotherapy

Recently, there has been growing attention to *cultural ruptures* in group psychotherapy, specifically the enactment of *microaggressions* (Belcher Platt, 2017; Cone-Uemura & Bentley, 2018; Kivlighan et al., 2021; Lefforge et al., 2020; Miles et al., 2021). Sue and Spanierman (2020) defined microaggressions as "verbal and nonverbal interpersonal exchanges in which a perpetrator causes harm to a target, whether intended or unintended" (p. 8). They went on to say that "these brief and commonplace indignities communicate hostile, derogatory, and/or negative slights to the target" (p. 8). Kivlighan and colleagues (2021) found that microaggressions are common in group psychotherapy, with 72 percent of their sample of racial and ethnic minority participants reporting having experienced at least one racial microaggression. Sue (2015) noted that the occurrence of a microaggression often provides an opening for dialogue, but that difficult dialogues about issues like race and racism are often avoided because they violate societal protocols related to politeness (because they may make people uncomfortable) and color-blind ideology (because they acknowledge racial differences and racism; Neville et al., 2013). The Racial Microaggressions in Counseling Scale (Constantine, 2007) is one tool for assessing the occurrence of microaggressions. This ten-item measure has been adapted for use in group psychotherapy (Kivlighan et al., 2021). The adapted instructions read "How often did each of the following situations occur?" and "If these situations occurred, how much did they bother you?" Example items include: "The group sometimes was insensitive about my cultural group when trying to understand or help with my concerns or issues" and "The group sometimes seemed unaware of the realities of race and racism."

Cone-Uemura and Bentley (2018) noted that the occurrence of a microaggression in group offers "a rich opportunity for deeper growth and connection" (p. 23), if it is addressed directly and appropriately by the group leader. They noted that group leader intervention will likely vary based on the type of group. The first step, regardless of type of group, however, is recognizing when a microaggression has occurred (Lefforge et al., 2020). Lefforge and colleagues described a training they developed to help group psychotherapists be able to recognize microaggressions and to build the abilities and willingness to intervene appropriately. Miles and colleagues (2021) also discussed strategies for addressing microaggressions in groups, including suggestions for proactively preparing the group for difficult dialogues related to cultural ruptures and adapting bystander intervention strategies developed by microaggressions researchers (Sue et al., 2019).

Fostering a Multicultural Group Orientation

The multicultural orientation, as originally conceived, is characterized by a therapist's 1) cultural humility (i.e., having a stance of openness and non-defensiveness in the face of cultural difference; Hook et al., 2013); 2) taking or missing opportunities to explore cultural issues as they arise in sessions; and 3) comfort with addressing these cultural issues (Owen, 2013). The multicultural orientation (MCO) framework compliments the traditional notion of multicultural competencies (i.e., knowledge, skills, and attitudes/awareness; Sue et al., 1992) by proposing a "way of being" (Owen et al., 2011, p. 274) with clients. In the therapy group, the task of intervening when a microaggression occurs does not fall on the group leader alone (a group leader might, in fact, be the one to commit the microaggression but also could be the target). Kivlighan and Chapman (2018) suggested that it is important to help foster a *group multicultural orientation*. Kivlighan and colleagues (2019) have extended the notion of the therapist's MCO by assessing how group therapy members experience the group-as-a-whole in terms of the dimensions of humility, taken or missed opportunities to explore cultural issues in the group and comfort with this exploration. These researchers report the development of a measure of a group's multicultural orientation, the Multi-cultural Orientation Inventory-Group Version, which asks participants to rate their group's level of comfort and their style (e.g., open versus closed to discussing cultural issues). For example, participants rate their agreement with the statements: "The other group members discussed my cultural background in a way that worked for me" and "The other group members avoided topics related to my cultural background." The MCO-G is discussed further with the other group process measures below. As a final note to consider regarding multicultural processes in group psychotherapy, broadly, we note that some psychologists have recently encouraged an expansion of the way in which issues related to culture and oppression are discussed. Specifically, Grzanka and colleagues (2019) proposed a centering of anti-oppressive work in our interventions, including helping clients from privileged social identity backgrounds to engage in difficult introspection and dialogues about their own racial and other cultural attitudes and behaviors and not reserving cultural work for min-oritized clients. We believe this holds for group psychotherapy, too.

Once again returning to our case example, in the fifth session, one of the two group members who are People of Color was talking about an experience of racism at his work-place. In response, a White group member unwittingly committed a racial microaggression by saying to that group member that he did not deserve that treatment at work because he is "so articulate." Because the group leaders had been regularly assessing the group multi-cultural orientation using the MCO-G, Stacy felt the group members perceived the group as having high levels of cultural humility and comfort exploring cultural issues and thus, she encouraged the group members in processing the microaggression and the impacts on the members of color and the group-as-a-whole.

The Relationship of Process to Outcome

Authors have long argued for the need to bridge group psychotherapy research and prac-tice (e.g., Lau et al., 2010; Lo Coco et al., 2015; Miles & Paquin, 2014; Ogrodniczuk et al., 2010) and the assessment of group process is one important means for building this bridge. Above, we discussed reasons why it is useful for practitioners to know about group dynamics and collect process data. The ongoing exploration, both through clinical observation and formal assessment, of what is happening in the group—its process—is aimed primarily at evaluating whether the group is "on task," that is, whether it is moving toward achieving its goals. Simply stated, group process, in addition to being linked to social structure, is also directly linked to outcome. A group whose processes reflect therapeutic values will likely lead to positive therapeutic outcomes whereas a group engaged in antitherapeutic or defensive dynamics will likely have less than optimal outcomes. The measures of process that have received the greatest scientific study in terms of its relationship to outcome are discussed in the following section.

Therapeutic Factors

The empirical literature on the relationship of therapeutic factors to treatment outcomes has been described as "mixed" in a review by Burlingame et al. (2004), especially since the results are very heterogeneous with regard to samples, types of groups, instruments, and research questions (Joyce et al., 2011; Tasca et al., 2016). The Burlingame et al. (2004) review concluded that the "advent of instruments and advanced methodology are a harbinger force for a better understanding of mechanisms of change" (p. 676). Perhaps the most promising of the instruments to date designed to capture Yalom's therapeutic factors is the development and ongoing refinement of the Therapeutic Factors Inventory. The work began (Lese & MacNair-Semands, 2000) with the construction of a 99-item inventory designed to capture group members' experiences of Yalom's 11 therapeutic factors in their groups. Since then, efforts have aimed at uncovering higher-order constructs that capture the essence of these factors and that reduce the number of items to be rated, particularly the Therapeutic Factors Inventory-Short form (TFI-S; MacNair-Semands et al., 2010) and the TFI-19 (Joyce et al., 2011), two measures that reflect four underlying dimensions that account for much of the variance in Yalom's original factors: social learning. secure emotional expression, installation of hope, and awareness of relational impact. An even shorter, 8-item version of this measure, the TFI-8, has recently been developed to provide an easy to administer measure that captures the essence of Yalom's therapeutic factors along one dimension which the authors describe as "feeling hopeful about the processes of emotional expression and relational awareness, which then translate into and promote social learning" (Tasca et al., 2016).

Cohesion

Arguably, the single group process construct that has received the greatest scientific attention is cohesion. While a number of conceptual and methodological issues plague this literature, particularly the inconsistent and varying definitions of cohesion and the correlational (as opposed to causal) nature of the findings, the most recent meta-analysis (Burlingame et al., 2018) entailing 55 studies and more than 6,000 group members yields a significant weighted average positive correlation between cohesion and outcome: $r = .26$ (95% CI $= .20, .31$), a moderate effect ($d = .56$) with high heterogeneity (79.3%). Among the variables that were found to moderate the size of this association was group orientation: Higher cohesion-outcome correlations were produced by interpersonally oriented groups ($r = .48$), followed by psychodynamic ($r = .27$) and CBT ($r = .22$) as well as supportive and eclectic approaches (both $r = .22$). Dose also produced a statistically significant pattern: groups with 20 or more sessions posted the highest relationship ($r = .41$), followed by those with 13–19 sessions ($r = .27$) and 12 or fewer sessions ($r = .21$). These findings, consistent with clinical wisdom, underscore the practical importance of monitoring cohesion in group therapy on a regular basis.

Member-leader Alliance

The concept of working alliance or therapeutic alliance derives from the individual psychotherapy literature and reflects the nature of the emotional bond between patient and therapist. This concept has been seen as relevant to the group therapy, although the nature of the emotional bonds of each member to other individual members and to the group-as-a-whole are also relevant relationship constructs. The relationship between member-leader alliance and outcome of group therapy was summarized in a recent meta-analysis (Alldredge et al., 2021). The 29 studies in this meta-analysis included 3,628 patients and yielded a significant weighted average correlation between alliance and outcome of $r = .17$, which was significantly lower compared to the correlation observed in individual treatment ($r = .28$). The authors suggested a possible explanation for this is the fact that the relationship between a patient and therapist is only one of several relational components in the therapy group while it makes up the entirety of the therapeutic relationship in individual therapy. Some moderators observed as a basis of the heterogeneity of study results were treatment orientation (lower correlation in CBT than other group treatments) and the reporting perspective (higher correlation for patient reported than mixed or observer reported alliance). It is important to differentiate (member-leader) alliance as one aspect of the therapeutic relationship in groups and group cohesion as a more group-related relationship construct. Both factors will have a different importance depending on the goal of the group and the amount of leader activity.

Anti-Therapeutic Processes, Attendance, and Dropout

In addition to the core positive group processes of therapeutic factors, cohesion, and alliance, groups also experience and enact processes that have the potential to disrupt the group, challenge the leader and members, and adversely impact outcomes (Greene & Kaklauskas, 2020a). Greene and Kaklauskas (2020a) suggest it is "the challenge of the group therapist to 'harness' these potentially disruptive forces in the service of the work of the group" (p. 71). Some of the more familiar of these processes include the emerging of dysfunctional subgrouping and deviant roles, and scapegoating dynamics. Clearly some of these processes involve one member or a subset of group individuals, which has implications for the assessment and interpretation of group process data. For example, a group deviant can be understood as someone who "does not fit into a group" in a way that "interferes with the group task" (Yalom & Leszcz, 2020, p. 305). This person may be an outcast in terms of behavior and/or experience of the group and, therefore, an outlier in the group process data. As Gold and Kivlighan (2018) illustrate, divergences in group process data profiles or patterns between an individual member and the rest of the group may signal a scapegoating or polarizing process and thus can alert the therapist of the need to harness this kind of disruptive process before further deterioration occurs.

Practical Issues

The primary consideration in administering process measures is how to do it in a way that promotes rather than interferes with the clinical work of the group (Miller et al., 2015; Solstad et al., 2019; Solstad, Kleiven, Castonguay, & Moltu et al., 2021; Solstad, Kleiven, & Moltu, 2021). As these recent reports reveal, the group therapist needs to explore patients' interest in and commitment to completing the measures. They suggest that resistances and suspicions about the use of the data from these measures can be addressed, in part, by providing a clear rationale for their use and by providing feedback about the findings that the patients can receive without defensiveness. Frequency of administration, the number and kinds of measures to administer, and the timing needed to complete them must all be carefully considered to avoid fatigue, to ensure that there is adequate time for the here-and-now clinical work, and to have the measures be experienced as relevant to the clinical work.

Recent works (Burlingame, Alldredge et al., 2021; Gleave et al., 2017; Gold & Kivlighan, 2018; Griner et al., 2018; Whitcomb, Woodland et al., 2018; Yalom & Leszcz, 2020) reveal that there is no one prescribed way for choosing and administering measures, analyzing the data and providing feedback. Each therapist, as manager of the unique social system being conducted, needs to assess the how, what, and when of process measure implementation and feedback to optimize their utility and minimize adverse reactions. One approach, following Yalom and Leszcz (2020), is for the therapist to start each session with a report and review of the salient processes in the previous session, as gleaned from measurement data. However, there are many alternative ideas in the literature regarding the choice of instruments, the timing of administration, and how feedback is offered to the members. As detailed in Chapter 1, regardless of the specific administrative procedures employed, the very decision to use these kinds of tools defines measurement-based care and, as such, can serve to correct, adjust, and refocus the trajectory of the group to ultimately optimize treatment outcome (cf. Lewis et al., 2019).

With regard to data analysis, a group therapist might examine individual group members' responses to the GCQ to see if all of the group members are experiencing the emotional climate within and across sessions in about the same way or if there is an outlier or divergent subgroup that reports a substantially different experience. Therapists might also look at data from the group-as-a-whole to examine patterns of group climate development (e.g., is engagement increasing over time? Is the group stuck in some ongoing conflict?) or compare patterns of climate development across groups that they lead to get a sense of when a group may be exhibiting an unexpected pattern. In general, we suggest examining process data and providing feedback that highlight **several kinds of patterns**:

1   Significant divergences between an individual member and the rest of the group or some established norm that reveal 'outlier' status of that individual. Here the therapist explores what is contributing to the deviant member's experience, for example, scapegoating.
2   Changes, either deterioration or improvement, of a patient's scores over time. With these data, the therapist can assess whether the individual patient is improving or deteriorating on important process dimensions such as Engagement.
3   Divergences or "splits" in a member's relationship to two different structural components of the group, such as other members and the leader. By comparing a member's relationship to different structural components of the group, the therapist can explore whether some defensive processes, such as splitting or devaluing, are being used by a patient.
4   A general consensus in the responses of all of the members suggesting cohesion or distinct patterns in various subgroups suggesting splitting processes. Here the therapist assesses the degree of harmony in the group-as-a-whole or whether subgrouping is occurring.
5   Comparison of the present group to other groups run by the therapist or to established norms. The therapist explores this comparison to assess whether the group-as-a-whole is on track.

Cultural Issues Related to Group Process Measures

The field of group psychotherapy has been heavily influenced by "Judeo-Christian, White-European, heterocentric, gender binary, and patriarchal traditions of the Western world" (Kaklauskas & Nettles, 2020, p. 25). As a result, it is influenced by the biases of these perspectives, like any domain of psychology or science. This is also true when it comes to assessment, so it is important for group therapists to attend to cultural issues in the administration of group process measures.

For example, Mio and colleagues (2020) discuss how assessment in psychology often uses a "White [European] standard" to which all individuals are compared, regardless of race or ethnicity. The impact of this is the potential pathologizing of individuals who do not meet this White standard, when the difference observed actually reflects cultural difference, not pathology. This means therapists need to be aware of cultural differences in worldviews and communication styles and how they may impact clients' behaviors in group, including receptivity to and responses on self-report process measures. Given historical mistreatment and exploitation (e.g., the infamous Tuskegee study in the US), those from marginalized groups may have a warranted mistrust when it comes to participating in treatment and providing data to healthcare providers (Mio et al., 2020). Consequently, group therapists need to be transparent in how they use the process data they collect and to seek to engage members in the process with fully informed consent, especially in contexts that do not have client privacy protections.

A final consideration relates to the language of assessment instruments. Fortunately, some of the most commonly used process measures have been translated and validated into multiple languages. For example, the TFI-19 has been translated into Italian (Landi et al., 2020), Czech (Dubovska et al., 2019), German (Mander et al., 2016), Japanese (Kageyama et al., 2016), and other languages, and has been used around the globe. Group therapists need to take care to note that translated versions of measures reflect various forms of equivalence in variables, including functional, conceptual, and linguistic equivalence (Mio et al., 2020). Linguistic equivalence is the form of equivalence that deals with the actual translation, and it is recommended that back translation (the process of translating a measure into the new language and then translating it back to ensure it retains its intended meaning) is used (Mio et al., 2020).

Evidence-based Practice versus Formal Process Research

The focus of this volume relates to *evidence-based practice* or *measurement-based care*, using validated measures to track treatment process and progress and demonstrate outcome in a particular group of interest. In a sense, the group psychotherapist using such an approach is a "local clinical scientist" employing a conceptual framework about therapeutic change and helping the members' appreciate and explore how process in the group can serve or interfere with therapeutic progress. The focus on collecting process data in one's group is aimed at exploring what is going on at a particular time and in a particular group and comparing the present data to data collected at other times in the group or to other groups or norms. Looking at the patterns that can be gleaned in the data, within individual members, subgroups and the group-as-a-whole over time, can vitally help the therapist better comprehend the trajectories of the individual members and the entire group and help formulate timely and well-aimed interventions.

There is, of course, a second major use of process measures, namely in formal research designed to discover more universal cause-and-effect truths about what happens, not in a particular group, but in groups in general, in the service of theory-building. Tasca (2016) points out that meaningful process research requires sophisticated statistical methods to reflect the actuality and complexity of group life. In particular, the nested nature of group data (i.e., sessions are "nested" within members who are nested within groups) means that these data are "non-independent" and need to be handled differently than individual-level data to avoid the risk of errors in data analysis, especially obtaining a significant effect when none actually exists (Baldwin et al., 2005; Janis et al., 2016). For researchers, this means using multi-level or hierarchical linear modeling approaches to handle the non-independence in the data (Lo Coco et al., 2015). In addition to more complex statistical handling of the data, formal research is likely to rely not just on paper-and-pencil self-report measures, as typically used in clinical contexts, but also rater observations of process (e.g., Tasca et al., 2011). While a thorough description of current trends is beyond our scope, we refer readers interested in more depth to recent reviews of this research literature (Tasca, 2016, 2021). The average practitioner may or may not have interest or resources for conducting some of the complex data analytic techniques but an awareness of these techniques can help practitioners think about the myriad ways that group process data can be analyzed (Heppner et al., 2016). Awareness of these techniques might also inspire practitioner-researcher collaborations to answer more complex questions that benefit both the practical and scientific understanding of group process.

Group Process Measures

Recently, Orfanos and colleagues (2020) systematically summarized different self-report measures for the assessment of therapeutic group process. The review resulted in a total of 13 different group process measures. The authors discriminated six therapeutic group process measures:

1   Three versions of the TFI (TFI-19, Joyce et al., 2011; TFI, Lese & MacNair-Semands, 2000; TFI-S, MacNair-Semands et al., 2010)
2   The Group Cohesiveness scale (Wongpakaran et al., 2013)
3   The Group Cohesion scale (Treadwell et al., 2001)
4   The Group Attitudes Scale (Evans & Jarvis, 1986)
5   The Curative Climate Instrument (Fuhriman et al., 1986)
6   The Scale for the Evaluation of Group Counseling (Murillo et al., 1981)

and seven measures more broadly covering overall group process:

1   The Group Observational Measurement of Engagement (Cohen-Mansfield et al., 2017)
2   The Factors Aspecific and Specific in Group Therapy (Marogna & Caccamo, 2014)
3   The Social Exchange Scale (Brown et al., 2014)
4   The Ferrara Group Experiences Scale (Caruso et al., 2013)
5   The Group Questionnaire (Krogel et al., 2013)
6   The Group Sessions Rating Scale (Quirk et al., 2013)
7   The GCQ (two versions, Mackenzie 1981; 1983)

Using a variety of mainly psychometric criteria (e.g., content validity, internal consistency, construct validity), Orfanos and colleagues (2020) classified the Group Cohesiveness Scale as one of the best therapeutic group process measures (followed by two short versions of the TFI: TFI-19 and TFI-S). Among the overall group process measures, the GQ and the Group Sessions Rating Scale (GSRS) revealed the highest scores in the classification system.

Our own evaluation of the extant measures gives weight to those instruments that not only have received considerable validation but reflect higher order, clinically robust, and multiple dimensions of group process that are likely to be more comprehensive and encompassing regarding therapeutic group process than single dimension measures, such as measures of group cohesion.

While we believe there are benefits to using multidimensional measures of process such as those detailed above, we also acknowledge that some clinicians may have a particular theoretical or clinical interest in tapping single dimensional aspects of group process (cf.

Hornsey et al., 2012; Woodland et al., 2022). Clearly, the most numerous and popular of these measures are those that tap cohesion. The Orfonos et al. (2020) review identifies two of them (Treadwell et al., 2001; Wongpakaran et al. 2013) while others continue to appear in the literature (e.g., Hornsey et al., 2012; Woodland et al., 2022). While such measures can be useful in assessing a process domain of particular interest for the therapist, they do leave open a number of conceptual and empirical questions, primarily whether the extant measures are indeed assessing the same theoretical construct. Greene (2017) has suggested three approaches to address this question: 1) analyzing whether cohesion can be deconstructed into narrower constituent components, as Hornsey et al. (2009) recommend; 2) systematically exploring the empirical overlap and unique contributions of the measures; and 3) embedding the cohesion construct into more abstract and higher order concepts, as exemplified by the development of the GQ and short forms of the TFI.

The Group Questionnaire

The ongoing development of Group Questionnaire (GQ) is a prime example of research efforts designed to discover higher order dimensions of group process and hence bring greater conceptual and empirical clarity regarding therapeutic relationships in groups (cf. Burlingame et al., 2004). The pioneering study by Johnson et al. (2005) explored the conceptual and empirical overlap of four commonly used measures of cohesion, climate, working alliance and empathy measures by having 662 members of 111 counseling center and personal growth groups complete a copy of each. The researchers report a two-dimensional model that captures the associations among these four measures with the *quality* of relationship defined by three broad factors: 1) *positive bond* (e.g., "I felt that I could trust the group leaders during today's session"); 2) *positive work* (e.g., "The other group members and I agree on what is important to work on"); and 3) *negative relationship* (e.g., "There was friction and anger between the members"); and the *structure* of relationship defined by two commonly accepted facets: *member-to-member* and *member-to-leader*. Bormann and Strauss (2007) replicated and extended the Johnson et al. model. They found the same three factors of the quality dimension but a third structural factor: member-to-group (in addition to member-to-leader and member-to member). Several additional studies across distinct group orientations (personal growth, counseling center, outpatient analytic and inpatient psychodynamic) and countries have now been conducted which provide further validation and refinement of this instrument (Bakali et al., 2009; Janis et al., 2018; Krogel, 2008; Krogel et al., 2013; Bormann et al. 2011; Thayer & Burlingame, 2014) Table 3.1 contains the source, description, properties, and administration considerations for the GQ, along with sample references.

Recent papers (Burlingame, Alldredge et al., 2021; Griner et al., 2018) demonstrate how the GQ can be used in clinical practice to detect deterioration effects and alliance ruptures in group therapy and help the therapist formulate interventions that aim to improve therapeutic relationships. In sum, the GQ offers a clinically and theoretically useful measure of the quality of relationships in the group and, as Thayer and Burlingame (2014) remind us, "group relationships that both support and challenge group members have been consistently linked to positive treatment outcome and low dropout rates (p. 319).

Group Climate Questionnaire

Though it is incorporated into the GQ a separate discussion of the Group Climate Questionnaire (GCQ), developed by K. Roy MacKenzie (1983), warranted, as it is arguably the most used process measure in research and practice (c.f. Bakali et al., 2013). The GCQ is a

Table 3.1 Group Questionnaire

Item	Information
Name of Instrument	Group Questionnaire (GQ)
Authors	Krogel et al. (2013); Janis et al. (2018)
Source	Krogel, J., Burlingame, G. B., Chapman, C., Renshaw, T., Gleave, R., Beecher, M., MacNair-Semands, R. (2013). The group questionnaire: A clinical and empirically derived measure of group relationship. *Psychotherapy Research, 23*(3), 344–354.
Brief Description	The GQ was developed based upon an empirical study demonstrating the conceptual and empirical overlap of four commonly used relationship constructs in group research: cohesion, climate, working alliance and empathy (Johnson et al., 2005). Using data obtained with common measures of these constructs, several studies with different samples and from different countries derived a 2-dimensional model with the *quality* of relationship defined by three factors (*positive bond, positive working and negative relationship*), and the *structure* of relationship defined by two commonly accepted facets *(member-to-member and member-to-leader)*. Accordingly, the 30 items of the GQ are based on the three-factor model of the therapeutic relationship within groups. All three factors comprise first-order factors reflecting the level of the relationship, i.e., member-leader, member-member, and two factors for the member-group relationship. The GQ comprises 30 items describing personal relationship experiences in "your therapy group" using a 7-point Likert scale ranging from 1 (*not true*) to 7 (*all to very true*).
Time Issues	10–15 minutes
Subscales and Scoring	The GQ measures three domains: • *Positive Bonding* is defined as the sense of belonging or attraction that a member has to the group, its members, and its leader(s) that creates a positive atmosphere which allows members to feel genuinely understood and appreciated. • *Positive Working* is defined as the ability of the group to agree upon and work toward treatment goals in an effective manner. • *Negative Relationship* is defined as lack of trust, genuineness, and understanding as well as friction and distance that might exist between the group, its members, or its leaders. Additional substructure: Member-Member-Relationship (Cohesion, tasks/goals, empathic failure), Member-Leader-Relationship (Alliance, tasks/goals, alliance rupture), Member-Group-Relationship (Climate, conflict).
Psychometric Properties	Internal consistency was determined in different samples with alpha coefficients ranging between .87 and .91 for the bonding, .90 and .95 for the working subscale and .71 and .86 for the negative relationship scale (lower alpha scores of this scale were due to a restriction of range in two subsamples)
Norms and any normative data re: diversity for each instrument	No norms re. diversity so far, statistical data from different countries
Translations	English, Spanish, French, German, Italian, Norwegian and Polish
Sensitivity to Change	Has been demonstrated where the GQ was used as a continuously administered instrument in feedback studies (cf. Chapter x)
Sample references	Janis et al., 2018
Website Resources	US version: OQ measures www.oqmeasures.com

Item	Information
How to Obtain/Cost	English version: OQ measures L.L.C.; other language versions: Authors Cost: All OQ group measures – the OQ®-GQ, OQ®-GRQ and GCQ – are bundled together for the price of one instrument, and pricing for use of these bundled group measures depends on the type of license needed. Contact sales@oqmeasures.com to request a quote.
Administration Types	Originally pencil and paper; can be used via App, Web, Tablet
Analytics	Yes, GQ was used in feedback studies based upon reliable change indices and alerts.
Benchmarking	Comparative samples available: counseling center clients (US), inpatients (European), outpatients with personality disorders (Norway), SMI inpatient (US), non-clinical (US): total ~3000 individuals; Norms probably needed for different populations (Janis et al., 2018)

12-item self-report measure (described in Table 3.2) assessing group members' perceptions of the group climate or emotional tone of the group, assessed along three robust domains of the social-emotional quality of the relationships in the group. The Engagement scale (e.g., "The members liked and cared about each other") reflects cohesion and willingness of the members to be a part of the group, Avoidance (e.g., "The members avoided looking at important issues going on between themselves") taps a reluctance or resistance to take responsibility for using the group as an instrument for change or to explore what is going on in the here-and-now and Conflict (e.g., "There was friction and anger between the members") assesses the experience of the group as conflictual, aggressive, and distrustful. MacKenzie's instrument is closely linked to his four-stage model of group development (MacKenzie, 1997) of engagement, differentiation, interpersonal work, and termination.

The GCQ-S has been used across a wide range of groups and has reached popularity based on good psychometric properties, ease of use, the clinical meaningfulness of the three relatively independent scales (cf. Burlingame et al., 2006), and its significant association to outcome in group therapy (cf. Janis et al., 2018). Returning to our case example, when she was explaining her rationale and procedures for administering group process measures, Stacy explains to Mike that if she wants to collect group process data but is worried about the time burden on her group members, she will often just administer the GCQ-S to get a "quick pulse" of the emotional climate of the group because it is relatively brief but useful.

Therapeutic Factors Inventory

The development of comprehensive systems of therapeutic factors has a long history (Bloch et al., 1981; Bloch et al., 1979; Corsini, & Rosenberg, 1955; Yalom & Leszcz, 2020). The original Therapeutic Factors Inventory (TFI), a 99-item self-report measure, was an initial attempt to systematically assess all these factors as perceived by group members (Lese & MacNair-Semands, 2000). Like the research done with the GQ, important subsequent research on the TFI has aimed at developing shorter versions, not only for increasing ease of use, but also identifying higher order factors associated with the eleven therapeutic factors. The TFI-19 in particular is a short version (designed by including the highest factor loading items on each therapeutic factor from the original TFI in a series of factor analytic studies) identifying and tapping *four broad therapeutic factors*: Instillation of Hope (e.g., "Things seem more hopeful since joining group"), Secure Emotional Expression (e.g., " I get to vent my feelings in group"), Awareness of Interpersonal Impact (e.g., "By getting honest

Table 3.2 Group Climate Questionnaire

Item	Information
Name of Instrument	Group Climate Questionnaire (GCQ-S)
Authors	Original version: K. Roy MacKenzie (1983). The clinical application of a group climate measure. In: R. R. Dies & K. R. MacKenzie (Eds) *Advances in group psychotherapy* (pp. 159–179). Int. Univ. Press.
Source	www.oqmeasures.com/gcq-sgcq-s
Brief Description	The GCQ-S consists of 12 items (of originally 32 items) forming three factor-analytically derived subscales used to describe the group atmosphere: Engagement describes the positive working group atmosphere. Conflict reflects tension and anger in the group. Avoidance describes the behavior indicating avoidance of personal responsibility of group work by the members. Items are related on a 7-point Likert scale ranging from 0 (*not at all*) to 6 (*extremely*)
Time Issues	Usually, it does not take more than 5 minutes to complete the GCQ-S.
Subscales and Scoring	Scales scores are determined by calculating the mean of the relevant items. If a scale has missing items, then divide by the number of items actually rated. If the overall GCQ-S has more than 4 items missing, then the test should be considered invalid. Round the mean for each scale to the nearest integer. Scale 1: Engaged Items $(1 + 2 + 4 + 8 + 11)/ 5$ This describes the positive working group atmosphere. Scale 2: Conflict Items $(6 + 7+ 10 + 12)/ 4$ This reflects anger and tension in the group. Scale 3: Avoiding Items $(3 + 5 + 9)/ 3$ This describes the avoidance of constructive involvement and responsibility in the group.
Psychometric Properties	Several studies tried to replicate the factor structure of the GCQ-S with similar results. One item (12) describing tension and anxiety sometimes has been shown to load on the avoidance factor. Coefficient alphas for the subscales are normally ranged between .88 and .94 (e.g., Kivlighan & Goldfine, 1991), but sometimes lower (e.g., Johnson et al., 2006: .40 to .75). The avoidance factor seemed to be the "weakest" in some studies (e.g., Bonsaksen et al., 2013; Bakhali et al., 2013) Construct validity has been shown in numerous studies linking GCQ scores with outcome and process variables in group treatments.
Norms and any normative data re: diversity for each instrument	N/A
Translations	English, Farsi, German, Italian, Norwegian, Portuguese, and Spanish
Sensitivity to Change	The GCQ-S has been used in several longitudinal studies (cf. below), there are some doubts related to its use as a process measure, owing to its shortness and the fact that the factor structure was not always completely supported (Johnson, 2013).
Sample references	Bakali et al., 2013; Bonsaksen et al., 2013; Kivlighan & Kivlighan, 2013
Website Resources	OQ-Family (cf. source) Can also be obtained at no cost by downloading from: https://www.routledge.com/Core-Principles-of-Group-Psychotherapy-An-Integrated-Theory-Research/Kaklauskas-Greene/p/book/9780367203092 (using the button entitled Support Materials and choosing the folder entitled Process 1–4). GCQ-S: Process #2.
How to Obtain/Cost	Since the items of the GCQ have been published several times (e.g., Burlingame et al., 2006), the instrument is generally available and ready to use.

Item	Information
Administration Types	Originally conceptualized as a pencil and paper instrument, the GCQ can also be administered via app, tablet or internet.
Analytics	No
Benchmarking	Except the OQ-family database, there are no official norms of the GCQ. On the other hand, in view of its wide use, a researcher will find GCQ reference scores related to many clinical and non-clinical, though rather small samples.

feedback from members and facilitators, I've learned a lot about my impact on other people"), and Social Learning (e.g., "Group has shown me the importance of other people in my life" (Joyce et al., 2011). These four subscales tap important therapeutic processes that, when regularly assessed, can enhance the awareness of the group leader about what is happening in the group and with individual members. In a more recent study, Tasca and colleagues (2016) further reduced the number of items on the TFI to an 8-item version, with items selected to represent each of the four factors of the TFI-19. The authors classified the TFI-8 as a brief, reliable, and valid measure of a single *higher-order group therapeutic factor*, which they conceptualize as a feeling of hopefulness about experiencing the processes of emotional expression and relational awareness in the group, which then promotes social learning.

The TFI studies have also shown significant relationships to several dimensions of outcome, including improvement in symptoms, quality of life experiences, and interpersonal distress. Though the TFI-8 has also been used in empirical studies and translated into Italian (Landi et al., 2020), we provide the source, description, properties, and administration considerations for the TFI-19 (see Table 3.3) because it may be most accessible, globally given that it also exists in several other languages (e.g., Czech, Dubovska et al., 2019; Japanese, Kageyama et al., 2016; and German, Mander et al., 2016). Table 3.3 contains the source, description, properties, and administration considerations for the TFI-19 and TFI-S, along with sample references.

Table 3.3 Therapeutic Factors Inventory – 19 and Short Form

Item	Information
Name of Instrument	Therapeutic Factors Inventory (TFI-19) and (TFI-S) Short Form
Authors	Original Version: Lese, K. P. & MacNair-Semands, R. R. (2000)
Source	TFI-S: MacNair-Semands et al. (2010) and TFI-19: Joyce et al. (2011)
Brief Description	The TFI-S was developed on the bases of an original Therapeutic Factors Inventory using Yalom´s (2005) descriptions finally comprising 99 items forming 11 subscales. The first TFI-S version was a 44-item self-report measure representing 11 therapeutic factors, i.e., instillation of hope, universality, imparting information, altruism, corrective recapitulation of the primary family group, development of socializing techniques, imitative behavior, interpersonal learning, group cohesiveness, catharsis, and existential learning. Items are rated using a 7-point Likert scale ranging from 1 (*strongly disagree*) to 7 (*strongly agree*). In a factor analysis (MacNair-Semands et al., 2010) 4 subscales were derived with the following denominations: • Instillation of hope • Secure emotional expression • Awareness of interpersonal impact • Social learning. The 4 subscales have been replicated in a study by Joyce et al. (2011) who further reduced the questionnaire to 23 items from which 19 are used to form the four subscales.

Item	Information
Time Issues	It takes between 10 and 15 minutes to complete the TFI-S, a recently developed 8-item version (combining items from the 4 subscales; cf. Tasca et al., 2016) needs a maximum of 5 minutes to be completed.
Subscales and Scoring	Instillation of hope (Items 2, 6, 10, 14, 17) Secure emotional expression (Items 3, 7, 11, 15, 18, 21, 23) Awareness of interpersonal impact (Items 4, 8, 12, 16, 19, 22) Social learning (Items 1, 5, 9, 13). Details of the scoring are shown in the appendix of Joyce et al.'s (2011) publication.
Psychometric Properties	Joyce et al. (2011) reported the most recent internal consistency coefficients ranging between alpha =.66 (social learning) and alpha =.90 (instillation of hope). The same authors support the instrument's good sensitivity to change, its discriminant (scale scores largely independent of social desirability and initial disturbance), convergent (correlations with GCQ-S scales) and predictive validity (related to post treatment outcome).
Norms and any normative data re: diversity for each instrument	Norms are available but no norms re. diversity so far; statistical data exists from different countries
Translations	German, Japanese, Czech, Brazilian Portuguese, Spanish, Danish and other language versions: Contact Authors. It has also been used in Australia, the UK, Canada, England, Ireland, and Switzerland.
Sensitivity to Change	See above
Sample references	The TFI has been used in samples of distinct therapy groups
Website Resources	Can be obtained at no cost by downloading from: www.routledge.com/Core-Principles-of-Group-Psychotherapy-An-Integrated-Theory-Research/Kaklauskas-Greene/p/book/9780367203092 (using the button entitled Support Materials and choosing the folder entitled Process 1–4). TFI-19: Process #3; TFI-8: Process #4. Also found in https://doi.org/10.1037/a0024677
How to Obtain/Cost	The recent TFI-S is available in the article of Joyce et al. (2011) including a description of its scoring at no cost.
Administration Types	Originally conceptualized as a pencil and paper instrument, the TFI-S can also be administered via app, tablet or internet
Analytics	N/A
Benchmarking	N/A

Group Session Rating Scale

A more recent development among the process measures is the Group Session Rating Scale (GSRS) (see Table 3.4 for a description), an "ultra-brief alliance measure" (Quirk et al., 2012; p. 195) for group treatment. The GSRS comprises four items derived from the Session Rating Scale (SRS; Duncan et al., 2003) using bipolar visual analogue scales to assess: the *relationship* ("Feeling understood, accepted and respected by the leader and the group"), the *goals and topics* of the group work ("Working and talking about what I wanted to work on"), the acceptability of the *approach or method* ("Feeling that the leader and group's approach is a good fit for me") and a rating of the *overall* fit of the group for the individual member ("Felt like a part of the group"). A therapist may choose this very brief measure to help gain perspective on foundational group processes, in addition to using measures like the TFI to assess emerging processes. In the one article with a clinical sample (Quirk et al., 2013), the GSRS was shown to have good reliability

Table 3.4 Group Session Rating Scale

Item	Information
Name of Instrument	Group Session Rating Scale (GSRS)
Authors	Duncan, B. L., & Miller, S. D. (2007).
Source	Duncan, B. L., & Miller, S. M. (2007). *The Group Session Rating Scale.* Jensen Beach, FL: Author.
Brief Description	The GSRS is a four-item measure of group cohesion (i.e., "member's relationship to the group, including leaders, rather than just the relationship between client and therapist" (Slone et al., 2015). It assesses four areas related to the working alliance: relationship, goals, approach/method, and overall, each rated on a bipolar continuum (e.g., "The 'relationship' aspect was assessed on a continuum of 'I felt understood, respected, and accepted by the leader and the group' to 'I did not feel understood, respected, and/or accepted by the leader and/or the group'" (Quirk et al., 2013, p. 196).
Time Issues	The GSRS takes about two minutes to complete at the end of a session (Quirk et al., 2013).
Subscales and Scoring	The GSRS has four bipolar items assessing relationship, goals and topics, approach or method, and overall perceptions. Respondents place an "X" on a continuum between the bipolar items that most characterizes their experience in the preceding session. Measurements of where the "X" falls on each 10 cm line are added for a total score, with scores ranging from 0 to 40.
Psychometric Properties	Quirk et al. (2013) found all four items loaded onto a single factor. They also found concurrent validity through positive correlations with the GCQ, the cohesion scale of the TFI, and client and therapist responses to the Working Alliance Inventory. The GSRS has been shown to have good reliability: Chapman and Kivlighan (2019) reported a Chronbach's alpha of .90.
Norms and any normative data re: diversity for each instrument	N/A
Translations	Afghanistan, Afrikaans, Chinese, Creole, Finnish, French, German, Hungarian, Italian, Japanese, Korean, Norwegian, Spanish, Vietnamese, and Welsh (all available at https://betteroutcomesnow.com [see below])
Sensitivity to Change	N/A
Sample references	Chapman, N., & Kivlighan, D. M., III. (2019). Does the cohesion–outcome relationship change over time? A dynamic model of change in group psychotherapy. *Group Dynamics: Theory, Research, and Practice, 23*(2), 91–103. http://dx.doi.org/10.1037/gdn0000100 Quirk, K., Miller, S., Duncan, B., & Owen, J. (2013). Group session rating scale: Preliminary psychometrics in substance abuse group interventions. *Counselling & Psychotherapy Research, 13*(3), 194–200. http://dx.doi.org/10.1080/14733145.2012.744425 Slone, N. C., Reese, R. J., Mathews-Duvall, S., & Kodet, J. (2015). Evaluating the efficacy of client feedback in group psychotherapy. *Group Dynamics: Theory, Research, and Practice, 19*(2), 122–136. http://dx.doi.org/10.1037/gdn0000026
Website Resources	https://betteroutcomesnow.com
How to Obtain/Cost	The GSRS is available at https://betteroutcomesnow.com. It is free to individual users for download upon agreeing to the license and registering with your email (along with all other Partners for Change Outcome Management System (PCOMS) measures).

Item	Information
Administration Types	Pencil and paper; online (The online version of the PCOMS, called Better Outcomes Now (BON), administers the measures and provides graphs of scores to use with clients and information about other data for use by therapists, programs, and organizations. The BON is available for an additional annual fee that varies depending on the number of users).
Analytics	No
Benchmarking	N/A

(internal consistency with an alpha between .86 and .90 over four sessions), medium-to-high test-retest correlations, and significant and expected correlations with other process measures (e.g., GCQ, Working Alliance Inventory and TFI Cohesiveness scale). The authors of this initial study point to some methodological limitations of this work and we suggest future research is needed for further refinement and validation of this promising measure and exploration of the conceptual and empirical overlap of this measure to others before its regular use in practice.

Critical Incidents Measure

The Critical Incidents measure (CI) is based on the Most Important Event Questionnaire (Bloch et al., 1979) to assess members' experiences of therapeutic processes (see Table 3.5 for source, description, and administration considerations of the CI). Unlike most self-report inventories that entail ratings, this measure is open ended, asking the respondent to describe in narrative form some recent impactful event in the group. It starts with the instruction: "Of the events which occurred in this session (or during this phase), which one do you feel was the most important to/ for you personally. Describe the event (what took place, which members were involved, how was your reaction, why was it important?)." These responses are then judged by independent raters as reflective of one or more therapeutic factors. Probably owing to the time necessary to fill out the measure (e.g., up to 20 minutes, depending on the depth of written answers of group members) and to classify the responses, the measure is not very often used. However, it can be an extremely useful qualitative measure to add context and richness to the otherwise quantitative data collected from the other measures described here. It is also easy to administer and group members can write as much (or little) as they choose. The CI could, for example, be an attractive tool for the therapist as well as group members to reflect on the basis of an individual narrative what critical moments, interactions, or interventions were important in a session and how these could eventually explain changes or "alerts" in process related self-reports. Bloch et al. (1979) provide an illustrative example of a group member who said:

> I think that the most important event during the last three meetings was when I became the centre of attention of the group. I was asked by other members of the group to say what I was thinking and to tell them what my feelings towards them were—which I hadn't really done at all up to this point. Although I found this difficult I think I had some measure of success. Not saying what I am thinking, and not expressing my feelings towards people is one of the major difficulties I have.
>
> (p. 258)

A more recent study (Erby, 2019) examined critical incident reports of students participating in an experiential group as a part of a multicultural counseling course to understand the specific experiences that helped and hindered difficult conversations about issues like race

Table 3.5 Critical Incident Measure

Item	Information
Name of Instrument	Critical Incident measure (CI)
Authors	Bloch et al. (1979)
Source	Bloch, S., Reibstein, J., Crouch, E., Holroyd, P., & Themen, J. (1979). A method for the study of therapeutic factors in group psychotherapy. *The British Journal of Psychiatry, 134*, 257–263. https://doi.org/10.1192/bjp.134.3.257
Brief Description	The CI (initially referred to as the "most important event questionnaire" by Bloch et al., 1979) is a qualitative measure designed to examine therapeutic factors in groups. Participants respond to the following prompts: "Of the events which occurred in the last session, which one do you feel was the most important for you personally? Describe the event: what actually took place, the group members involved, and your own reaction. Why was it important to you?" Responses are then assigned by trained raters to one of 10 therapeutic factors.
Time Issues	The CI takes about 15 minutes after a session.
Subscales and Scoring	Bloch et al. (1979) developed a list of 10 therapeutic factors: catharsis, self-disclosure, learning from interpersonal actions, universality, acceptance, altruism, guidance, self-understanding, vicarious learning, and instillation of hope. Raters read the CI reports and assign them to one of the 10 therapeutic factors. Bloch et al. provided a detailed guide for coding as an appendix.
Psychometric Properties	While Bloch et al. (1979) did not report on validity, they did report satisfactory inter-rater reliabilities, with kappas ranging from .52 to .62 for pairs of raters in their study.
Norms and any normative data re: diversity for each instrument	N/A
Translations	N/A
Sensitivity to Change	N/A
Sample references	Kivlighan, D. M., Jr. (2011). Individual and group perceptions of therapeutic factors and session evaluation: An actor–partner interdependence analysis. *Group Dynamics: Theory, Research, and Practice, 15*(2), 147–160. http://dx.doi.org/10.1037/a0022397
Website Resources	Can be obtained at no cost by downloading from: www.routledge.com/Core-Principles-of-Group-Psychotherapy-An-Integrated-Theory-Research/Kaklauskas-Greene/p/book/9780367203092 (using the button entitled Support Materials and choosing the folder entitled Process 1–4). CI: Process #1
How to Obtain/Cost	A full description of the measure and coding is available in the source paper cited above (Bloch et al., 1979)
Administration Types	Can be administered via pencil and paper or electronically.
Analytics	N/A
Benchmarking	N/A; The measure has been used across an extremely wide variety of clinical and non-clinical groups, though.

and social class, which could provide additional depth and context for understanding other quantitative measures, like the Multicultural Orientation Inventory-Group Version (Kivlighan et al., 2019).

Multicultural Orientation Inventory – Group Version

A group's MCO refers to its cultural humility, ability and willingness to explore differences in cultures represented in the group, and its comfort in doing so (Kivlighan & Chapman, 2018). The group's MCO can be assessed through a 27-item measure developed by Kivlighan and colleagues (2019), the Multicultural Orientation Inventory-Group Version (MCO-G) (see Table 3.6). The MCO-G was adapted from three measures assessing cultural humility (the Cultural Humility Scale, Hook et al., 2013), Cultural Missed Opportunities (Owen et al., 2016), and therapist cultural comfort (the Therapist Comfort Scale, Slone & Owen, 2015). Kivlighan and Chapman (2018) suggest that these pillars of the MCO framework can be useful for therapists, for example, in the early stages of group development as norms are being established. They suggest leaders can model their own cultural humility (e.g., expressing a sense of openness and curiosity as cultural issues come up in group) and a willingness and comfort in talking about versus avoiding them. This early work in developing the group MCO, they suggest, can prepare the group for impasses and ruptures related to culture that occur later in the group (e.g., the enactment of a racial microaggression by one group member toward another). Examining the relationship of the MCO-G to other process measures and outcomes, Kivlighan and colleagues (2019), for example, found that all three factors were associated with the TFI-8 (Tasca et al., 2016), and cultural humility and missed cultural opportunities, but not cultural comfort, were associated with a measure of improvement, suggesting the MCO-G is related to other group process measures and, at least partially, related to some measures of outcome. Interestingly, research on group MCO highlights how more traditional group processes interact with cultural processes. For example, Kivlighan and colleagues (2020) found that racial and ethnic minority clients' perceptions of their groups cultural comfort may serve to buffer the negative impact of racial microaggressions in the group on their perceptions of cohesion.

Table 3.6 Multicultural Orientation – Group Version

Item	Information
Name of Instrument	Multicultural Orientation – Group version (MCO-G)
Authors	Kivlighan et al. (2019)
Source	Kivlighan, D. M., Adams, M. C., Drinane, J. M., Tao, K. W., & Owen, J. (2019). Construction and validation of the multicultural orientation Inventory—Group version. *Journal of Counseling Psychology, 66*(1), 45–55. http://dx.doi.org/10.1037/cou0000294
Brief Description	The MCO-G is a 27-item instrument with three subscales assessing perceptions of: (1) the group's cultural humility (i.e., an orientation toward the other; a stance of openness in the face of cultural difference; Hook et al., 2013), (2) the extent to which the group misses (versus takes) opportunities to engage around cultural issues, and (3) the group's comfort in exploring cultural issues. Responses are given on a five-point Likert scale ranging from 1 (*strongly disagree*) to 5 (*strongly agree*).
Time Issues	Administration takes five minutes or less
Subscales and Scoring	The MCO-G has three subscales: cultural humility (12 items), cultural comfort (10 items), and cultural missed opportunities (5 items). Means are calculated for each subscale, with higher scores indicating higher levels of cultural humility, cultural comfort, and cultural missed opportunities, respectively.
Psychometric Properties	Kivlighan et al. (2019) confirmed the hypothesized three-factor structure (i.e., cultural humility, cultural comfort, and missed cultural opportunities). They also reported convergent validity in the form of significant associations with the TFI-8 (Tasca et al., 2016). Kivlighan and colleagues (2019) also reported acceptable to good reliabilities of the subscales, with Chronbach's alphas of .88, .88, and .73 for cultural humility, cultural comfort, and cultural missed opportunities, respectively.

Item	Information
Norms and any normative data re: diversity for each instrument	N/A
Translations	N/A
Sensitivity to Change	Unknown
Sample references	Grimes, J. L., & Kivlighan, D. M. (2021). Whose multicultural orientation matters most? Examining additive and compensatory effects of the group's and leader's multicultural orientation in group therapy. *Group Dynamics: Theory, Research, and Practice*. Advance online publication. http://dx.doi.org/10.1037/gdn0000153
	Kivlighan, D. M., & Chapman, N. A. (2018). Extending the multicultural orientation (MCO) framework to group psychotherapy: A clinical illustration. *Psychotherapy, 55*(1), 39–44. https://doi.org/10.1037/pst0000142
	Kivlighan, D. M., Drinane, J. M., Tao, K. W., Owen, J., & Liu, W. M. (2019). The detrimental effect of fragile groups: Examining the role of cultural comfort for group therapy members of color. *Journal of Counseling Psychology, 66*(6), 763–770. http://dx.doi.org/10.1037/cou0000352
	Kivlighan, D. M., Swancy, A. G., Smith, E., & Brennaman, C. (2021). Examining racial microaggressions in group therapy and the buffering role of members' perceptions of their group's multicultural orientation. *Journal of Counseling Psychology, 68*(5), 621–628. http://dx.doi.org/10.1037/cou0000531
Website Resources	N/A
How to Obtain/Cost	Full measure is published in the source article cited above/Free.
Administration Types	Paper and pencil
Analytics	No
Benchmarking	N/A

In summary, we note that group process measures like those reviewed above have great utility for group therapists. For example, measures like the GQ can alert group therapists to ruptures that need to be repaired in the group (e.g., Svien et al., 2021) by pointing to changes in relationship components (intrapersonal splits such as a member's divergent reactions to the group-as-a-whole versus to the leader) over time or between members (interpersonal splits such as divergent reactions of different members to the group-as-a-whole). And the Engagement scale of the GCQ-S and the TFI can help leaders detect changes in experiences in the group that may well be associated with group member outcome (McClendon & Burlingame, 2010). The MCO-G can also help leaders understand if group members feel the group is open and able to discuss cultural issues (Kivlighan & Chapman, 2018), which may relate to therapeutic factors experienced in the group. Finally, use of the qualitative CI can help provide context for quantitative changes observed, pointing to specific events within sessions that group members found meaningful. Next, we turn our focus to processes driven (and assessed) at the level of the group leader.

Measuring Leadership Style and Behaviors

While the measures reviewed above tend to assess process as a function of the group members or the group-as-a-whole, the leadership style and behavior of the group therapists also represent important processes with implications for group member outcomes (e.g., Riva et al., 2004). As a result, we review one potentially useful tool for assessing group leader behavior, the Group Psychotherapy Intervention Rating Scale (Chapman et al., 2010). We also review measures that may help assess group leader cultural and social justice competencies.

Group Psychotherapy Intervention Rating Scale

The Group Psychotherapy Intervention Rating Scale (GPIRS, Chapman et al., 2010) is an observer-rated tool to assess the quality of leader interventions, based on Burlingame and colleagues' (2002) empirically derived framework addressing group leader contributions to the development of cohesion (see Table 3.7 for a description and administration considerations). These contributions fall within three domains: group structuring behaviors (e.g., establishing norms and defining roles), verbal interactions (e.g., giving timely and appropriate feedback, making here-and-now process observations), and creating and maintaining a therapeutic climate (e.g., expressing openness and warmth). Trained observers code intervention "units" for the clarity and quantity of each intervention type, based on observable leader behavior, either in live sessions or from video recordings. Chapman and colleagues (2010) report good reliability and concurrent validity for the total measure.

Perhaps more importantly for practical purposes, initial studies of the GPIRS (c.f. Chapman et al., 2010) found both that the quality of group interventions was related to client perceptions of the group climate measured with the GCQ and verbal interaction, and that observer ratings on the GPIRS were correlated with therapist self-ratings. While the GPIRS may be resource intensive (e.g., requiring a trained rater), it can be useful for highlighting the specific contributions of group leaders to the group process (e.g., their contributions to the development of cohesion, Tucker et al., 2020).

Leader Multicultural Orientation

As discussed above, the MCO (Owen et al., 2011), which includes a therapist's cultural humility, taking/missing opportunities to address cultural issues, and cultural comfort has recently been adapted to assess members' experience of the multicultural orientation of the group (Kivlighan et al., 2019). Recall that some evidence suggests that the group MCO, specifically cultural comfort, may serve to buffer the negative impact of racial microaggressions on racial and ethnic minority (REM) clients' perceptions of cohesion (Kivlighan et al., 2020). Recent research, however, suggests that it is not just the group MCO that may be important, but the relationship between the group MCO and group therapist MCO. Specifically, research has shown that clients perceived the most improvement when the cultural humility of the group and the group leader were both perceived to be high or when either the group or the leader compensates for a high level of missed cultural opportunities in the other (e.g., the group, but not the leader, are high in missed opportunities) (Grimes & Kivlighan, 2021). Grimes and Kivlighan created a measure of group therapist MCO by modifying the MCO-G (see Table 3.6). They report, for example:

> "the instructions for the CHS of the MCO-G were adapted to read as follows: "Please indicate the extent to which you agree or disagree with the following statements about the leader(s) of your group. Regarding the core aspect(s) of my cultural background, the group leader(s)."
>
> (p. 6)

Group therapists may be interested in using the MCO in conjunction with the MCO-G to examine both how group members perceive the group in terms of its MCO, as well as how they view the therapist in these terms. If, for example, group members rate the therapist as high in missed cultural opportunities, the therapist may wish to listen more purposefully for these opportunities, explore this in supervision, and/or seek continuing education around specific cultural issues. In conjunction with the CI, the therapist may get a sense of the

Table 3.7 Group Psychotherapy Intervention Rating Scale

Item	Information
Name of Instrument	Group Psychotherapy Intervention Rating Scale (GPIRS)
Authors	Chapman et al.
Source	Chapman, C. L., Baker, E. L., Porter, G., Thayer, S. D., & Burlingame, G. M. (2010). Rating group therapist interventions: The validation of the group psychotherapy intervention rating scale. *Group Dynamics: Theory, Research, and Practice, 14*(1), 15–31. https://doi.org/10.1037/a0016628
Brief Description	The GPIRS is an observer-rated tool to assess the quality of leader interventions related to the development of cohesion within three domains: group structuring behaviors (e.g., establishing norms and defining roles), verbal interactions (e.g., giving timely and appropriate feedback, making here-and-now process observations), and creating and maintaining a therapeutic climate (e.g., expressing openness and warmth).
Time Issues	The GPIRS may involve a significant time investment in training raters (Chapman et al., 2010) reported a three-week training period. Administration also involves breaking down session material into intervention segments (which Chapman et al. described as "defined as leader verbalizations or specific purposeful leader behaviors aimed to improve group processes" [p. 25]) for coding. Timing of coding, then, depends on the number of intervention segments to be coded.
Subscales and Scoring	An updated version of the GPIRS includes 36 observer-rated items in three domains: group structuring (e.g., "Discussed group rules such as time, attendance, absences, tardiness, confidentiality, and participation"), verbal interactions (e.g., "Gave structured feedback exercise"), and creating and maintaining an emotional climate (e.g., "Encouraged active emotional engagement between group members") (Chapman et al., 2010). Items are scored on a 3-point Likert-type scale ranging from 0 (*intervention did not occur*) to 1 (*ambiguous—occurred but clarity could be improved*), to 2 (*intervention was performed with clarity*) (Tucker et al., 2020).
Psychometric Properties	Chapman et al. (2010) found a hypothesized positive relationshis between Engagement, as measured by the GCQ, and a hypothesized negative relationship with Conflict, also as measured by the GCQ.
Norms and any normative data re: diversity for each instrument	N/A
Translations	Dutch
Sensitivity to Change	N/A
Sample references	Tucker, J. R., Wade, N. G., Abraham, W. T., Bitman-Heinrichs, R., Cornish, M. A., & Post, B. C. (2020). Modeling cohesion change in group counseling: The role of client characteristics, group variables, and leader behaviors. *Journal of Counseling Psychology, 67*(3), 371–385. https://doi.org/10.1037/cou0000403
Website Resources	N/A
How to Obtain/Cost	The GPIRS is available directly from Gary Burlingame.
Administration Types	Paper and pencil
Analytics	N/A
Benchmarking	N/A

specific cultural opportunities that were meaningful for group members, but missed or avoided by the therapist.

Final Case Example

We return one more time to our case example, this time focusing on a specific group member, Stephen, who is a Black, cisgender, heterosexual man in his second year at the university. He was referred to Stacy and Mike's interpersonal psychotherapy group by his individual therapist at the counseling center. After the first administration of the process measures, ratings on the Engagement scale of the GCQ were universally high and ratings of Conflict were relatively low. Reports on the CI reflected generally positive interactions that the co-therapists interpreted as especially reflecting the therapeutic factor of Instillation of Hope. Scores on the MCO-G appeared fairly consistent across members and showed fairly high levels of Cultural Humility and Cultural Comfort, suggesting members felt the group expressed a sense of curiosity and comfort in addressing issues around culture when they come up in group. After the second administration of the process measures, the leaders noticed Stephen's (and two other group members') ratings on the Engagement subscale were lower than their own previous ratings and also lower than the other group members' ratings, and their ratings of Conflict and the group's Missed Cultural Opportunities were elevated relative to the other members. To Stacy, these divergences in Stephen's (and the other two group members') assessment data seemed noteworthy, so during supervision she suggested they examine the members' CIs for the most recent administration. Upon doing so, they noted Stephen's report that the most important event for him was when another member said to him with surprise he was "very articulate," a well-known racial microaggression that conveys the message that it is unusual that a Black person would be articulate. Stephen went on to note that no one, including the leaders reacted or checked in with him, leaving him feeling targeted and invalidated. Stacy said to Mike the next session might be difficult, but that it was important to process the unaddressed microaggression and the impact it had on the group in terms of perceptions of engagement and conflict. She suggested they model cultural humility and take responsibility for missing the cultural opportunity and in the hopes of helping repair the rupture.

This expression of cultural humility by the leaders and acknowledgement of his (and the two other members') experience of the climate allowed Stephen to open up about the familiar pain he experienced hearing the microaggression, given that the group had come to hold importance for him and felt like a "safe space." The group processed the impact of the microaggressive event, and the perpetrator of the microaggression took responsibility, with the help of the leaders' noting that intent and impact of a statement may be different particularly when relating to this type of cultural rupture. The leaders also helped the group reflect on how groups can operate as social microcosms that may (if even unintentionally) replicate oppressive societal dynamics that perpetuate inequity (e.g., through this type of microaggressions) if not illuminated and the rupture repaired. The leaders explained the concept of MCO, and the importance of cultural humility, specifically, and talked about how the group might foster humility and a willingness to engage in difficult dialogues about cultural issues. Group members engaged in a discussion of agreements they would like to have to bolster their ability to engage in these difficult dialogues, including acknowledging that intent and impact are different, and agreeing to support each other in unlearning of racism and other forms of oppression. While group members expressed trepidation, ultimately, ratings of Missed Opportunities declined and Cultural Comfort and Engagement increased.

Summary, Recommendations, and Conclusion

Our review of the group process literature and measures leads us to the following general recommendations:

- Group leaders should be familiar with conceptualizations of group process, both within the field of group psychotherapy and from other domains such as social and organizational psychology.
- Group leaders should be familiar with the literature on group process in terms of how process relates to the social structuring of the group, as well as to therapeutic outcomes.
- In deciding to implement group process measures, group leaders need to thoughtfully and sensitively address a number of procedural and logistical questions, including: (1) which measures are most applicable to my particular group, (2) how to present a rationale to the group members and solicit their commitment and compliance, (3) to whom is the feedback from the process measures given (the therapist? the supervisor? the members?) and how is this delivered?
- In collecting group process data, group leaders need to consider issues related to the level of the data (session, individual member, and group) as well as both the amount and consistency of assessed variables in their group.
- Group therapists need to be particularly attentive to divergences or changes in the process data that may signal deterioration and need for therapeutic intervention, as when an individual member's scores deviate significantly from previous ratings or from other group members, or when scores for the group-as-a-whole deviate markedly from previous scores or from normative values.
- Group leaders should recognize that cultural processes may play an important role in group process and outcome.
- Group leaders should consider processes related to the members and the group-as-a-whole, but also consider their own processes and how they impact the group.

We believe the GQ, TFI-19, GCQ, CI, and MCO-G are useful tools for assessing the group processes of group therapy, are illuminated in research and theory within the field of group psychotherapy and beyond (e.g., in social and organizational psychology) and have implications for thinking about the structuring of groups and therapeutic outcomes. Group development, group norms, therapeutic factors, and more general social psychological processes all operate within therapy groups to shape group member experiences and outcomes for the group-as-a-whole. We do not suggest that these measures replace clinical judgment (see Chapter 1) but compliment it. We also add the suggestion that the measures can work together (e.g., using the CI to provide context and richness to illuminate levels or changes in quantitative measures). Finally, we also note that assessment fatigue is a real issue for group members and group leaders have limited time to administer and review data. As a result, we suggest that some of these measures may be administered on an "as needed" basis.

One of the major shifts in this version of the CORE Battery is the attention focused on cultural issues in groups. Much has been written about multicultural issues in therapy, however, most of this tends to assume the discussion is of individual therapy and the cultural dynamics between therapist and a single client. Increased attention to cultural issues in group therapy in research and practice helps put the focus on how all groups are multicultural and, as social microcosms, have the potential to perpetuate oppressive situations or provide opportunities for corrective experiences. The MCO-G adds a way for group therapists to assess group members' perceptions of their group's cultural humility, and the extent to which they do and are comfortable in engaging with cultural issues in group. This adds a contextual level to the CORE Battery that acknowledges how individuals' identities and associate experiences with privilege and oppression may impact their experiences of and behaviors in group. In this updated CORE Battery, we also provide suggestions for assessing processes related to leadership, including the leadership profile and the group leader's multicultural orientation. Research using these measures suggests that leader behavior, cultural humility, and comfort in addressing cultural issues in group can interact with group processes in ways that have important implications for the group.

References

Alldredge, C. T., Burlingame, G. M., Yang, C., & Rosendahl, J. (2021). Alliance in group therapy: A meta-analysis. *Group Dynamics: Theory, Research, and Practice*, 25(1), 13–28. doi:10.1037/gdn0000135.

Bakali, J., Baldwin, S., & Lorentzen, S. (2009). Modeling group process constructs at three stages in group psychotherapy. *Psychotherapy Research*, 19, 332–343. doi:1kis.idm.oclc.org/10.1080/10503300902894430.

Bakali, J. V., Wilberg, T., Klungsøyr, O., & Lorentzen, S. (2013). Development of group climate in short- and long-term psychodynamic group psychotherapy. *International Journal of Group Psychotherapy*, 63(3), 367–393. doi:10.1521/ijgp.2013.63.3.366.

Baldwin, S. A., Murray, D. M., & Shadish, W. R. (2005). Empirically supported treatments or type I errors? problems with the analysis of data from group-administered treatments. *Journal of Consulting and Clinical Psychology*, 73(5), 924–935. doi:10.1037/0022-006X.73.5.924.

Beck, A. P. & Lewis, C. M. (Eds). (2000). *The process of group psychotherapy: Systems for analyzing change*. American Psychological Association. doi:10.1037/10378-000.

Belcher Platt, A. A. (2017). *Racial-cultural events and microaggression in group counseling as perceived by group counseling members of color* (Publication No. 10607840) [Doctoral dissertation, Fordham University]. ProQuest Dissertations & Theses Global: Social Sciences.

Bion, W. (1961). *Experiences in groups and other papers*. London: Tavistock.

Bloch, S., Crouch, E., & Reibstein, J. (1981). Therapeutic factors in group psychotherapy: A review. *Archives of General Psychiatry*, 38 (5), 519–526. doi:1kis.idm.oclc.org/10.1001/archpsyc.1980.01780300031003.

Bloch, S., Reibstein, J., Crouch, E., Holroyd, P., & Themen, J. (1979). A method for the study of therapeutic factors in group psychotherapy. *The British Journal of Psychiatry*, 134, 257–263. doi:10.1192/bjp.134.3.257.

Bormann, B., Burlingame, G., & B. Strauss (2011). Der Gruppenfragebogen (GQ-D). Instrument zur Messung von therapeutischen Beziehungen in der Gruppenpsychotherapie. *Psychotherapeut*, 56, 297–309. doi:10.1007/s00278-011-0841-4.

Bormann, B. & Strauss, B. (2007). Group climate, cohesion, alliance, and empathy as components of the therapeutic relationship within group psychotherapy – Test of a multilevel model. *Gruppenpsychotherapie und Gruppendynamik*, 43, 1–20.

Brown, L.D., Tang, X., & Hollman, R.L. (2014). The structure of social exchange in self-help support groups: Development of a measure. *American Journal of Community Psychology*, 53(2), 83–95. doi:10.1007/s10464-013-9621-3.

Brown, N. W. (2003). Conceptualizing process. *International Journal of Group Psychotherapy*, 53(2), 225–244. doi:10.1521/ijgp.53.2.225.42814.

Burlingame, G. M., Alldredge, C. T. & Arnold, R. A. (2021). Alliance rupture detection and repair in group therapy: Using the Group Questionnaire—GQ. *International Journal of Group Psychotherapy*, 71 (2), 338–370. doi:10.1080/00207284.2020.1844010.

Burlingame, G. M., Fuhriman, A., & Johnson, J. E. (2002). Cohesion in group psychotherapy. In J. C. Norcross (Ed.), *Psychotherapy relationships that work: Therapist contributions and responsiveness to patients*. (pp. 71–87). Oxford University Press.

Burlingame, G. M., MacKenzie, K. R., & Strauss, B. (2004). Small group treatment: Evidence for effectiveness and mechanisms of change. In M. J. Lambert (Ed.), *Bergin & Garfield's handbook of psychotherapy and behavior change* (5th ed., pp. 647–696). Wiley.

Burlingame, G. M., McClendon, D. T., & Alonso, J. (2011a). Cohesion in group therapy. *Psychotherapy*, 48(1), 34–42. doi:1kis.idm.oclc.org/10.1037/a0022063.

Burlingame, G. M., McClendon, D. T., & Alonso, J. (2011b). *Cohesion in group therapy*. In J. C. Norcross (Ed.), 2nd ed.; Psychotherapy relationships that work: Evidence-based responsiveness (2nd ed., pp. 110–131) Oxford University Press. doi:10.1093/acprof:oso/9780199737208.003.0005.

Burlingame, G. M., McClendon, D. T., & Yang, C. (2018). Cohesion in group therapy: A meta-analysis. *Psychotherapy*, 55(4), 384–398. doi:10.1037/pst0000173.

Burlingame, G. M. & Strauss, B. (2021). Efficacy of small group treatments: Foundation for evidence-based practice. In M. Barkham, W. Lutz, & L. G. Castonguay (Eds), *Bergin and Garfield's handbook of psychotherapy and behavior change: 50th anniversary edition*, (7th ed.) (pp. 583–624). Hoboken, NJ: John Wiley & Sons.

Burlingame, G., Strauss, B., Bormann, B., & Johnson, J. (2008). Are there common change mechanisms for all small group treatments? A conceptual model for change mechanisms inherent in small groups. *Gruppenpsychotherapie und Gruppendynamik*, 44(3), 177–241.

Burlingame, G. M., Strauss, B., & Joyce, A. S. (2013). Change mechanisms and effectiveness of small group treatments. *Bergin and Garfield's Handbook of Psychotherapy and Behavior Change* (6th ed.) (pp. 640–673). Wiley.

Burlingame, G. M., Strauss, B., Joyce, A., MacNair-Semands, R., MacKenzie, K. R., Ogrodniczuk, J., & Taylor, S. M. (2006). CORE Task Force (2006). *CORE Battery-Revised: An assessment tool kit for promoting optimal group selection, process and outcome*. American Group Psychotherapy Association.

Burlingame, G. M., Whitcomb, K. E., Woodland, S. C., Olsen, J. A., Beecher, M., & Gleave, R. (2018). The effects of relationship and progress feedback in group psychotherapy using the Group Questionnaire and Outcome Questionnaire-45: A randomized clinical trial. *Psychotherapy: Theory, Research, & Practice, 55(2)*, 116–131. doi:10.1037/pst0000133.

Caruso, R. et al. (2013). Exploration of experiences in therapeutic groups for patients with severe mental illness: Development of the Ferrara Group Experiences Scale (FE-GES). *BMC Psychiatry*, 13 (242). doi:10.1186/1471-244x-13-242.

Chapman, C. L., Baker, E. L., Porter, G., Thayer, S. D., & Burlingame, G. M. (2010). Rating group therapist interventions: The validation of the group psychotherapy intervention rating scale. *Group Dynamics: Theory, Research, and Practice*, 14(1), 15–31. doi:10.1037/a0016628.

Chapman, C. L., Burlingame, G. M., Gleave, R., Rees, F., Beecher, M., & Porter, G. S. (2012). Clinical prediction in group psychotherapy. *Psychotherapy Research*, 22(6), 673–681. doi:10.1080/10503307.2012.702512.

Chen, E. C., Thombs, B. D., & Costa, C. I. (2003). Building connection through diversity in group counseling: A dialogical perspective. In D. B.Pope-Davis, H. L. K.Coleman, W. M.Liu, & R. L. Toporek (Eds), *Handbook of multicultural competencies in counseling & psychology* (pp. 456–477). Sage Publications. doi:10.4135/9781452231693.n29.

Coché, E., Dies, R. R., & Goettelmann, K. (1991). Process variables mediating change in intensive group therapy training. *International Journal of Group Psychotherapy*, 41(3), 379–397.

Cohen-Mansfield, J., Hai, T., & Comishen, M. (2017). Group engagement in persons with dementia: The concept and its measurement. *Psychiatry Research*, 251, 237–243. doi:10.1016/j.psychres.2017.02.013.

Cole, E. R. (2020). Demarginalizing women of color in intersectionality scholarship in psychology: A Black Feminist critique. *Journal of Social Issues*, 76(4), 1036–1044. doi:10.1111/josi.12413.

Cone-Uemura, K. & Bentley, E. S. (2018). *Multicultural/diversity issues in groups*. In M. D. Ribeiro, J. D. Gross, & M. M. Turner (Eds), *The college counselor's guide to group psychotherapy* (pp. 19–35). Routledge.

Constantine, M. G. (2007). Racial microaggressions against African American clients in cross-racial counseling relationships. *Journal of Counseling Psychology*, 54(1), 1–16. doi:10.1037/0022-0167.54.1.1.

Corsini, R. J. & Rosenberg, B. (1955). Mechanisms of group psychotherapy: Processes and dynamics. *Journal of Abnormal and Social Psychology*, 51(3), 406–411. doi:10.1037/h0048439.

Curtin, N., Stewart, A. J., & Cole, E. R. (2015). Challenging the status quo: The role of intersectional awareness in activism for social change and pro-social intergroup attitudes. *Psychology of Women Quarterly*, 39(4), 512–529. doi:10.1177/0361684315580439.

DeMatteo, J. S., Eby, L. T., & Sundstrom, E. (1998). Team-based rewards: Current empirical evidence and directions for future research. In B. M.Staw & L.L. Cummings (Eds), *Research in organizational behavior, Vol. 20. An annual series of analytical essays and critical reviews* (pp. 141–183). Elsevier Science/JAI Press.

Diemer, M. A. et al. (2020). Development of the short critical consciousness scale (ShoCCS). *Applied Developmental Science*. Advance online publication. doi:10.1080/10888691.2020.1834394.

Diemer, M. A., Rapa, L. J., Park, C. J., & Perry, J. C. (2017). Development and validation of the Critical Consciousness Scale. *Youth & Society*, 49(4), 461–483. httdoi:10.1177/0044118X14538289.

Dubovská, E., Furstová, J., Růžička, J., & Tavel, P. (2019). Validity of the Czech version of the Therapeutic Factors Inventory—Short form (TFI-S). *International Journal of Group Psychotherapy*, 69(3), 308–327. doi:10.1080/00207284.2019.1584527.

Duncan, B. L., Miller, S. D., Reynolds, L., Sparks, J., Claud, D., Brown, J., & Johnson, L. D. (2003). The session rating scale: Psychometric properties of a "working" alliance scale. *Journal of Brief Therapy*, 3, 3–12.

Erby, A. N. (2019). Critical incidents in a brief multicultural counseling experiential group. *The Journal for Specialists in Group Work*, 44(4), 235–250. doi:10.1080/01933922.2019.1669754.

Evans, N. J & Jarvis, P. A. (1986). The Group Attitude Scale: A measure of attraction to group. *Small group behavior*, 17(2), 203–216. doi:10.1177/104649648601700205.

Fernandez, E., Salem, D., Swift, J. K., & Ramtahal, N. (2015). Meta-analysis of dropout from cognitive behavioral therapy: Magnitude, timing, and moderators. *Journal of Consulting and Clinical Psychology*, 83(6), 1108–1122. doi:10.1037/ccp0000044.

Forsyth, D. R. (2010). *Group dynamics* (5th ed.). Belmont, CA: Wadsworth, Cengage Learning.

Freire, P. (1970/2008). *Pedagogy of the oppressed*. Continuum International.

Fuhriman, A., Drescher, S., Hanson, E., Henrie, R., & Rybicki, W. (1986). Refining the Measurement of Curativeness: An empirical approach. *Small Group Research*, 17(2), 186–201. doi:10.1177/104649648601700204.

Fuhriman, A. & Burlingame, G. M. (Eds). (1994). *Handbook of group psychotherapy: An empirical and clinical synthesis*. Wiley.

Gantt, S. P. & Agazarian, Y. M. (2017). Systems-centered group therapy. *International Journal of Group Psychotherapy*, *67(Suppl1)*, S60–S70. doi:1kis.idm.oclc.org/10.1080/00207284.2016.1218768.

Gleave, R. L., Burlingame, G. M., Beecher, M. E., Griner, D., Hansen, K., & Jenkins, S., (2017). Feedback-informed group treatment: Application of the OQ–45 and Group Questionnaire (pp. 141–166). In D. S. Prescott, C. L., Maeschalck, & S. D. Miller (Eds), *Feedback-informed treatment in clinical practice: Reaching for excellence*. Washington, DC: American Psychological Association.

Gold, P. B. & Kivlighan, D. M. Jr. (2018). It's complicated: Using group member process-feedback to improve group therapist effectiveness. *Psychotherapy*, *55(2)*, 164–169. doi:1kis.idm.oclc.org/10.1037/pst0000146.

Greene, L. R. (2020). Group structure and level of analysis. In F. J. Kaklauskas & L. R. Greene (Eds), *Core principles of group psychotherapy: An integrated theory, research, and practice training manual* (pp. 49–55). New York: Taylor & Francis.

Greene, L. R. (2017). Group psychotherapy research studies that therapists might actually read: My top 10 list. *International Journal of Group Psychotherapy*, 67(1), 1–26. doi:10.1080/00207284.2016.1202678.

Greene, L. R., Barlow, S., & Kaklauskas, F. J. (2020). Therapeutic factors. In F. J. Kaklauskas & L. R. Greene (Eds), *Core principles of group psychotherapy: An integrated theory, research, and practice training manual* (pp. 56–70). Taylor & Francis.

Greene, L. R. & Kaklauskas, F. J. (2020a). Anti-therapeutic, defensive, regressive, and challenging group processes and dynamics. In F. J. Kaklauskas & L. R. Greene (Eds), *Core principles of group psychotherapy: An integrated theory, research, and practice training manual* (pp. 71–85). Taylor & Francis.

Greene, L. R. & Kaklauskas, F. J. (2020b). Group development. In F. J. Kaklauskas & L. R. Greene (Eds), *Core principles of group psychotherapy: An integrated theory, research, and practice training manual* (pp. 56–70). New York: Taylor & Francis.

Grimes, J. L. & Kivlighan, D. M. (2021). Whose multicultural orientation matters most? Examining additive and compensatory effects of the group's and leader's multicultural orientation in group therapy. *Group Dynamics: Theory, Research, and Practice*. Advance online publication. doi:10.1037/gdn0000153.

Griner, D., Beecher, M. E., Brown, L. B., Millet, A. J., Worthen, V., Boardman, R. D., Hansen, K., Cox, J. C., & Gleave, R. L. (2018). Practice-based evidence can help! Using the Group Questionnaire to enhance clinical practice. *Psychotherapy: Theory, Research, & Practice, 55(2)*, 196–202. doi:10.1037/pst0000136.

Grzanka, P. R., Gonzalez, K. A., & Spanierman, L. B. (2019). White supremacy and counseling psychology: A critical-conceptual framework. *The Counseling Psychologist*, 47(4). doi:10.1177/0011000019880843.

Heppner, P. P., Wampold, B. E., Owen, J., Thompson, M. N., & Wang, K. T. (2016). *Research design in counseling* (4th ed.). Cengage.

Hook, J. N., Davis, D. E., Owen, J., Worthington, E. L., Jr., & Utsey, S. O. (2013). Cultural humility: Measuring openness to culturally diverse clients. *Journal of Counseling Psychology*, 60(3), 353–366. httdoi:10.1037/a0032595\

Hornsey, M. J., Dwyer, L., Oei, T. P. S., & Dingle, G. A. (2009). Group processes and outcomes in group psychotherapy: Is it time to let go of 'cohesiveness'? *International Journal of Group Psychotherapy, Vol 59(2)*, 267–278. doi:1kis.idm.oclc.org/10.1521/ijgp.2009.59.2.267.

Hornsey, M. J., Olsen, S., Barlow, F. K., & Oei, T. P. S. (2012). Testing a single-item visual analogue scale as a proxy for cohesiveness in group psychotherapy. *Group Dynamics: Theory, Research, and Practice, 16*(1) 80–90.

Janis, R. A., Burlingame, G. M., & Olsen, J. A. (2018). Developing a therapeutic relationship monitoring system for group treatment. *Psychotherapy, Vol 55(2)*, June, 105–115. doi:10.1037/pst0000139.

Janis, R. A., Burlingame, G. M., & Olsen, J. A. (2016). Evaluating factor structures of measures in group research: Looking between and within. *Group Dynamics: Theory, Research, and Practice*, 20(3), 165–180. https://doi.org/10.1037/gdn0000043.

Johnson, J. E., Burlingame, G. M., Olsen, J. A., Davies, D. R., & Gleave, R. L. (2005). Group climate, cohesion, alliance, and empathy in group psychotherapy: Multilevel structural equation models. *Journal of Counseling Psychology*, 52(3), 310–321. doi:10.1037/0022-0167.52.3.310.

Johnson, J. E., Burlingame, G. M., Strauss, B., Bormann, B. (2008). Die therapeutischen Beziehungen in der Gruppenpsychotherapie. *Gruppenpsychotherapie und Gruppendynamik*. 44, 52–89.

Joyce, A. S., MacNair-Semands, R., Tasca, G. A., & Ogrodniczuk, J. S. (2011). Factor structure and validity of the Therapeutic Factors Inventory–Short Form. *Group Dynamics: Theory, Research, and Practice*, 15(3), 201–219. doi:10.1037/a0024677.

Kageyama, M., Nakamura, Y., Kobayashi, S., & Yokoyama, K. (2016). Validity and reliability of the Japanese version of the therapeutic factors Inventory–19: A study of family peer education self-help groups. *Japan Journal of Nursing Science*, 13(1), 135 146. doi:10.1111/jjns.12098.

Kaklauskas, F. J. & Nettles, R. (2020). Towards multicultural and diversity proficiency as a group psychotherapist. In In F. J.Kaklauskas & L. R. Greene (Eds), *Core principles of group psychotherapy: An integrated theory, research, and practice training manual* (pp. 22–45). New York: Taylor & Francis.

Kivlighan, D. M., Jr. & Holmes, S. E. (2004). The importance of therapeutic factors: A typology of therapeutic factors studies. In J. L. DeLucia-Waack, D. A. Gerrity, C. R. Kalodner, & M. T. Riva (Eds), *Handbook of group counseling and psychotherapy* (pp. 23–36). Sage Publications.

Kivlighan, D. M., Jr. & Kivlighan, D. M., III. (2010). Are group leader knowledge structures related to member satisfaction with the leader? *Small Group Research*, 41(2), 175–197.

Kivlighan, D. M., III, Adams, M. C., Drinane, J. M., Tao, K. W., & Owen, J. (2019). Construction and validation of the multicultural orientation Inventory—Group version. *Journal of Counseling Psychology*, 66(1), 45–55. doi:10.1037/cou0000294.

Kivlighan, D. M. III, Ali, R. W., & Garrison, Y. L. (2020). Is there an optimal level of positive and negative feedback in group therapy? A response surface analysis. *Psychotherapy*, 57(2), 174–183. doi:10.1037/pst0000244.

Kivlighan, D. M. & Chapman, N. A. (2018). Extending the multicultural orientation (MCO) framework to group psychotherapy: A clinical illustration. *Psychotherapy*, 55(1), 39–44. doi:10.1037/pst0000142.

Kivlighan, D. M., III & Kivlighan, D. M., Jr. (2016). Examining between-leader and within-leader processes in group therapy. *Group Dynamics: Theory, Research, and Practice*, 20(3), 144–164 doi:10.1037/gdn0000050.

Kivlighan, D. M., III, Swancy, A. G., Smith, E., & Brennaman, C. (2021). Examining racial microaggressions in group therapy and the buffering role of members' perceptions of their group's multicultural orientation. *Journal of Counseling Psychology*, 68 (5), 621–628. doi:10.1037/cou0000531.

Krogel, J. (2008). The Group Questionnaire: A new measure of the group relationship. *Dissertation Abstracts International: Section B: The Sciences and Engineering*, 69(6-B), 3851.

Krogel, J., Burlingame, G. M., Chapman, C., Renshaw, T., Gleave, R., Beecher, M., & MacNair-Semands, R. (2013). The Group Questionnaire: A clinical and empirically derived measure of group relationship. *Psychotherapy Research*, 23(3), 344–354. doi:10.1080/10503307.2012.729868.

Landi, G. et al. (2020). Therapeutic factors in a psychiatric group therapy: A preliminary validation of Therapeutic Factors Inventory-8, Italian version. *Psychiatric Quarterly*. doi:10.1007/s11126-020-09834-2.

Lau, M. A., Ogrodniczuk, J., Joyce, A. S., & Sochting, I. (2010). Bridging the practitioner-scientist gap in group psychotherapy research. *International Journal of Group Psychotherapy*, 60(2), 177–196. doi:10.1521/ijgp.2010.60.2.177.

Lefforge, N. L., Mclaughlin, S., Goates-Jones, M., & Mejia, C. (2020). A training model for addressing microaggressions in group psychotherapy. *International Journal of Group Psychotherapy*, 70(1), 1–28. doi:10.1080/00207284.2019.1680989.

Lese, K. P. & MacNair-Semands, R. R. (2000). The Therapeutic Factors Inventory: Development of a scale. *Group*, 24, 303–317.

Lewicki, R. J., Saunders, D. M., Barry, B., & Lewicki, R. J. (2006). *Negotiation*. McGraw-Hill Irwin.

Lewis, J. A., Mendenhall, R., Harwood, S. A., & Browne Huntt, M. (2016). "Ain't I a woman?": Perceived gendered racial microaggressions experienced by black women. *The Counseling Psychologist*, 44(5), 758–780. doi:10.1177/0011000016641193.

Lo Coco, G., Gullo, S., Prestano, C., & Burlingame, G. M. (2015). Current issues on group psychotherapy research: An overview. In O. C. G. Gelo, A. Pritz & B. Rieken (Eds), *Psychotherapy research: Foundations, process, and outcome; psychotherapy research: Foundations, process, and outcome* (pp. 279–292, Chapter IX). Springer-Verlag Publishing. doi:10.1007/978-3-7091-1382-0_14.

Lo Coco, G., Tasca, G., Hewitt, P., Mikail, S., & Kivlighan, D. (2019). Ruptures and repairs of group therapy alliance. An untold story in psychotherapy research. *Research in Psychotherapy: Psychopathology, Process and Outcome*, 22(1), 58–70.

Lewis, C. C., Boyd, M., Puspitasari, A., Navarro, E., Howard, J., Kassab, H., Hoffman, M., Scott, K., Lyon, A., Douglas, S., Simon, G., & Kroenke, K. (2019). Implementing measurement based care in behavioral health: A review. *JAMA Psychiatry*, 76(3), 324–335. https://doiorg.tcsedsystem.idm.oclc.org/10.1001/jamapsychiatry.2018.332.

MacKenzie, K. R. (1981). Measurement of group climate. *International Journal of Group Psychotherapy*, 31, 287–295.

MacKenzie, K. R. (1983). The clinical application of a group climate measure. In R. R. Dies & K. R. MacKenzie (Eds), *Advances in group psychotherapy: Integrating research and practice* (pp. 159–170). International Universities Press.

MacKenzie, K. R. (1997). Clinical application of group development ideas. *Group Dynamics: Theory, Research, and Practice* 1, 275–287.

MacNair-Semands, R.R., Ogrodniczuk, J., & Joyce, A. (2010). Structure and initial validation of a short form of the Therapeutic Factors Inventory. *International Journal of Group Psychotherapy*, 60(2), 245–281. doi:10.1521/ijgp.2010.60.2.245.

Mander, J., Vogel, E., & Wiesner, V. et al. (2016). Yalom's Wirkfaktoren in der Gruppentherapie. *Psychotherapeut*, 61, 384–392. doi:10.1007/s00278-016-0119-y.

Marogna, C. & Caccamo, F. (2014). Analysis of the process in brief psychotherapy group: the role of therapeutic factors. *Research in Psychotherapy: Psychopathology, Process and Outcome*, 17(1), 43–51. doi:10.4081/ripppo.2014.161.

McClendon, D. T. & Burlingame, G. M. (2010). Group climate: Construct in search of clarity. In R. K. Conyne (Ed.), *The Oxford handbook of group counseling* (pp. 164–181). Oxford University Press.

Mio, D. S., Barker, D. A., Rodríguez, M. D., & Gonzalez, J. (2020). *Multicultural Psychology* (5th ed.). Oxford University Press.

Miles, J. R., Anders, C., Kivlighan III, D. M., & Belcher Platt, A. (2021). Cultural ruptures: Addressing microaggressions in group therapy. *Group Dynamics: Theory, Research, and Practice*, 25(1), 744–788. doi:10.1037/gdn0000149.

Miles, J. R. & Kivlighan, D. M., Jr. (2010). Co-leader similarity and group climate in group interventions: Testing the co-leadership team cognition-team diversity model. *Group Dynamics: Theory, Research, and Practice*, 14(2), 114–122. doi:10.1037/a0017503.

Miles, J. R. & Paquin, J. D. (2014). Best practices in group counseling and psychotherapy research. In J. L. Delucia-Waack, C. R. Kalodner, & M. Riva (Eds), *The handbook of group counseling and psychotherapy* (2nd ed.) (pp. 178–192). Sage Publications.

Miller, S. D., Hubble, M. A., Chow, D., & Seidel, J. (2015). Beyond measures and monitoring: Realizing the potential of feedback-informed treatment. *Psychotherapy*, *52(4)*, 449–457. doi:10.1037/pst0000031.

Moradi, B. & Grzanka, P. R. (2017). Using intersectionality responsibly: Toward critical epistemology, structural analysis, and social justice activism. *Journal of Counseling Psychology*, 64(5), 500–513. doi:10.1037/cou0000203.

Mosley, D. V., Hargons, C. N., Meiller, C., Angyal, B., Wheeler, P., Davis, C., & Stevens-Watkins, D. (2021). Critical consciousness of anti-black racism: A practical model to prevent and resist racial trauma. *Journal of Counseling Psychology*, 68(1), 1–16. doi:10.1037/cou0000430.

Muller, J. T. & Miles, J. R. (2017). Intergroup dialogue in undergraduate multicultural psychology education: Group climate development and outcomes. *Journal of Diversity in Higher Education*, 10(1), 52–71. doi:10.1037/a0040042.

Murillo, N., Shaffer, P., & Michael, W. B. (1981). The development and validation of a preliminary measure for student evaluation of group counseling experiences. *Educational and Psychological Measurement*, 41(2), 463–472. doi:10.1177/001316448104100225.

Neville, H. A., Awad, G. H., Brooks, J. E., Flores, M. P., & Bluemel, J. (2013). Color-blind racial ideology: Theory, training, and measurement implications in psychology. *American Psychologist*, 68(6), 455–466. doi:10.1037/a0033282.

Obeid, N., Carlucci, S., Brugnera, A., Compare, A., Proulx, G., Bissada, H., & Tasca, G. A. (2018). Reciprocal influence of distress and group therapeutic factors in day treatment for eating disorders: A progress and process monitoring study. *Psychotherapy*, 55(2), 170–178. doi:10.1037/pst0000138.

Ogrodniczuk, J. S., Cheek, J., & Kealy, D. (2021). Group therapy development: Implications for nontherapy groups. In C. D. Parks & G. A. Tasca (Eds), *The psychology of groups: The intersection of social psychology and psychotherapy research* (pp. 231–248). American Psychological Association.

Ogrodniczuk, J. S., Piper, W. E., Joyce, A. S., Lau, M. A., & Sochting, I. (2010). A survey of Canadian group psychotherapy association members' perceptions of psychotherapy research. *International Journal of Group Psychotherapy*, 60(2), 159–176. doi:10.1521/ijgp.2010.60.2.159.

O'Neill, R. M., Gantt, S. P. Burlingame, G. M., Mogle, J., Johnson, J., & Silver, R. (2013). Developing the systems-centered functional subgrouping questionnaire-2. *Group Dynamics: Theory, Research, and Practice*, 17(4), 252–269. doi:1kis.idm.oclc.org/10.1037/a0034925.

Orfanos, S., Burn, E., Priebe, S., & Spector. A. (2020). A systematic review and quality assessment of therapeutic group process questionnaires. *International Journal of Group Psychotherapy*, 70(3), 425–454. doi:10.1080/00207284.2020.1755292.

Owen, J. (2013). Early career perspectives on psychotherapy research and practice: Psychotherapist effects, multicultural orientation, and couple interventions. *Psychotherapy*, 50(4), 496–502. doi:10.1037/a0034617.

Owen, J., Tao, K. W., Drinane, J. M., Hook, J., Davis, D. E., & Kune, N. F. (2016). Client perceptions of therapists' multicultural orientation: Cultural (missed) opportunities and cultural humility. *Professional Psychology: Research and Practice*, 47(1), 30–37. doi:10.1037/pro0000046.

Owen, J. J., Tao, K., Leach, M. M., & Rodolfa, E. (2011). Clients' perceptions of their psychotherapists' multicultural orientation. *Psychotherapy*, 48(3), 274–282. doi:10.1037/a0022065.

Parks, C. D. & Tasca, G. A. (2021). *The psychology of groups: The intersection of social psychology and psychotherapy research*. The American Psychological Association. hdoi:10.1037/0000201-000.

Parks, C. D. & Tasca, G. A. (2021). *Introduction: Groups as vehicles for change, growth, and productivity*. In C. D.Parks & G. A. Tasca (Eds), *The psychology of groups: The intersection of social psychology and psychotherapy research* (pp. 3–9). American Psychological Association. doi:10.1037/0000201-001.

Pascual-Leone, A. & Andreescu, C. (2013). Repurposing process measures to train psychotherapists: Training outcomes using a new approach. *Counselling & Psychotherapy Research*, 13(3), 210–219. doi:1kis.idm.oclc.org/10.1080/14733145.2012.739633.

Quirk, K., Miller, S., Duncan, B., & Owen, J. (2013). Group session rating scale: Preliminary psychometrics in substance abuse group interventions. *Counselling & Psychotherapy Research*, 13(3), 194–200. doi:10.1080/14733145.2012.744425.

Ruiz, M. A., Pincus, A. L., Borkovec, T. D., Echemendia, R. J., Castonguay, L. G., & Ragusa, S. A. (2004). Validity of the Inventory of Interpersonal Problems for predicting treatment outcome: An investigation with the Pennsylvania Practice Research Network. *Journal of Personality Assessment, 83*, 213–222. https://dx.doi.org/10.1027/s15327752jpa8303_05

Riva, M. T., Wachtel, M., & Lasky, G. B. (2004). Effective leadership in group counseling and psychotherapy: Research and practice. In J. L. DeLucia-Waack, D. A. Gerrity, C. R. Kalodner & M. T. Riva (Eds), *Handbook of group counseling and psychotherapy* (pp. 37–48). Sage Publications.

Shin, R. Q., Ezeofor, I., Smith, L. C., Welch, J. C., & Goodrich, K. M. (2016). The development and validation of the contemporary critical consciousness measure. *Journal of Counseling Psychology*, 63(2), 210–223. doi:10.1037/cou0000137.

Shin, R. Q., Smith, L. C., Lu, Y., Welch, J. C., Sharma, R., Vernay, C. N., & Yee, S. (2018). The development and validation of the contemporary critical consciousness measure II. *Journal of Counseling Psychology*, 65(5), 539–555. doi:10.1037/cou0000302.

Slone, N. C.& Owen, J. (2015). Therapist alliance activity, therapist comfort, and systemic alliance on individual psychotherapy outcome. *Journal of Psychotherapy Integration*, 25(4), 275–288. doi:10.1037/a0039562.

Slone, N. C., Reese, R. J., Mathews-Duvall, S., & Kodet, J. (2015). Evaluating the efficacy of client feedback in group psychotherapy. *Group Dynamics: Theory, Research, and Practice*, 19(2), 122–136. doi:10.1037/gdn0000026.

Solstad, S. M., Castonguay, L. G., & Moltu, C. (2019). Patients' experiences with routine outcome monitoring and clinical feedback systems: A systematic review and synthesis of qualitative empirical literature. *Psychotherapy Research*, 29, 157–170. doi:10.1080/10503307.2017.1326645.

Solstad, S. M., Kleiven, G. S., Castonguay, L. G., & Moltu, C. (2021). Clinical dilemmas of routine outcome monitoring and clinical feedback: A qualitative study of patient experiences. *Psychotherapy Research*, 31, 200–210, doi:10.1080/10503307.2020.1788741.

Solstad, S. M. , Kleiven, G. S., & Moltu, C. (2021) Complexity and potentials of clinical feedback in mental health: an in-depth study of patient processes. *Quality of Life Research*, 30, 3117–3125, doi:10.1007/s11136-020-02550-1.

Stock, D. & Thelen, H. A. (1958). Member perceptions as a factor in subgrouping: Introduction. In D. Stock & H. A. Thelen, *Emotional dynamics and group culture: Experimental studies of individual and group behavior* (pp. 67–70). New York: New York University Press.

Strauss, B. (2021). "You can't make an omelet without breaking eggs". Studies on side effects and adverse effects in group psychotherapy. *International Journal of Group Psychotherapy*, 71(3), 472–480. doi:10.1080/00207284.2021.1890089.

Sue, D. W. (2015). *Race talk and the conspiracy of silence: Understanding and facilitating difficult dialogues on race.* Hoboken, NJ: John Wiley & Sons Inc.

Sue, D. W., Alsaidi, S., Awad, M. N., Glaeser, E., Calle, C. Z., & Mendez, N. (2019). Disarming racial microaggressions: Microintervention strategies for targets, white allies, and bystanders. *American Psychologist, 74(*1), 128–142. doi:10.1037/amp0000296.

Sue, D. W., Arredondo, P., & McDavis, R. J. (1992). Multicultural counseling competencies and standards: A call to the profession. *Journal of Multicultural Counseling and Development*, 20(2), 64–88. doi:10.1002/j.2161-1912.1992.tb00563.x.

Sue, D. W. & Spanierman, L. B. (2020). *Microaggressions in everyday life* (2nd ed.). John Wiley & Sons.

Svien, H., Burlingame, G. M., Griner, D., Beecher, M. E., & Alldredge, C. T. (2021). Group therapeutic relationship change: Using routine outcome monitoring to detect the effect of single versus multiple ruptures. *Group Dynamics: Theory, Research, and Practice*, 25(1), 45–58. doi:10.1037/gdn0000148.

Tasca, G. (2021). Twenty-five years of *Group Dynamics: Theory, research and practice*: Introduction to the special issue. *Group Dynamics: Theory, Research, and Practice*, 25, 205–212. doi:10.1037/gdn0000167.

Tasca, G. A. (2016). Statistical methods in group psychology and group psychotherapy: Introduction to the special issue. *Group Dynamics: Theory, Research, and Practice*, 20(3), 121–125. doi:10.1037/gdn0000054.

Tasca, G. A., Cabrera, Ch., Kristjansson, E., MacNair-Semands, R., Joyce, A. S., & Ogrodniczuk, J. S. (2016). The therapeutic factor inventory-8: Using item response theory to create a brief scale for continuous process monitoring for group psychotherapy, *Psychotherapy Research*, 26(2), 131–145. doi:10.1080/10503307.2014.963729.

Tasca, G. A., Foot, M., Leite, C., Maxwell, H., Balfour, L., & Bissada, H (2011) Interpersonal processes in psychodynamic-interpersonal and cognitive behavioral group therapy: A systematic case study of two groups. *Psychotherapy, 48(3)*, 260–273. doi:10.1037/a0023928.

Thayer, S. D. & Burlingame, G. M. (2014). The validity of the Group Questionnaire: Construct clarity or construct drift? *Group Dynamics: Theory, Research, and Practice*, 18(4), 318–332. doi:1kis.idm.oclc.org/10.1037/gdn0000015.

Treadwell, T., Lavertue, N., Kumar, V. K, & Veeraraghavan, V. (2001). The Group Cohesion Scale-Revised: Reliability and validity. *Journal of Group Psychotherapy, Psychodrama and Sociometry*, 54(1), 3.

Tucker, J. R., Wade, N. G., Abraham, W. T., Bitman-Heinrichs, R., Cornish, M. A., & Post, B. C. (2020). Modeling cohesion change in group counseling: The role of client characteristics, group variables, and leader behaviors. *Journal of Counseling Psychology*, 67(3), 371–385. doi:10.1037/cou0000403.

Tuckman, B. W. & Jensen, M. A. (1977). Stages of small-group development revisited. *Group & Organization Studies*, 2, 419–427. doi:10.1177/105960117700200404.

Vera, E. M. & Speight, S. L. (2003). Multicultural competence, social justice, and counseling psychology: Expanding our roles. *The Counseling Psychologist*, 31(3), 253–272. doi:10.1177/0011000003031003001.

Wheelan, S. A. (2005). *Group process: A developmental perspective* (2nd ed.). Allyn & Bacon.

Whitcomb, K. E., O'Neill, R. M., Burlingame, G. M., Mogle, J. Gantt, S. P., Cannon, J. A. N., & Roney, T. (2018). Measuring how systems-centered® members connect with group dynamics: FSQ-2 construct validity. *International Journal of Group Psychotherapy*, 68 (2), 163–183. doi:1kis.idm.oclc.org/10.1080/00207284.2017.1381024.

Whitcomb, K. E., Woodland, S. C., & Burlingame, G. M. (2018). Do clinicians really use feedback-monitoring systems? A qualitative analysis of 16 group leaders. *Psychotherapy*, 55(2), 132–143. doi:10.1037/pst0000141.

Wongpakaran, T., Wongpakaran, N., Intachote-Sakamoto, R., & Boripuntakul, T. (2013). The group cohesiveness scale (GCS) for psychiatric inpatients. *Perspectives in psychiatric care*, 49(1), 58–64. doi:10.1111/j.1744-6163.2012.00342.x.

Woodland, S., Gilliland, R., & Blue Star, J. (2022). Cohesion and chronic pain: A case for assessing an overlooked process variable. *Psychotherapy*, 59(2), 271–283. doi:10.1037/pst0000405.

Yalom, I. D. & Leszcz, M. (2020). *The theory and practice of group psychotherapy* (6th ed.) Basic Books.

4 Assessing Outcomes in Group Psychotherapy

Martin Kivlighan and Giorgio A. Tasca

In this chapter, we address the question of measuring outcomes in group psychotherapy. Many stakeholders could be interested in the effectiveness of a group intervention. Clients may want an objective sense of how they are doing in a therapy group, or how previous clients have fared before they commit to a particular course of treatment. Therapists may be interested in their own outcomes to guide future treatment decisions, to indicate where to focus their continuing education, to inform future clients of the effectiveness of the group therapy, or to justify compensation for their work. By the same token, agencies or third-party payers may want to know if their funds are being used well to provide treatment to clients. And more broadly, the public, politicians, and the research community have a stake in whether the mental health problems in a population are treated optimally.

What defines an appropriate outcome for group treatment depends on several factors, including the goals of the treatment. Ideally, goals for group therapy should be agreed upon by clients and therapists. The collaborative agreement between client and therapist on the goals of therapy should be one of the first tasks as they begin therapeutic work. The agreement on goals is a key component of a therapeutic alliance (Fluckiger et al., 2018) which is an important predictor of outcomes in group therapy (Alldredge et al., 2021; Lo Coco et al., 2022). Disagreement or lack of clarity on goals indicates clients and therapists are working at cross purposes, which will negatively affect client outcomes. The type and focus of the treatment should also align with the client's goals. Thus, the outcome measures should reflect the client's goals and what the treatment targets. For example, if the treatment's focus is on providing education about a certain client condition (like depression or anxiety), then the goal for this aspect of the treatment might be to increase the client's knowledge of their condition. In this case, the outcome measurement should emphasize the client's uptake and retention of the information (and not necessarily a reduction in symptoms, although reduced symptoms may also occur). A broader goal for group therapy might be to improve a client's quality of relationships. In that case, a component of the treatment should focus on interpersonal conflicts or style, and an outcome measure might assess change in interpersonal functioning. On the other hand, if clients and therapists agree that symptom reduction is the goal and if the focus of the group therapy is on the client's symptoms (e.g., anxiety, depression), then the appropriate outcome to measure are the symptoms targeted by the group therapy.

One of the aims of this chapter is to help clinicians to select psychometrically sound outcome measures to assess client change in group psychotherapy. However, we first address the questions of why this is necessary. The assessment of outcomes from psychotherapy is a complex process made more complicated by the group context. Judgments of patient mental health outcomes require the therapist to make several determinations, including: a) an accurate assessment of the level of the client's symptoms (e.g., depression) and whether the symptoms are clinically elevated (i.e., within the range typical of clinically

DOI: 10.4324/9781003255482-4

depressed people) at the start of group therapy; b) that the client's level of depression improved (i.e., symptoms reduced) due to group therapy; and c) that the client's level of depression at the end of therapy is within the range typical of non-depressed people. Making such accurate judgments involves knowing the signs of depression in the client, knowing what a clinical level of depression is, estimating how much reduction in particular symptoms is meaningful, and knowing the base rates or common levels of symptoms among the population of depressed and non-depressed individuals. Further complicating matters are potential conscious and unconscious biases that may occur when making clinical judgements in an emotionally charged context such as group therapy. Clients may not want to appear ungrateful when asked if they were helped, and therapists may not want to be perceived as less effective than ideal. No wonder psychotherapists are notoriously poor at identifying clients who deteriorate in psychotherapy (Lambert, 2017), and therapists often over-estimate their own effectiveness relative to peers (Walfish et al., 2012).

Validated psychometric tests provide tools that aid clinicians in making these complex judgments about client progress. Psychometric assessment is not meant to diminish the role of clinical judgement, expertise, and experience, but rather to enhance clinical decision-making skills. Such instruments provide useful information about what is a clinical or non-clinical level of a symptom or set of symptoms, and how much change is clinically meaningful. In the development phase, these instruments are often given to large samples of those representing clinical and non-clinical populations (e.g., depressed and/or non-depressed individuals). Sometimes the data that researchers gather about the instruments are further subdivided by sex, ethnicity, race, age, language, and other meaningful individual factors. These data allow the clinician to make more fine-tuned determinations about the client's outcomes that may be affected by these individual client factors. The process of validating a scale also provides information about what is a clinically elevated score relative to the population (a clinical cut-off score), and how much change in that score is a reliable indicator of improvement or deterioration. For example, a score of greater than 15 on the Patient Health Questionnaire (PHQ-9; Kroenke et al., 2010) indicates moderately severe depression, and a score of less than 5 indicates no clinically meaningful depression. These cut-off scores are based on thousands of individuals who are clinically depressed or not depressed. A reduction of 5 points or more in PHQ-9 scores from pre- to post-treatment (for example a score going from 16 to 4) indicates that the client's depressive symptoms reliably improved. If a PHQ-9 score is below 5 at post-treatment *and* reduced by 5 points or more from pre-treatment, then one could say that the client reliably recovered. As illustrated by this example, a psychometrically valid scale can provide an invaluable aid in helping the clinician to make complex judgments about client improvement and recovery that is not only based on their own personal history with depressed patients but is also informed by data from large studies in the general and clinical populations.

Progress Monitoring

We make a distinction between progress monitoring and outcome monitoring. In progress monitoring, typically the client completes a brief measure of symptoms or functioning after every session or after every few sessions. The information about the client's progress relative to their previous session and relative to clinical and non-clinical norms is provided to therapists. If the client is progressing as expected, then the therapists may use this information to continue the therapy as is. However, if the client is showing higher levels of distress or is deteriorating relative to their previous levels and relative to the norm, then the therapist might change some process in therapy to correct course.

There is now substantial research on the utility of progress monitoring used in this manner. In a meta-analysis, Lambert et al. (2018) reviewed 24 studies and found that two-thirds of the studies reported that psychotherapy with progress monitoring was superior to treatment-as-usual offered by the same practitioners. Mean standardized effect sizes indicated that the effects ranged from small to moderate. Most importantly, progress monitoring and feedback to the therapist reduced client deterioration rates and nearly doubled rates of clinically reliable change in clients who otherwise would have had a poor outcome.

There are a few examples of the effects of progress monitoring and feedback in group therapy. For example, Schuman et al. (2015) used the Partners for Change Outcome Management System (PCOMS) (Miller et al., 2005) which includes the Outcome Rating Scale (ORS) (Duncan et al., 2015) in a group substance abuse program for active-duty soldiers. Participants were randomly assigned to a feedback condition in which therapists received feedback about patient progress (n = 137) or treatment as usual (n = 126). Soldiers of therapists in the feedback condition achieved significantly better outcomes than those in treatment as usual. In another study (Slone et al., 2015), clients in a university counseling center (n = 84) were randomly assigned to a feedback condition or treatment as usual. Those in the feedback condition had better outcomes and attended more group therapy sessions.

Outcome Monitoring

By contrast, outcome monitoring refers to collecting data to assess patient functioning (e.g., symptoms, quality of life, psychosocial adaptation), usually at pre-treatment and at post-treatment. In this manner, clinicians can assess the impact of group therapy on mental disorders and related conditions. These procedures have been the cornerstone of demonstrating the efficacy of group therapy for several decades. Recently, a number of meta-analyses showed that group therapy is more effective than no treatment and as effective as individual therapy for most common conditions (see Burlingame et al., 2016; Janis et al., 2020; Grenon et al., 2017).

Is collecting outcomes in routine clinical practice feasible? Hunsley and Lee (2007) reviewed 35 studies evaluating pre- and post-treatment outcomes in routine psychological practices. Hunsley and Lee illustrated how such outcome monitoring is possible in real world settings, and how the outcomes are comparable to those achieved in clinical trials. However, one of the challenges to collecting outcome data is that up to 40 percent of patients in clinical practices may drop out of treatment and thus do not provide post-treatment data to assess outcomes (Swift & Greenberg, 2012). One solution is to measure outcomes repeatedly during treatment, thus providing outcome values closer to the last session attended by a client. Such a strategy brings this clinical practice closer to progress monitoring especially if the clinician has access to the client's scores at previous sessions and to normative or clinical population data.

Reasons to Engage in Outcome Monitoring

We focused earlier on the reasons for assessing outcomes that include informing the therapy and providing an alternative perspective in addition to clinical observation, providing information to the client so they can make informed choices, and responsibility to third party payers. Another important reason includes the continuing development of therapist skills in a professional or training context. For example, research indicates that on average therapists tend to be very skilled or effective with approximately two patient problem domains (e.g., depression, anxiety), and reliably ineffective on average for approximately one patient problem domain (Constantino et al., 2021). Therapists and prospective clients may not be aware of those areas for which a therapist is particularly effective or ineffective. However, outcome monitoring can give therapists much needed information about their effectiveness in various areas of client functioning. Therapists who assess their outcomes with a range of client problems by using valid psychometric instruments can identify areas that require further training and supervision.

This brings us to some ethical considerations. Professional regulatory bodies increasingly require registrants to be more accountable for ongoing professional development. Some professional codes of ethics indicate an ethical obligation to evaluate services provided and work within one's boundaries of competence (American Psychological Association, 2017), and scholars have underscored the utility of outcome monitoring to uphold ethical standards (Muir et al., 2019; Pinner & Kivlighan, 2018). Progress and outcome monitoring help fulfill these obligations to the profession and to clients. Progress and outcome monitoring are also integral parts of evidence-based practice (Dozois et al., 2014; Tasca et al., 2019).

Nevertheless, there is a well-documented research-practice gap in many areas of health care including psychotherapy (Ionita & Fitzpatrick, 2014; Solstad et al., 2017). Clinicians may see brief questionnaires as too superficial for complex contexts like group therapy, and others may express concerns about progress monitoring being used primarily for performance audits rather than to inform clinical decision making (Tasca et al., 2019). Research indicates that clinicians are more likely to use progress monitoring when the measures fit their approaches (Knoll et al., 2016), when they have direct clinical experience with the measures (Gyani et al., 2015), when it is not perceived as an extra burden, and when they receive adequate training in their use (Persons et al., 2016). Another concern expressed by therapists is that clients will respond negatively to filling out questionnaires. However, research indicates that clients feel empowered by the process of assessing their outcomes and that using the measures facilitated collaboration with the therapist (Solstad et al., 2017).

In the end, which outcome measure to select will depend in part on the context of the therapy and values of the therapist, client, or third-party payer. The choice of outcome measure may be linked to theory (e.g., measuring change in cognitive distortions based on a cognitive-behavioral model of depression, or measuring a reduction in interpersonal problems in a psychodynamic therapy), mechanisms of change (e.g., that Socratic questioning results in reduced cognitive distortions and improved depressive affect, or that transference interpretations reduce patterns of interpersonal distress), client or therapist values (e.g., their collaborative agreement on the goals of therapy), or what the insurance company or agency values (e.g., return to work, reduced readmissions). As mentioned, a therapist's intention to use outcome measures will depend in part on whether the therapist perceives the measure to be useful and the measure's fits with the therapist's clinical values (Knoll et al., 2016).

How to Select an Outcome Measure

The task of selecting an outcome measure may seem complicated, and there are several issues that a clinician must consider. One might be tempted to create a homemade measure as a means of documenting change in a therapy group. We advise clinicians against this. For example, a clinician asks all clients attending a group for depression to complete a one-question measure that asks, "on a scale of 1 (very low) to 10 (very high), how sad do you feel right now?" Intuitively, this seems to tap into a depressive affect – a level of sadness. But how does one interpret a score of "6" on this scale? Does this level represent more or less sadness than someone who is clinically depressed or someone who is not depressed? If the client started group therapy with a score of "8" on this scale, does a score of "6" at the end of treatment indicate reliable improvement? Also, the question only taps into one aspect of the construct of depression which also might include disturbed sleep, change in appetite, low self-esteem, poor concentration, and impaired social and work functioning. Does feeling sad alone really mean "depression"?

Another challenge is the issue of what is meant by "psychometrically sound." The concept of psychometric soundness refers to the reliability and the validity of the scale, and to the availability of standardized norms to aid in interpreting scores. In the next section, we will review the notion of psychometric soundness only in the context of client self-report measures, as clinicians most frequently use these to assess client outcomes.

Reliability of Outcome Measures

Reliability in psychometrics refers to the consistency of the items or the scores, indicating the measure's stability. A common assessment of reliability includes the *internal consistency* of a measure, which refers to how stable items are within a scale or the unidimensionality of the scale items. That is, do the items of a scale relate to each other and thus to a common construct? Metrics for internal consistency include the Cronbach's alpha coefficient and the mean inter-item correlation. Typically, for clinical applications, a Cronbach's alpha coefficient of .80 or higher or a mean inter-item correlation between .15 and .50 indicates adequate internal consistency (Clark & Watson, 2019). Another common indicator of reliability is the *test-retest stability*, which indicates how consistent a scale score is across time or re-assessments. One would expect that a scale score related to some common mental health outcomes (depression, anxiety) should be stable or consistent at least in the short term. A typical metric for test-retest stability is the Pearson correlation coefficient, and a test-retest correlation of .80 or higher for repeated testing that occurs two weeks later indicates good stability of a scale (Clark & Watson, 2019).

Validity of Outcome Measures

Validity in psychometrics generally refers to the degree to which a scale measures the construct it is purported to measure. A common concept used in this regard is *construct validity* which encompasses various types of metrics. We will focus only on a few that are of particular interest to client self-report of outcome measurement. The first is *content validity*, which refers to the extent to which the scale items reflect the construct being measured. This was illustrated in the example above in which only sadness was measured to indicate depression, but low self-esteem, problems with sleep and eating, reduced concentration, and impaired functioning were not assessed. The single item on sadness had limited content validity because it did not represent all of what encompasses depression. The second type of validity is *predictive validity*, which, in the case of the depression example, refers to the extent to which the scale differentiates those who are depressed from those who are not depressed. A third indicator of construct validity refers to the *factor structure* of a scale. Typically, authors will use a factor analysis to see if items of a scale representing a construct are related to each other while at the same time remaining largely unrelated to items representing other constructs. For example, one might expect those items indicating depression would be related to each other to a greater degree than to items indicating panic disorder. Finally, *concurrent validity* is sometimes reported by researchers. This usually refers to the degree to which a scale is correlated with another scale measuring the same construct. For example, if we develop a self-report scale of depression, then its score should correlate at least moderately with another valid clinician-rated scale of depression.

Standardized Norms

A key issue of useful psychometric measures is that they should have standardized norms. Norms allow clinicians to assess whether a client's score on a scale is within the range of scores typical for someone with the disorder or problem, or whether the score is within the range typical of someone who does not have the disorder or problem. Published norms for a scale are based on hundreds, if not thousands of people in the clinical and non-clinical populations. Some well-validated outcome measures include published clinical cut-off scores intended to help a clinician to decide about a patient's condition. In addition to norms indicating the clinical level of a condition or symptom, some measures also indicate the degree of change in scores that is necessary to indicate that the change is reliable and meaningful, and also whether the reliable change resulted in the client no longer being symptomatic (i.e., recovered).

Cross-Cultural Uses and Implications

Often, psychometric measures are developed for an English-speaking population. And at times, the sample of patients or participants on which the scale norms and clinical cut-offs are based can be limited. For example, if the standardized norms are from a primarily White English-speaking sample of patients from the United States, then these norms may not generalize to patients of other cultural and ethnic groups. In their review of issues raised by applying psychometric scales cross-culturally, Bader and colleagues (2021) identified several potential causes of bias or error when applying scales cross-culturally. For example, translations across languages may be inconsistent resulting in differences caused by the translation. Also, there may be actual differences between cultural groups on the constructs of interest. Furthermore, when a scale developed in English is given to a non-native English speaker, the findings might be due to misunderstanding or issues with language comprehension. Bader and colleague's review highlights that the very meaning of the scale's scores themselves may be affected. In other words, one may not be able to interpret scale scores in the same way across cultures and languages.

We encourage clinicians to use scales that were adequately validated for the population of which the individual patient or group is a member. In the sections below in which we describe useful scales for measuring group therapy progress and outcomes, we also identify if the scale has been validated for diverse groups. However, in the absence of such cross-cultural validation data, and when feasible, the clinician might consider partnering with a researcher who is knowledgeable in psychometrics to do some of the preliminary psychometric work for a particular population. This might involve collecting a sample of patient data from a specific cultural, ethnic, or linguistic group, and evaluating if the factor structure and the internal consistency of the scales are similar to those reported for the original validation sample. Otherwise, we urge clinicians to use scales that were not validated for a particular population of patients with caution as the interpretation of the scale scores may be biased due to the unknown validity for that population.

Where to Find Valid and Reliable Outcome Measures

There are a number of accessible and free scales that are brief and user-friendly. Clinicians should look for scales that are valid and reliable, that offer clinical cut-offs based on normative and clinical data. A clinical cut-off refers to a score that is high or low relative to the norm and that identifies a clinically important level of a symptom. For example, someone who is clinically depressed is much more likely to score 15 or above on the PHQ-9 than someone who is not clinically depressed. Thus, a score of 15 or higher on the PHQ-9 represents its clinical cut-off. Also, outcome measures should provide some indication of how much of a difference in scores from pre- to post-treatment indicates a reliable index of meaningful change (Jacobson & Truax, 1991). On the PHQ-9, a change of 5 points or more indicates reliable improvement and not just chance fluctuation in scores. We also encourage clinicians to use scales that provide clinical cut-offs and reliable change indices specific to individual client factors like sex, gender, race, ethnicity, age, and sexual orientation when indicated and feasible. That is, clinical cut-off scores and reliable change indices might differ across populations. Better psychometric scales provide these indices for a variety of populations.

There are several good resources that clinicians can use to identify appropriate scales for outcome measurement. Hunsley and Mash's (2018) book *A Guide to Assessments that Work* includes both technical and practical help to select measures, including lists of measures and their description. Beidas and colleagues (2015) provide a list of free and validated measurements including how to access these measures (see: www.ncbi.nlm.nih.gov/pmc/arti cles/PMC4310476/pdf/nihms-589127.pdf). The Society of Clinical Psychology of the American Psychological Association is currently working on an assessment repository that promises to house numerous valid measures (see https://div12.org/assessment-repository/). The Joint Commission's Behavioral Healthcare Instruments Listing provides a comprehensive description of many scales, references to the scales, and how to obtain them (see: https://manual.jointcommission.org/BHCInstruments/WebHome?_ga=2.265414857.712589292.1615323669-1992168669.1615323669). Currently, two sites provide immediate access to free scales. Psychologytools.com lists numerous useful scales for a variety of purposes many of which are free (see: www.psychologytools.com/download-scales-and-measures). HealthMeasures.net comprises four comprehensive systems for measuring mental health, physical health, and quality of life. The site is searchable and provides some free to use scales (see: www.healthmeasures.net/index.php).

Recommended Outcome Measures

We recommend using outcome measures for group practice that are a) brief and user-friendly; b) valid and reliable; and c) provide clinical cut-off scores and reliable indices of meaningful change based on normative and clinical data. Given these criteria, we identified the following outcome measures: Outcome Questionnaire – 45.2 (OQ-45.2) (Lambert et al., 2004), Youth Outcome Questionnaire – 30.2 (YOQ-30.2) (Burlingame et al., 2005), Patient Health Questionnaire – 9 (PHQ-9) (Kroenke et al., 2001), Generalized Anxiety Disorder – 7 (GAD-7) (Spitzer et al., 2006), and the Outcome Rating Scale (ORS) (Duncan & Reese, 2015). Most of these outcome measures assess psychological symptoms, however, we recognize that group therapy goals might also include diverse areas of client functioning and domains (i.e., affect regulation, interpersonal functioning, well-being, etc.). For these areas, we recommend several additional outcome measures despite not meeting all the recommended criteria above. These measures include the Inventory of Interpersonal Problems – 32 (IIP-32) (Barkham et al., 1996), Difficulties in Emotion Regulation Scale (DERS) (Gratz & Roemer, 2004), WHO Quality of Life Measure – Brief version (WHOQOL-BREF) (World Health Organization, 1996), and the Experiences in Close Relationships Scale (ECR-12; Lafontaine et al., 2015). Below we provide a brief description of the measures we recommend for outcome monitoring in group therapy with attention to the psychometric properties, normed data, and use and scoring of each measure.

Outcome Questionnaire – 45.2 (OQ-45.2) (Lambert et al., 2004)

The Outcome Questionnaire (OQ-45) is a self-report instrument designed for repeated measurement of adult patient progress over the course of therapy, at termination and beyond. It was designed to assess three key areas of functioning: symptomatic distress (e.g., *I feel hopeless about the future*), interpersonal functioning (e.g., *I feel lonely*), and social role performance (e.g., *I feel stressed at work/school*). Items are rated on a 5-point Likert-type scale (0

= Never to 4 = Almost Always), yielding a possible range of scores of 0 to 180, with higher scores indicating greater pathology. The OQ-45.2 provides subscale scores for all three areas of functioning, as well as an overall total score. The Symptom Distress subscale assesses symptoms from the most frequently diagnosed mental disorders. Its items emphasize depression and anxiety symptoms and also include items for the detection of substance dependence. The Interpersonal Relations subscale includes items that assess problems with friendships, family life, and marriage. Other items address issues associated with isolation, feelings of inadequacy, withdrawal, and interpersonal conflict. The Social Role Performance subscale includes items that gauge the patient's level of dissatisfaction, conflict, or distress in their employment, family roles, and leisure activities. The OQ-45 total score that is derived from all of the items from the three subscales represents a metric of global distress across all three areas of functioning.

Administration of the OQ-45.2 requires about 5–7 minutes and scoring takes about 3–5 minutes. The OQ-45.2 can be easily scored by hand, although computer administration and scoring software are available (www.oqmeasures.com). The OQ-45.2 is a psychometrically sound measure (Lambert et al., 2004). Based on normative samples collected from sites across the United States and Germany, internal consistency and test-retest reliability estimates range from .70 to .93 and .66 to .86, respectively. Studies reveal high correlations with specific measures of depression, anxiety, interpersonal functioning, and social adjustment. Using normative data from patients and non-patients, the following criteria were developed to indicate clinically significant change and reliable change on the OQ-45. *Clinically significant change* refers to a patient's score moving from a dysfunctional range at pre-treatment to a functional range of scores at post-treatment or follow up. That is, the patient's score is no longer in the clinically elevated range at post-treatment. For the OQ-45, the clinically significant cut-off score is 63. Scores above this cut-off are considered dysfunctional, while scores below are considered functional. A patient must move from a score above the cut-off of 63 to below in order to make clinically significant change. *Reliable change* refers to change that exceeds the natural variation in scores due to error. The reliable change criterion for the OQ-45 is 14. Thus, for a patient to make reliable change on the OQ-45, their score must change by at least 14 points from pre- to post-treatment. Clinically significant change and reliable change should be considered together. Thus, if a patient who begins therapy with a score of 64 or greater ends treatment with a score below 64 and has at least a 14-point change in their OQ-45 score, they then can be considered to have achieved meaningful clinical change (i.e., recovered). Using these two criteria, patient change can be classified into one of four categories: improvement (scores reduced by 14 points or more but still in the clinical range [above 64]), deterioration (scores increased by 14 points or more), no change (scores did not change by 14 points or more), and recovery (scores reduced by 14 points or more and no longer falling in the clinical range [below 64]). Although widely used, the OQ-45.2 does have the disadvantage of offering global rather than disorder-specific symptom scales.

Although the OQ-45.2 was originally normed with majority US-based White samples, a large amount of research has examined the validity and psychometric properties of the OQ-45.2 across different cultures and languages. The OQ-45.2 has been translated and validated in Dutch (de Jong et al., 2007), Portuguese (De Francisco Carvalho & Rocha, 2009), Hebrew and Arabic (Raz Gross et al., 2015), German (Lambert et al., 2002), Italian (Lo Coco et al., 2008), Spanish (Iraurgi & Penas, 2021), and Chinese (She et al., 2017). Although this is not an exhaustive list of all research that has considered translation bias of the OQ-45.2, it is evident that the OQ-45.2 has been validated in many different languages. In addition, researchers have also examined the validity of the OQ-45.2 across various cultural and racial groups, such as African American, Asian, Pacific Islander, Latino/a, and Native American populations (Lambert et al., 2006). See Table 4.1 for more information on the OQ-45.

Table 4.1 Outcome Questionnaire – 45.2 (OQ-45.2)

Item	Information
Name of Instrument	**Outcome Questionnaire – 45.2 (OQ-45.2)**
Authors	Michael J. Lambert & Gary M. Burlingame
Source	Lambert, M. J., Morton, J. J., Hatfield, D., Harmon, C., Hamilton, S., Reid, R. C., & Burlingame, G. M. (2004). Administration and scoring manual for the Outcome Questionnaire-45. Salt Lake City, UT: OQ Measures.
Brief Description	The Outcome Questionnaire (OQ-45) is a self-report instrument designed for repeated measurement of adult patient progress through the course of therapy and at termination. It was designed to assess three key aspects of the patient's life: a) subjective discomfort; b) interpersonal relationships; and c) social role performance. Items on this instrument address commonly occurring problems across a wide variety of disorders and assess the symptoms most likely to occur.
Time Issues	Administration: < 5 min Scoring: < 7 min
Subscales and Scoring	Items are rated on a 5-point Likert-type scale (0 = Never to 4 = Almost Always), yielding a possible range of scores of 0 to 180, with higher scores indicating greater pathology. The OQ-45.2 provides subscale scores for all three areas of functioning, as well as an overall total score. The Symptom Distress subscale assesses symptoms from the most frequently diagnosed mental disorders. Its items emphasize depression and anxiety symptoms and also includes items for the detection of substance dependence. The Interpersonal Relations subscale includes items that assess problems with friendships, family life, and marriage. Other items address issues associated with isolation, feelings of inadequacy, withdrawal, and interpersonal conflict. The Social Role Performance subscale includes items that gauge the patient's level of dissatisfaction, conflict, or distress in their employment, family roles, and leisure activities. The OQ-45 total score that is derived from all of the items from the three subscales represents a metric of global distress across all three areas of functioning.
Psychometric Properties	The OQ-45.2 is a psychometrically sound measure (Lambert et al., 2004). Based on normative samples collected from sites across the United States and Germany, internal consistency and test-retest reliability estimates range from .70 to. 93 and .66 to. 86, respectively. Studies reveal high correlations with specific measures of depression, anxiety, interpersonal functioning, and social adjustment.
Norms and any normative data re: diversity for each instrument	Although the OQ-45.2 was originally normed with majority US-based White samples, a large amount of research has examined the validity and psychometric properties of the OQ-45.2 across different cultures and languages. Researchers have examined the validity of the OQ-45.2 across various cultural and racial groups, such as African American, Asian, Pacific Islander, Latino/a, and Native American populations (Lambert et al., 2006).
Translations	The OQ-45.2 has been translated and validated in Dutch (de Jong et al., 2007), Portuguese (Carvalho & Rocha, 2009), Hebrew and Arabic (Raz Gross et al., 2015), German (Lambert et al., 2002), Italian (Lo Coco et al., 2008), Spanish (Iraurgi & Penas, 2021), and Chinese (She et al., 2017). Although this is not an exhaustive list of all research that has considered translation bias of the OQ-45.2, it is evident that the OQ-45.2 has been validated in many different languages.

Item	Information
Sensitivity to Change	Using normative data from patients and non-patients, the following criteria were developed to indicate clinically significant change and reliable change on the OQ-45. For the OQ-45, the clinically significant cut-off score is 63. Scores above this cut-off are considered dysfunctional, while scores below are considered functional. The reliable change criterion for the OQ-45 is 14. Thus, for a patient to make reliable change on the OQ-45, their score must change by at least 14 points from pre- to post-treatment.
Sample references	Boswell, D. L., White, J. K., Sims, W. D., Harrist, R. S., & Romans, J. S. (2013). Reliability and validity of the Outcome Questionnaire–45.2. Psychological Reports, 112(3), 689–693. Rice, K. G., Suh, H., & Ege, E. (2014). Further evaluation of the Outcome Questionnaire–45.2. Measurement and Evaluation in Counseling and Development, 47(2), 102–117.
Website Resources	www.oqmeasures.com
How to Obtain/Cost	Proprietary-sample copy provided herein. License required with no per use cost.
Administration Types	Paper and Pencil/Electronic
Analytics	Administration, scoring and interpretive portfolio software identifying treatment failure cases.
Benchmarking	N/A

Youth Outcome Questionnaire – 30.2 (YOQ-30.2) (Burlingame et al., 2004)

The YOQ-30.2 is the youth and adolescent version of the Outcome Questionnaire. This measure is a 30-item outcome instrument that can either be completed by the patient (YOQ-30.2 SR) or a parent/guardian (YOQ-30.2 PR) for youth and adolescents ages 4–17 in treatment. Items are rated on a 5-point Likert-type scale (0 = Never to 4 = Almost Always). In addition to the total score, which provides an overall indication of patient functioning, the Y-OQ also provides six subscale scores, Intrapersonal Distress, Somatic, Interpersonal Relations, Social Problems, Behavioral Dysfunction, and Critical Items. The Intrapersonal Distress scale is a measure of emotional distress that the patient is experiencing, including symptoms of anxiety, depression, fearfulness, hopelessness, and self-harm. The Somatic scale assesses bodily distress, such as headaches, dizziness, stomach aches, nausea, and bowel difficulties. The Interpersonal Relations scale assesses issues relevant to the patient's relationships with parents, other adults, and peers. The Social Problems scale reflects problematic behaviors that are socially related, such as aggressiveness, delinquency, truancy, sexual problems, running away, and substance use. The Behavioral Dysfunction scale assesses the patient's ability to organize tasks, complete assignments, concentrate, handle frustration, and manage impulses. In addition, Critical Items describe features often found in inpatient services, such as paranoia, obsessive-compulsive behaviors, hallucination, suicide, mania, and eating disorders. Each item of the YOQ-30.2 is scored on a 5-point scale (0–4), yielding a possible range of scores from 0 to 240, with higher scores indicating greater distress.

Administration of the YOQ-30.2 requires approximately 5–7 minutes and scoring takes approximately 3–5 minutes. The YOQ-30.2 can be easily scored by hand, although computer administration and scoring software is available (www.oqmeasures.com). The YOQ-30.2 is a psychometrically sound measure (Burlingame et al., 2004). Based on four large normative samples, internal consistency estimates ranged from.51 to.90 for the subscales and.93 to.95 for the total score.

Using normative data from patients and non-patients, the following criteria were developed for indicating clinically significant change and reliable change on the Y-OQ. For the YOQ-30.2, the clinically significant cut-off score is 46. Scores above this mark are considered within the dysfunctional (clinically elevated) range, while scores below are considered in the functional range. A patient must move from a score of 46 or above to a score that is below the cut-off of 46 in order to make clinically significant change. The reliable change criterion is 13. Thus, for a patient to make reliable change on the Y-OQ, their score must change by at least 13 points. As with the OQ-45, clinically significant change and reliable change should be considered together. Thus, a patient who begins therapy with a score of 46 or greater, ends treatment with a score below 46, and has at least a 13-point change in their Y-OQ score can be considered to have achieved meaningful clinical change, that is, they may be considered as "recovered."

Similar to the OQ-45.2, the YOQ-30.2 was originally validated with majority US-based White samples. Unfortunately, less attention has been paid to the cross-cultural validity of the YOQ-30.2. As a result, group practitioners and researchers should be mindful of the possibility of cultural and translational bias when using this measure with populations that have not been included in previous samples. See Table 4.2 for more information on the YOQ-30.2.

Table 4.2 Youth Outcome Questionnaire – 30.2 (YOQ-30.2)

Item	Information
Name of Instrument	Youth Outcome Questionnaire – 30.2 (YOQ-30.2)
Authors	Gary M. Burlingame, Gawain Wells, & Michael J. Lambert
Source	Burlingame, G. M., Dunn, T., Hill, M., Cox, J., Wells, M. G., Lambert, M. J., & Brown, G.S. (2004). Administration and Scoring Manual for the YOQ-30.2 (Youth Outcome Questionnaire-30 Version 2.0). Salt Lake City, UT: American Professional Credentialing Services.
Brief Description	The YOQ-30.2 is the youth and adolescent version of the Outcome Questionnaire. This measure is a 30-item outcome instrument that can either be completed by the patient (YOQ-30.2 SR) or a parent/guardian (YOQ-30.2 PR) for youth and adolescents ages 4–17 in treatment.
Time Issues	Administration: < 5 min Scoring: < 7 min
Subscales and Scoring	Items are rated on a 5-point Likert-type scale (0 = Never to 4 = Almost Always). In addition to the total score, which provides an overall indication of patient functioning, the Y-OQ also provides six subscale scores, Intrapersonal Distress, Somatic, Interpersonal Relations, Social Problems, Behavioral Dysfunction, and Critical Items. The Intrapersonal Distress scale is a measure of emotional distress that the patient is experiencing, including symptoms of anxiety, depression, fearfulness, hopelessness, and self-harm. The Somatic scale assesses bodily distress, such as headaches, dizziness, stomachaches, nausea, and bowel difficulties. The Interpersonal Relations scale assesses issues relevant to the patient's relationships with parents, other adults, and peers. The Social Problems scale reflects problematic behaviors that are socially related, such as aggressiveness, delinquency, truancy, sexual problems, running away, and substance use. The Behavioral Dysfunction scale assesses the patient's ability to organize tasks, complete assignments, concentrate, handle frustration, and manage impulses. In addition, Critical Items describe features often found in inpatient services, such as paranoia, obsessive-compulsive behaviors, hallucination, suicide, mania, and eating disorders. Each item of the YOQ-30.2 is scored on a 5-point scale (0–4), yielding a possible range of scores from 0 to 240, with higher scores indicating greater distress.

Item	Information
Psychometric Properties	The YOQ-30.2 is a psychometrically sound measure (Burlingame et al., 2004). Based on four large normative samples, internal consistency estimates ranged from.51 to.90 for the subscales and.93 to.95 for the total score.
Norms and any normative data re: diversity for each instrument	Similar to the OQ-45.2, the YOQ-30.2 was originally validated with majority US-based White samples. Unfortunately, less attention has been paid to the cross-cultural validity of the YOQ-30.2. As a result, group practitioners and researchers should be mindful of the possibility of cultural and translational bias when using this measure with populations that have not been included in previous samples.
Translations	N/A
Sensitivity to Change	Using normative data from patients and non-patients, the following criteria were developed for indicating clinically significant change and reliable change on the Y-OQ. For the YOQ-30.2, the clinically significant cut-off score is 46. Scores above this mark are considered within the dysfunctional (clinically elevated) range, while scores below are considered in the functional range. The reliable change criterion is 13. Thus, for a patient to make reliable change on the Y-OQ, their score must change by at least 13 points.
Sample references	Burlingame, G. M., Wells, M. G., Lambert, M. J., & Cox, J. C. (2014). Youth outcome questionnaire. In The use of psychological testing for treatment planning and outcomes assessment (pp. 235–274). Routledge. Ridge, N. W., Warren, J. S., Burlingame, G. M., Wells, M. G., & Tumblin, K. M. (2009). Reliability and validity of the youth outcome questionnaire self-report. Journal of Clinical Psychology, 65(10), 1115–1126.
Website Resources	www.oqmeasures.com
How to Obtain/Cost	Proprietary-sample copy provided herein. License required with no per use cost.
Administration Types	Paper and Pencil/Electronic
Analytics	Administration, scoring and interpretive portfolio software identifying treatment failure cases.
Benchmarking	N/A

Patient Health Questionnaire – 9 (PHQ-9) (Kroenke et al., 2001)

The PHQ-9 is a multipurpose instrument for screening, diagnosing, monitoring and measuring the severity of depression. The PHQ-9 is brief, useful in clinical practice, can be completed by the client in minutes, and is rapidly scored by the clinician. This brief 9-item self-report tool was developed by incorporating DSM-5 depression diagnostic criteria to rate the frequency of several depressive symptoms.

Items are rated on a 4-point Likert scale (0 = not at all to 3 = nearly every day) assessing the frequency of depressive symptoms. A total score is calculated by adding all items, with higher scores representing greater depressive symptom severity. Item 9 of the PHQ-9 measures the presences and duration of suicidal ideation. The diagnostic validity of the PHQ-9 was established across multiple samples, and the PHQ-9 demonstrates good psychometric properties of reliability (Kroenke et al., 2001).

Based on normed data, the clinical cut-off scores for mild, moderate, moderately severe, and severe depressive symptoms are 5, 10, 15, and 20, respectively. This means that patients who score between 5 and 9 endorsed mild depressive symptoms, patients who score between 10 and 14 endorsed moderate symptoms, patients who score between 15 and 19 endorsed moderately severe depressive symptoms, and patients who score above 20 endorsed severe depressive symptoms. Patients must move from one clinical cut-off area to another in order to experience clinically meaningful change. The reliable change index for the PHQ-9 is 5, meaning that to make reliable change on the PHQ-9, a patient's score must change by at least 5 points. Thus, to be considered "recovered" on the PHQ-9, a patient must change from a clinically elevated score at pre-treatment to a score below 5 at post-treatment, and that change must be greater than 5 points.

Considering the cross-cultural validity of the PHQ-9, researchers have attempted to account for both translation bias and cultural bias of the PHQ-9. Regarding translation bias, the PHQ-9 has been translated and validated in many languages (Moriarty et al., 2015). Similarly, a large number of studies have examined the cross-cultural validity and reliability of the PHQ-9 using measurement invariance approaches and other techniques (see Harry et al., 2021 as an example). See Table 4.3 for more information on the PHQ-9.

Table 4.3 Patient Health Questionnaire-9

Item	Information
Name of Instrument	Patient Health Questionnaire-9
Authors	Kurt Kroenke, Robert L. Spitzer, and Janet B. W. Williams
Source	Kroenke, K., Spitzer, R. L., & Williams, J. B. W. (2001). The PHQ-9. Journal of General Internal Medicine: JGIM, 16(9), 606–613.
Brief Description	The PHQ-9 is a multipurpose instrument for screening, diagnosing, monitoring and measuring the severity of depression. The PHQ-9 is brief, useful in clinical practice, can be completed by the client in minutes, and is rapidly scored by the clinician. This brief 9-item self-report tool was developed by incorporating DSM-5 depression diagnostic criteria to rate the frequency of several depressive symptoms.
Time Issues	Administration: 2 min Scoring: < 2 min
Subscales and Scoring	Items are rated on a 4-point Likert scale (0 = not at all to 3 = nearly every day) assessing the frequency of depressive symptoms. A total score is calculated by adding all items, with higher scores representing greater depressive symptom severity. Item 9 of the PHQ-9 assesses the presences and duration of suicidal ideation. Based on normed data, the clinical cut-off scores for mild, moderate, moderately severe, and severe depressive symptoms are 5, 10, 15, and 20, respectively.
Psychometric Properties	The diagnostic validity of the PHQ-9 was established across multiple samples, and the PHQ-9 demonstrates good psychometric properties of reliability (Kroenke et al., 2001).
Norms and any normative data re: diversity for each instrument	The PHQ-9 is an internationally used measure of depression and has been used and validated with diverse cultural groups. Considering the cross-cultural validity of the PHQ-9, researchers have attempted to account for both translation bias and cultural bias of the PHQ-9. Regarding translation bias, the PHQ-9 has been translated and validated in many languages (Moriarty et al., 2015). Similarly, a large number of studies have examined the cross-cultural validity and reliability of the PHQ-9 using measurement invariance approaches and other techniques (see Harry et al., 2021 as an example).
Translations	The PHQ-9 has been globally disseminated and translated into more than 100 languages.
Sensitivity to Change	The reliable change index for the PHQ-9 is 5.

Item	Information
Sample references	Kroenke, K., Spitzer, R. L., & Williams, J. B. W. (2001). The PHQ-9. *Journal of General Internal Medicine: JGIM*, 16(9), 606–613. https://doi.org/10.1046/j.1525-1497.2001.016009606.x Kroenke, K. (2021). PHQ-9: global uptake of a depression scale. *World Psychiatry*, 20(1), 135–136. https://doi.org/10.1002/wps.20821
Website Resources	N/A
How to Obtain/Cost	The PHQ-9 is free and publicly accessible.
Administration Types	Paper and Pencil
Analytics	No
Benchmarking	N/A

Generalized Anxiety Disorder – 7 (GAD-7; Spitzer et al., 2006)

The GAD-7 is a valid and efficient tool for screening for generalized anxiety disorder and assessing the severity of anxiety symptoms in clinical practice (Spitzer et al., 2006). This is a 7-item self-report measure of anxiety symptoms. Items are rated on a 4-point Likert scale (0 = not at all to 3 = nearly every day) assessing the frequency of anxiety symptoms. A total score is calculated by summing all items with higher scores representing higher levels of anxiety.

Based on normed data, the clinical cut-off scores for mild, moderate, and severe anxiety symptoms are 5, 10, and 15, respectively. This means that patients who score between 5 and 9 endorsed mild anxiety symptoms, patients who score between 10 and 14 endorsed moderate anxiety symptoms, and patients who score above 15 endorsed severe anxiety symptoms. Patients must move from one clinical cut-off area to another in order to experience clinically meaningful change. The reliable change index for the GAD-7 is 6, meaning that to make reliable change on the GAD-7, a patient's score must change by at least 6 points. Thus, to be considered recovered on the GAD-7, a patient's score must change from a clinically elevated range to a score below 5 and that change must be greater than 6 points.

The GAD-7 was developed and normed with majority White US-based individuals, and therefore research on the cross-cultural use should be considered when using this measure with populations outside of previous samples used for norming purposes. Fortunately, research has examined the cross-cultural application and validity of the GAD-7 (see Parkerson et al., 2015 as an example), as well as the validity of translating the GAD-7 for use with non-English speakers (see He et al., 2010 for an example). See Table 4.4 for more information on the GAD-7.

Table 4.4 Generalized Anxiety Disorder-7

Item	Information
Name of Instrument	Generalized Anxiety Disorder-7
Authors	Robert L. Spitzer, Kurt Kroenke, Janet B. W. Williams, and Bernd Lowe
Source	Spitzer, R., Kroenke, K., Williams, J. B. W., & Löwe, B. (2006). A Brief Measure for Assessing Generalized Anxiety Disorder: The GAD-7. *Archives of Internal Medicine* (1960), 166(10), 1092–1097. https://doi.org/10.1001/archinte.166.10.1092
Brief Description	The GAD-7 is a valid and efficient tool screening, diagnosing, and monitoring Generalized Anxiety Disorder and anxiety symptoms. Items reflect the GAD symptom criteria from the *Diagnostic and Statistical Manual of Mental Disorders, Fourth Edition (DSM-IV)* and four additional items based on reviewing existing anxiety scales.
Time Issues	Administration: 2 min Scoring: < 2 min

Item	Information
Subscales and Scoring	Items are rated on a 4-point Likert scale (0 = not at all to 3 = nearly every day) assessing the frequency of anxiety symptoms. A total score is calculated by summing all items with higher scores representing higher levels of anxiety. Based on normed data, the clinical cut-off scores for mild, moderate, and severe anxiety symptoms are 5, 10, and 15, respectively.
Psychometric Properties	The GAD-7 is a psychometrically sound measure with evidence of good internal consistency, reliability, and validity.
Norms and any normative data re: diversity for each instrument	The GAD-7 was developed and normed with majority White US-based individuals, and therefore research on the cross-cultural use should be considered when using this measure with populations outside of previous samples used for norming purposes. Fortunately, research has examined the cross-cultural application and validity of the GAD-7 (see Parkerson et al., 2015 as an example), as well as the validity of translating the GAD-7 for use with non-English speakers (see He et al., 2010) for an example.
Translations	The GAD 7 has been translated in several languages such as Arabic, Chinese, Hindi, Korean, Russian, Spanish, and Urdu.
Sensitivity to Change	The reliable change index for the GAD-7 is 6.
Sample references	Spitzer, R., Kroenke, K., Williams, J. B. W., & Löwe, B. (2006). A Brief Measure for Assessing Generalized Anxiety Disorder: The GAD-7. Archives of Internal Medicine (1960), 166(10), 1092–1097. https://doi.org/10.1001/archinte.166.10.1092
Website Resources	N/A
How to Obtain/Cost	The GAD-7 is free and publicly accessible.
Administration Types	Paper and Pencil
Analytics	No
Benchmarking	N/A

Outcome Rating Scale (ORS; Duncan & Reese, 2015)

The ORS is a brief self-report instrument designed for repeated measurement of adult patient progress over the course of therapy, at termination and beyond. The ORS is a four-item visual analogue scale that assesses client distress on four domains: social role functioning, interpersonal functioning, individual (personal) well-being, and overall well-being. These four domains of functioning are presented visually as four 10 cm lines (i.e., 10-point scale). Clients complete the ORS by placing a hash on each of the four 10 cm lines, where 0 represents the lowest level of functioning and 10 represents the highest level of functioning. A total score (i.e., general sense of well-being) is then created by adding the four ratings, and so the total score ranges from 0–40. Administration and scoring of the ORS typically occurs during the first several minutes of the therapy appointment. Patients are provided a paper or electronic version of the ORS and complete the measure with the therapist present. Completing of the ORS takes approximately 1 minute or less. The therapist will then score the ORS by measuring the hash line on each item and totaling the score across all four items. This scoring method is completed in front of the client and the score is then discussed between the client and therapist to monitor progress or deterioration. The ORS can also be administered, scored, and monitored using an electronic system (https://betteroutcomesnow.com).

The ORS has demonstrated adequate reliability and validity (Miller et al., 2003). Based on normed clinical data, the clinical cut-off score for the mean of ORS scores is 25. Scores above this cut-off are considered in the dysfunctional (clinically elevated) range, while scores below are considered in the functional range. A patient must move from a score above the cut-off of 25 to below 25 in order to make clinically significant change. The reliable change criterion is 6. Thus, for a patient to make reliable change on the ORS, their score must change by at least 6 points (Duncan & Reese, 2015). Thus, to be considered recovered on the ORS, a patient's score must change from a clinically elevated range to a score below 25 and that change must be greater than 6 points.

Attention to the cross-cultural validity of the ORS is limited, with some notable exceptions. For example, Hafkenscheid and colleagues (2010) translated and validated the ORS with a sample of Dutch patients, demonstrating evidence for the utility and psychometric properties of the ORS Dutch version. Additional studies have demonstrated strong psychometric evidence for the Chinese version of the ORS (She et al., 2017; She et al., 2018). Outside of these studies, the ORS has been translated into additional languages for cross-cultural use (Duncan, 2012). See Table 4.5 for more information on the ORS.

Table 4.5 Outcome Rating Scale

Item	Information
Name of Instrument	Outcome Rating Scale
Authors	Barry L. Duncan and Robert J. Reese
Source	Duncan, B. L. & Reese, R. J. (2015). The Partners for Change Outcome Management System (PCOMS) Revisiting the Client's Frame of Reference. Psychotherapy (Chicago, Ill.), 52(4), 391–401. https://doi.org/10.1037/pst0000026
Brief Description	The ORS is a brief self-report instrument designed for repeated measurement of adult patient progress over the course of therapy, at termination and beyond. The ORS is a four-item visual analogue scale that assesses client distress on four domains: social role functioning, interpersonal functioning, individual (personal) well-being, and overall well-being.
Time Issues	Administration: 2 min Scoring: < 2 min
Subscales and Scoring	The four items of the ORS are presented visually as four 10 cm lines (i. e., 10-point scale). Clients complete the ORS by placing a hash on each of the four 10 cm lines, where 0 represents the lowest level of functioning and 10 represents the highest level of functioning. A total score (i.e., general sense of well-being) is then created by adding the four ratings, resulting in a total score range from 0–40. Based on normed clinical data, the clinical cut-off score for the mean of ORS scores is 25.
Psychometric Properties	The ORS has demonstrated adequate reliability and validity (Miller et al., 2003).
Norms and any normative data re: diversity for each instrument	The development and validation of the ORS was based on majority White US-based samples. However, additional research has attempted to examine the cross-cultural relevance of the ORS. Hafkenscheid et al. (2010) translated and validated the ORS with a sample of Dutch patients, demonstrating evidence for the utility and psychometric properties of the ORS Dutch version. Additional studies have demonstrated strong psychometric evidence for the Chinese version of the ORS (She et al., 2017; She et al., 2018).
Translations	Available in Spanish, Chinese, Korean, Arabic, Hebrew, French, Dutch, Russian, Portuguese
Sensitivity to Change	The reliable change criterion for the ORS is 6.

Item	Information
Sample references	Duncan, B. L., & Reese, R. J. (2015). The Partners for Change Outcome Management System (PCOMS) revisiting the client's frame of reference. *Psychotherapy*, *52*(4), 391–401. https://doi-org.proxy.lib.uiowa.edu/10.1037/pst0000026 Miller, S.D., Duncan, B.L., Brown, J., Sparks, J., Claud, D.A. (2003). The outcome rating scale: A preliminary study of the reliability, validity, and feasibility of a brief visual analog measure. *Journal of Brief Therapy* 2 (2), 91–100.
Website Resources	www.myoutcomes.com/outcome-rating-scale
How to Obtain/Cost	A license to use the ORS and SRS in paper and pencil format is available for free to individual practitioners from the website above. Licenses for paper and pencil use of the ORS and SRS are provided to group practices, agencies and behavioral health organizations for a fee. Web-based format available for a fee.
Administration Types	Paper and Pencil
Analytics	Yes
Benchmarking	N/A

Inventory of Interpersonal Problems – 32 (IIP-32) (Barkham et al., 1996; Horowitz et al., 2000)

The Inventory of Interpersonal Problems (IIP) is a self-report instrument designed to assess problems in interpersonal interactions that either are reflected by difficulties in engaging in a particular behavior (*It is hard for me to…*), or difficulties in exercising restraint (*I do… too much*). The instrument is based upon common interpersonal theories of behavior that have a long tradition in personality and social psychology (e.g., Sullivan, 1953; Leary, 1957; Kiesler, 1996).

The IIP is available in two versions of differing lengths (64 items, 32 items). The IIP-32 measure has 8 subscales, each reflecting a different dimension of interpersonal function: Domineering-controlling; Vindictive-self-centered; Cold-distant; Socially inhibited; Non-assertive; Overly accommodating; Self-sacrificing; and Intrusive-needy. The IIP-32 consists of 4 items per scale that are rated on a 5-point scale (0–4). The subscales can be scored by calculating the mean rating of the four items. In addition to the subscales, the IIP provides a total score which is a sum of all the items. The IIP-32 can be scored by hand or by using a simple computer program.

The IIP has strong psychometric properties (Barkham et al., 1996) and is a commonly used instrument in psychotherapy outcome research (e.g., Horowitz, 1993; Horowitz et al., 2000; Strupp et al., 1997). The scale structure has been confirmed in several factor analytic studies and seems to be stable in different countries (e.g., Horowitz et al., 2000). There is also good evidence that the IIP is particularly sensitive in capturing the effects of long-term psychotherapeutic interventions (e.g., Strauss & Burgmeier-Lohse, 1994). Despite these psychometric properties, one of the disadvantages of the IIP-32 is that there is no clinical cut-off or reliable change index available for the IIP-32 based on normed data.

The IIP-32 was originally developed and validated with majority White US-based samples. However, since then, the IIP-32 has been translated into several languages, including Dutch (Vanheule et al., 2006), German (Puschner et al., 2004), Spanish (Salazar et al., 2010), Italian (Lo Coco et al., 2018), Portuguese (Faustino et al., 2020), and Hebrew (Wiseman et al., 2006). In addition, the psychometric properties of the IIP-32 have been examined cross-culturally. See Table 4.6 for more information on the IIP-32.

Table 4.6 Inventory of Interpersonal Problems – 32 (IIP-32)

Item	Information
Name of Instrument	Inventory of Interpersonal Problems - 32
Authors	L.M. Horowitz and M. Barkham
Source	Barkham, M., Hardy, G. E., & Startup, M. (1996). The IIP-32: A short version of the Inventory of Interpersonal Problems. *British Journal of Clinical Psychology, 35*(1), 21–35. https://doi.org/10.1111/j.2044-8260.1996.tb01159.x
Brief Description	The Inventory of Interpersonal Problems – 32 (IIP-32) is a self-report instrument designed to assess problems in interpersonal interactions that either are reflected by difficulties in engaging in a particular behavior (*It is hard for me to…*), or difficulties in exercising restraint (*I do… too much*). The IIP-32 consists of 4 items per scale that are rated on a 5-point scale (0–4).
Time Issues	Administration: 5 min Scoring: < 5 min
Subscales and Scoring	The IIP-32 has 8 subscales, each reflecting a different dimension of interpersonal functioning: Domineering-controlling; Vindictive-self-centered; Cold-distant; Socially inhibited; Non-assertive; Overly accommodating; Self-sacrificing; and Intrusive-needy. The IIP-32 consists of 4 items per scale that are rated on a 5-point scale (0–4). The subscales can be scored by calculating the mean rating of the four items. In addition to the subscales, the IIP provides a total score which is a sum of all the items indicating overall interpersonal distress or problems.
Psychometric Properties	The IIP-32 has good psychometric properties. The scale structure has been confirmed in several factor analytic studies and seems to be stable in different countries (e.g., Horowitz, Strauss, & Kordy, 2000). There is also good evidence that the IIP is particularly sensitive in capturing the effects of long-term psychotherapeutic interventions (e.g., Strauss & Burgmeier-Lohse, 1994).
Norms and any normative data re: diversity for each instrument	The original researchers (Barkham et al., 1996; Horowitz et al., 2000) developed and validated the IIP-32 primarily with majority White samples. However, some research has been done with Chinese and Bangla samples suggesting good validity. There is no clinical cut-off or reliable change index available for the IIP-32 based on normed data. The longer IIP-64 (Horowitz et al., 2000) does provide clinical cut-off values based on population norms.
Translations	Various version of the IIP have been translated into Chinese, Italian, French, German, Dutch, and Bangla.
Sensitivity to Change	Not available.
Sample references	Barkham, M., Hardy, G. E., & Startup, M. (1996). The IIP-32: A short version of the Inventory of Interpersonal Problems. *British Journal of Clinical Psychology, 35*(1), 21–35. https://doi.org/10.1111/j.2044-8260.1996.tb01159.x Horowitz, L. M., Alden, L. E., Wiggins, J. S., et al. (2000). *IIP - Inventory of Interpersonal Problems Manual*. San Antonio, TX: The Psychological Corporation.
Website Resources	N/A
How to Obtain/Cost	Contact authors to obtain permission for use.
Administration Types	Paper and Pencil. Mind Garden provides an online administration and scoring for a fee at: www.mindgarden.com.
Analytics	No
Benchmarking	N/A

Difficulties in Emotion Regulation Scale (DERS) (Gratz & Roemer, 2004)

The Difficulties in Emotion Regulation Scale (DERS) is a widely used, theoretically driven, and psychometrically sound self-report measure of emotion regulation difficulties. The DERS is a 36-item self-report questionnaire designed to assess multiple aspects of emotional dysregulation. Items are rated on a 5-point Likert scale (1 = almost never to 5 = almost always). The measure yields a total score as well as six subscales: non-acceptance of emotional responses, difficulties engaging in goal directed behavior, impulse control difficulties, lack of emotional awareness, limited access to emotion regulation strategies, and lack of emotional clarity.

Total scores are calculated by summing all the items, and subscale scores are calculated by summing the items corresponding to the scale. Total scores on the DERS can range from 36–180, where higher scores represent greater problems with emotion regulation. The DERS is most commonly administered and scored by hand as there is no electronic system to administer and score the DERS. Administering and scoring the DERS takes approximately 5–10 minutes. In addition to the full DERS assessment tool, a brief 16-item version of the DERS exists (Bjureberg et al., 2016). The DERS-16 yields a total score and scores on six subscales: non-acceptance of negative emotions, inability to engage in goal-directed behaviors when distressed, difficulties controlling impulsive behaviors when distressed, limited access to emotion regulation strategies perceived as effective, and lack of emotional clarity. Like the original DERS, patients rate the extent to which each item applies to them on a 5-point Likert-type scale from 1 (almost never) to 5 (almost always). Total scores on the DERS-16 can range from 16 to 80, with higher scores reflecting greater levels of emotion dysregulation.

The DERS has good psychometric properties. Specifically, the DERS has been found to demonstrate good test-retest reliability and adequate construct and predictive reliability (Bardeen et al., 2012; Gratz & Roemer, 2004). Despite the reliability and validity of the DERS, one disadvantage is that the DERS does not have clinical cut-off scores or a reliable change index based on normed data.

Although the DERS was developed and validated with majority White US-based samples, researchers have translated and tested the validity and reliability of the DERS in several languages, including Italian (Giromini et al., 2012; Sighinolfi et al., 2010), Portuguese (Coutinho et al., 2010), Chinese (Li et al., 2018), and Turkish (Ruganci & Gencoz, 2010). Moreover, cross-cultural bias of the DERS has been examined across several cultural groups. See Table 4.7 for more information on the DERS.

Table 4.7 Difficulties in Emotion Regulation Scale

Item	Information
Name of Instrument	Difficulties in Emotion Regulation Scale
Authors	Kim Gratz and Lizabeth Roemer
Source	Gratz, K. L., & Roemer, L. (2004). Multidimensional assessment of emotion regulation and dysregulation: Development, factor structure, and validation of the difficulties in emotion regulation scale. *Journal of psychopathology and behavioral assessment, 26*(1), 41–54. https://doi.org/10.1023/B:JOBA.0000007455.08539.94
Brief Description	The Difficulties in Emotion Regulation Scale (DERS) is a widely used, theoretically driven, and psychometrically sound self-report measure of emotion regulation difficulties. The DERS is a 36-item self-report questionnaire designed to assess multiple aspects of emotional dysregulation. Items are rated on a 5-point Likert scale (1 = almost never to 5 = almost always).

Item	Information
Time Issues	Administration: 3 min Scoring: < 2 min
Subscales and Scoring	The measure yields a total score as well as six subscales: non-acceptance of emotional responses, difficulties engaging in goal directed behavior, impulse control difficulties, lack of emotional awareness, limited access to emotion regulation strategies, and lack of emotional clarity. Total scores are calculated by summing all the items, and subscale scores are calculated by summing the items corresponding to the scale. Total scores on the DERS can range from 36–180, where higher scores represent greater problems with emotion regulation.
Psychometric Properties	The DERS has good psychometric properties. Specifically, the DERS has been found to demonstrate good test-retest reliability and adequate construct and predictive reliability (Bardeen et al., 2012; Gratz & Roemer, 2004).
Norms and any normative data re: diversity for each instrument	Gratz and Roemer (2004) developed and validated the DERS primarily with White US-based samples. Cross-cultural bias of the DERS has been examined across several cultural groups.
Translations	The DERS-16 has been translated into several languages, including Italian, Portuguese, Chinese, and Turkish, Arabic, Russian, Spanish, Persian, and Finnish.
Sensitivity to Change	Not available.
Sample references	Bjureberg, Ljótsson, B., Tull, M. T., Hedman, E., Sahlin, H., Lundh, L.-G., Bjärehed, J., DiLillo, D., Messman-Moore, T., Gumpert, C. H., & Gratz, K. L. (2015). Development and Validation of a Brief Version of the Difficulties in Emotion Regulation Scale: The DERS-16. Journal of Psychopathology and Behavioral Assessment, 38(2), 284–296. https://doi.org/10.1007/s10862-015-9514-x Bjureberg, J., Ljótsson, B., Tull, M. T., Hedman, E., Sahlin, H., Lundh, L.- G., Bjärehed, J., DiLillo, D., Messman-Moore, T., Gumpert, C. H., & Gratz, K.L. (2016). Development and Validation of a Brief Version of the Difficulties in Emotion Regulation Scale: The DERS-16. *Journal of Psychopathology and Behavioral Assessment*, 1–13. http://doi.org/10.1007/s10862-015-9514-x
Website Resources	N/A
How to Obtain/Cost	Contact authors to obtain permission for use.
Administration Types	Paper and Pencil
Analytics	No
Benchmarking	N/A

WHO Quality of Life Measure – Brief version (WHOQOL-BREF; World Health Organization, 1996)

The WHOQOL is a broad instrument to assess health beyond symptom reduction, as well as a quality of life measure to be used cross-culturally in health care. The WHOQOL-BREF is a 26-item version of the WHOQOL-100 assessment (Skevington et al., 2004). The WHOQOL-BREF consists of four domains of quality of life: physical, psychological, social, and environment. The physical health domain consists of facets such as activities of daily living, pain, energy and fatigue, and mobility. The psychological domain assesses facets of psychological health such as negative and positive feelings, self-esteem, and spirituality and personal beliefs. The social domain assesses facets such as personal relationships and social support. Finally, the environment domain assesses facets such as financial resources, home environment, and freedom, physical safety and security.

Items are scored on a 5-point Likert scale, with higher scores indicating greater quality of life. A total score is calculated by averaging the responses across items, and the developers provide procedures for converting WHOQOL-BREF scores to scores from the WHOQOL-100 (World Health Organization, 1996). Parties interested in using the WHOQOL-BREF should consult with the WHOQOL Group prior to use (www.who.int/tools/whoqol). Administration and scoring of the WHOQOL takes approximately 3–5 minutes, and the measure should be administered as indicated in the WHOQOL manual, which can be found online (www.who.int/mental_health/media/en/76.pdf).

The WHOQOL-BREF has good to excellent psychometric properties of reliability and performs well in preliminary tests of validity (Skevington et al., 2004; World Health Organization, 1996). Most importantly, the WHOQOL was developed in consultation with WHO Centers across the world and represents a cross-cultural measure of quality of life. The WHOQOL is available in 19 different languages. There is no clinical cut-off or reliable change index available for the WHOQOL-BREF. See Table 4.8 for more information on the WHOQOL.

Table 4.8 World Health Organization Quality of Life (WHOQOL)-BREF

Item	Information
Name of Instrument	WHO Quality of Life (WHOQOL)-BREF
Authors	World Health Organization
Source	World Health Organization. (1996). *WHOQOL-BREF: introduction, administration, scoring and generic version of the assessment: field trial version, December 1996* (No. WHOQOL-BREF). World Health Organization.
Brief Description	The WHOQOL is a broad instrument to assess health beyond symptom reduction, as well as a quality of life measure to be used cross-culturally in health care. The WHOQOL-BREF is a 26-item version of the WHOQOL-100 assessment (Skevington et al., 2004). The WHOQOL-BREF consists of four domains of quality of life: physical, psychological, social, and environment. The physical health domain consists of facets such as activities of daily living, pain, energy and fatigue, and mobility. The psychological domain assesses facets of psychological health such as negative and positive feelings, self-esteem, and spirituality and personal beliefs. The social domain assesses facets such as personal relationships and social support. Finally, the environment domain assesses facets such as financial resources, home environment, and freedom, physical safety and security.
Time Issues	Administration: 3–5 min Scoring: 3–5 min
Subscales and Scoring	Items are scored on a 5-point Likert scale, with higher scores indicating greater quality of life. A total score is calculated by averaging the responses across items, and the developers provide procedures for converting WHOQOL-BREF scores to scores from the WHOQOL-100 (World Health Organization, 1996).
Psychometric Properties	The WHOQOL-BREF has good to excellent psychometric properties of reliability and performs well in preliminary tests of validity (Skevington et al., 2004; World Health Organization, 1996).
Norms and any normative data re: diversity for each instrument	The WHOQOL was developed in consultation with WHO Centers across the world and represents a cross-cultural measure of quality of life.
Translations	The WHOQOL is available in 19 different languages.

Item	Information
Sensitivity to Change	N/A
Sample references	www.who.int/publications/i/item/WHO-HIS-HSI-Rev.2012.03
	www.who.int/publications/i/item/WHO-HIS-HSI-Rev-2012
	www.who.int/publications/i/item/WHOQOL-BREF
Website Resources	WHOQOL Manual:
	www.who.int/mental_health/media/en/76.pdf
How to Obtain/Cost	Parties interested in using the WHOQOL-BREF should consult with the WHOQOL Group prior to use. www.who.int/tools/whoqol
Administration Types	Paper and Pencil
Analytics	No
Benchmarking	N/A

Experiences in Close Relationships Scales (ECR-12) (Lafontaine et al., 2015)

The ECR is one of the most commonly used measures of attachment insecurity. The ECR assesses attachment anxiety related to concerns about rejection or abandonment in close relationships, and attachment avoidance related to concerns about intimacy and inter-dependence (Lafontaine et al., 2015). The attachment anxiety dimension is associated with viewing oneself as needing others but being vulnerable to rejection. The attachment avoidance dimension is associated with a working model of others as overly needy, and with a strong desire to remain independent and self-reliant (Lafontaine et al., 2015).

The Experiences in Close Relationships-12 (ECR-12) (Lafontaine et al., 2015) is a 12-item self-report measure of attachment to romantic partners. The ECR-12 measures two dimensions of attachment, namely Attachment Avoidance (six items) and Attachment Anxiety (six items). Items are scored on a 7- point Likert scale, with higher scores indicating greater attachment avoidance and attachment anxiety with romantic partners. Attachment Anxiety scores are cal-culated by averaging the item values. Attachment Avoidance scores are calculated by first reverse scoring five of the items (except item #9), and then averaging the scores.

The ECR has high reliability and validity, demonstrated in many correlational and experimental studies. Convergent validity of the ECR has been demonstrated with mea-sures of relationship satisfaction, psychological distress, fear of intimacy, romantic depen-dence, accommodation strategies, and self-esteem (Lafontaine et al., 2015). High test-retest reliability has also been demonstrated for the ECR (Tasca et al., 2018; Lafontaine et al., 2015). Given the strong psychometric properties of the ECR, this measure has been used world-wide and translated to several languages, including Chinese, Dutch, Hebrew, French, Japanese, Spanish, and Italian (see Mallinckrodt et al., 2004 as an example). There is no clinical cut-off or reliable change index available for the ECR-12. See Table 4.9 for more information on the ECR-12.

Table 4.9 Experiences in Close Relationships-12

Item	Information
Name of Instrument	Experiences in Close Relationships-12
Authors	Marie-France Lafontaine, Audrey Brassard, Yvan Lussier, Pierre Valois, Philip R. Shaver, and Susan M. Johnson
Source	Lafontaine, M.F., Brassard, A., Lussier, Y., Valois, P., Shaver, P. R., & Johnson, S. M. (2016). Selecting the Best Items for a Short-Form of the Experiences in Close Relationships Questionnaire. European Journal of Psychological Assessment: Official Organ of the European Association of Psychological Assessment, 32(2), 140–154. https://doi.org/10.1027/1015-5759/a000243

Item	Information
Brief Description	The ECR assesses attachment anxiety related to concerns about rejection or abandonment in close relationships, and attachment avoidance related to concerns about intimacy and interdependence (Lafontaine et al., 2015). The attachment anxiety dimension is associated with viewing oneself as needing others but being vulnerable to rejection. The attachment avoidance dimension is associated with a working model of others as overly needy, and with a strong desire to remain independent and self-reliant (Lafontaine et al., 2015).
	The Experiences in Close Relationships-12 (ECR-12; Lafontaine et al., 2015) is a 12-item self-report measure of attachment to romantic partners. The ECR-12 measures two dimensions of attachment, namely Attachment Avoidance (six items) and Attachment Anxiety (six items). Items are scored on a 7- point Likert scale, with higher scores indicating greater attachment avoidance and attachment anxiety with romantic partners.
Time Issues	
Subscales and Scoring	Attachment Anxiety scores are calculated by averaging the item values. Attachment Avoidance scores are calculated by first reverse scoring five of the items (except item #9), and then averaging the scores.
Psychometric Properties	The ECR has high reliability and validity, demonstrated in many correlational and experimental studies. Convergent validity of the ECR has been demonstrated with measures of relationship satisfaction, psychological distress, fear of intimacy, romantic dependence, accommodation strategies, and self-esteem (Lafontaine et al., 2015). High test-retest reliability has also been demonstrated for the ECR (Tasca et al., 2018; Lafontaine et al., 2015).
Norms and any normative data re: diversity for each instrument	The ECR has been used world-wide and validated across diverse cultures.
Translations	Chinese, Dutch, French, Hebrew, Italian, Japanese, and Spanish
Sensitivity to Change	N/A
Sample references	Lafontaine, M.-F., Brassard, A., Lussier, Y., Valois, P., Shaver, P. R., & Johnson, S. M. (2015, February 27). Selecting the Best Items for a Short-Form of the Experiences in Close Relationships Questionnaire. *European Journal of Psychological Assessment, 32*, 140−154. http://dx.doi.org/10.1027/1015-5759/a000243
	Tasca G. A., Brugnera, A., Baldwin, D., Carlucci, S., Compare, A., Balfour, L., Proulx, G., Gick, M., & Lafontaine, M. (2018). Reliability and validity of the Experiences in Close Relationships Scale-12: Attachment dimensions in a clinical sample with eating disorders. The International Journal of Eating Disorders, 51(1), 18−27. https://doi.org/10.1002/eat.22807
	Wei, M., Russell, D. W., Mallinckrodt, B., & Vogel, D. L. (2007). The Experiences in Close Relationships (ECR) Scale-short form: Reliability, validity, and factor structure. Journal of Personality Assessment, 88, 187–204.
Website Resources	N/A
How to Obtain/Cost	Contact authors to obtain permission for use.
Administration Types	Paper and Pencil
Analytics	No
Benchmarking	N/A

Multicultural and Diversity Considerations

Recently scholars have noted the importance and utility of group therapy for addressing social justice and diversity issues (Burnes & Ross, 2010). Indeed, small group interventions have the power to promote cross-cultural relations, increase ethnocultural empathy, and progress social justice and racial equity (Merta, 1995; Ribeiro, 2020; White et al., 2019). Scholars have also noted how all groups are multicultural consisting of members who hold various social and cultural identities and lived experiences. These cultural factors inevitably inform and influence the processes and outcomes of group-based treatments for all members (Chen et al., 2008; Kivlighan & Chapman, 2018). As a result, group leaders and organizations can also consider utilizing outcome measures designed specifically to assess diversity and cultural domains of functioning, particularly for group-based interventions that have the primary goal of advancing social justice and addressing racial and other sociocultural injustices.

As an example, intergroup dialogue programs utilize small group interventions to increase diversity experiences, foster cross-cultural awareness, and foster social justice and change (Dessel et al., 2006; Gurin et al., 2013). Leaders of these groups may be interested in evaluating the effectiveness of these group-based interventions through the use of outcome measures that assess areas of culture and diversity. Moreover, many agencies and private practices offer identity-based group services for members of marginalized and historically oppressed cultural groups. Thus, the use of culturally relevant outcome measures may be useful in these contexts to understand how these group-based services are or are not addressing diversity issues. As a result, we recommend the following measures of diversity and culture for outcome monitoring for group psychotherapy: Scale of Ethnocultural Empathy (SEE) (Wang et al., 2003) and Critical Consciousness Scale–Short (CCS–S) (Rapa et al., 2020). Below we provide a description of these measures for monitoring diversity outcomes in group-based interventions with attention to the psychometric properties, normed data, and use and scoring of each measure.

Scale of Ethnocultural Empathy (SEE) (Wang et al., 2003)

The SEE is a 31-item self-report measure of ethnocultural empathy. Ridley and Lingle (1996) defined cultural empathy as a learned skill and is multidimensional and interpersonal by nature. The SEE was developed to assess empathy directed toward members of racial and ethnic groups different from one's own. The topic of ethnocultural empathy is critical given psychology's emphasis on diversity and multiculturalism as professional and scholarly issues. The SEE consists of four subscales: Empathic Feeling and Expression (15 items), Empathic Perspective Taking (7 items), Acceptance of Cultural Differences (5 items), and Empathic Awareness (4 items). Empathic Feeling and Expression consists of items that assess concerns about communication of discriminatory or prejudiced attitudes or beliefs and emotional responses to the experiences of people from racial or ethnic groups different from one's own. Empathic Perspective Taking consists of items that assess one's effort to understand the experiences and emotions of people from different racial and ethnic backgrounds. Acceptance of Cultural Differences consists of items that assess the understanding, acceptance, and valuing of cultural traditions and customs of individuals from differing racial and ethnic groups. Finally, Empathic Awareness consists of items that assess awareness or knowledge that one has about the experiences of people from racial or ethnic groups different from one's own (Wang et al., 2003).

Items of the SEE are rated on a 6-point Likert-type scale (1 = strongly disagree that it describes me to 6 = strongly agree that it describes me). Scores for the SEE are obtained by summing all items within each scale, with higher scores indicating higher levels of ethnocultural empathy (Wang et al., 2003). This measure can be administered and scored within approximately 5–8 minutes. The SEE is administered and scores by hand as no electronic system exists to aid in administration, scoring, or monitoring scores over time.

The SEE has demonstrated good reliability (Albiero & Matricardi, 2013; Wang et al., 2003). Specifically, Wang and colleagues (2003) demonstrated convergent validity of the SEE as evidenced by significant associations between the SEE and measures of general empathy and attitudes toward people's similarities and differences. High internal consistency and test–retest reliability estimates were also found across the three studies (Wang et al., 2003). Currently there are no clinical cut-off or reliable change index available for the SEE.

The SEE was developed and validated with a majority US-based White sample. However, researchers have examined the cross-cultural use of the SEE. For example, Albiero and Matricardi (2013) further validated the SEE Italian version for use with Italian-speaking samples. In addition, Spanish (Albar et al., 2015), Swedish (Rasoal et al., 2011), and Turkish versions (Özdikmenli-Demir & Demir, 2014) of the SEE have also been developed and further tested for use. See Table 4.10 for more information on the SEE.

Table 4.10 Scale of Ethnocultural Empathy

Item	Information
Name of Instrument	Scale of Ethnocultural Empathy
Authors	Yu-Wei Wang, M. Meghan Davidson, Oksana F. Yakushko, Holly Bielstein Savoy, Jeffrey A. Tan, and Joseph K. Bleier
Source	Wang, Y.W., Davidson, M. M., Yakushko, O. F., Savoy, H. B., Tan, J. A., & Bleier, J. K. (2003). The Scale of Ethnocultural Empathy. Journal of Counseling Psychology, 50(2), 221–234. https://doi.org/10.1037/0022-0167.50.2.221
Brief Description	The SEE is a 31-item self-report measure of ethnocultural empathy. Ridley and Lingle (1996) defined cultural empathy as a learned skill and is multidimensional and interpersonal by nature. The SEE was developed to assess empathy directed toward members of racial and ethnic groups different from one's own. The topic of ethnocultural empathy is critical given psychology's emphasis on diversity and multiculturalism as professional and scholarly issues. Items of the SEE are rated on a 6-point Likert-type scale (1 = strongly disagree that it describes me to 6 = strongly agree that it describes me).
Time Issues	Administration: 5–8 min Scoring: 5–8 min
Subscales and Scoring	The SEE consists of four subscales: Empathic Feeling and Expression (15 items), Empathic Perspective Taking (7 items), Acceptance of Cultural Differences (5 items), and Empathic Awareness (4 items). Empathic Feeling and Expression consists of items that assess concerns about communication of discriminatory or prejudiced attitudes or beliefs and emotional responses to the experiences of people from racial or ethnic groups different from one's own. Empathic Perspective Taking consists of items that assess one's effort to understand the experiences and emotions of people from different racial and ethnic backgrounds. Acceptance of Cultural Differences consists of items that assess the understanding, acceptance, and valuing of cultural traditions and customs of individuals from differing racial and ethnic groups. Finally, Empathic Awareness consists of items that assess awareness or knowledge that one has about the experiences of people from racial or ethnic groups different from one's own (Wang et al., 2003). Scores for the SEE are obtained by summing all items within each scale, with higher scores indicating higher levels of ethnocultural empathy (Wang et al., 2003).

Item	Information
Psychometric Properties	The SEE has demonstrated good reliability (Albiero & Matricardi, 2013; Wang et al., 2003). Specifically, Wang et al. (2003) demonstrated convergent validity of the SEE as evidenced by significant associations between the SEE and measures of general empathy and attitudes toward people's similarities and differences. High internal consistency and test–retest reliability estimates were also found across the three studies (Wang et al., 2003).
Norms and any normative data re: diversity for each instrument	The SEE was developed and validated with a majority US-based White sample, however researchers have examined the cross-cultural use of the SEE.
Translations	Swedish, Turkish, Spanish, Portuguese
Sensitivity to Change	N/A
Sample references	Wang, Y.W., Davidson, M. M., Yakushko, O. F., Savoy, H. B., Tan, J. A., & Bleier, J. K. (2003). The Scale of Ethnocultural Empathy. Journal of Counseling Psychology, 50(2), 221–234. https://doi.org/10.1037/0022-0167.50.2.221
Website Resources	N/A
How to Obtain/Cost	Contact authors to obtain permission for use.
Administration Types	Paper and Pencil
Analytics	No
Benchmarking	N/A

Critical Consciousness Scale–Short (CCS–S) (Rapa et al., 2020)

The CCS-S is a 14-item self-report measure of critical consciousness. Critical consciousness has been posited as an antidote to oppression and is defined as a developmental asset that enables individuals to identify and challenge societal inequities (Diemer et al., 2006; Watts et al., 1999). Diemer and colleagues (2006) argue that critical consciousness may serve as a protective factor that engenders greater adaptive development and enhances well-being, both for individuals and groups experiencing marginalization and oppression. As a result, the CCS-S was developed to assess Watts and colleagues' (2011) tripartite conceptualization of critical consciousness (Rapa & Geldhof, 2020). The CCS-S consists of four subscales: Critical Reflection – Perceived Inequality, Critical Reflection – Egalitarianism, Critical Motivation, and Critical Action – Sociopolitical Participation (Rapa et al., 2020). Critical Reflection – Perceived Inequality consists of items that assess one's knowledge or awareness of the constraints on opportunity across gender, ethnic-racial, and socioeconomic lines. The Critical Reflection – Egalitarianism subscale consists of items that assess the belief that all groups of people should be treated as equals in society. Critical Motivation consists of items that assess one's commitment and agency to make a difference in society and correct racial and economic inequalities. Lastly, the Critical Action subscale consists of items that assess one's participation in activities to promote equality and social justice.

Items are rated on a 6-point Likert scale, ranging from 1 (strongly disagree) to 6 (strongly agree). Scores for all four subscales are calculated by averaging all items for a given subscale. Higher scores reflect a higher degree of critical consciousness. The CCS is administered and scored by hand, as no electronic system exists to automate the administration, scoring, and monitoring of scores over time. It takes approximately 5–7 minutes to administer and score the CCS. Rapa and colleagues (2020) demonstrated good reliability and validity of the CCS-S. Rapa and colleagues (2020) provide evidence supporting measurement invariance (i.e., that the scales function similarly) across ethnic-racial identification, age, and gender groups. There is no clinical cut-off or reliable change index available for the CCS-S based on normed data.

The CCS-S was developed and validated with racially diverse non-clinical US-based samples, providing preliminary evidence for the use of this measure with racially diverse US samples, however, given the recent development of this scale, cultural and translation bias of the CSS has not yet been examined internationally. Group practitioners and researchers should be mindful of this when using this measure with populations outside of the sample used to develop and norm this measure. See Table 4.11 for more information on the CCS-S.

Table 4.11 Critical Consciousness Scale

Item	Information
Name of Instrument	Critical Consciousness Scale
Authors	Luke J. Rapa, Candice W. Bolding, and Faiza M. Jamil
Source	Rapa, Bolding, C. W., & Jamil, F. M. (2020). Development and initial validation of the short critical consciousness scale (CCS-S). Journal of Applied Developmental Psychology, 70, 101164. https://doi.org/10.1016/j.appdev.2020.101164
Brief Description	The CCS-S is a 14-item self-report measure of critical consciousness. Critical consciousness has been posited as an antidote to oppression (Watts et al., 1999). Diemer and colleagues (2006) argue that critical consciousness may serve as a protective factor that engenders greater adaptive development and enhances well-being, both for individuals and groups experiencing marginalization and oppression. As a result, the CCS-S was developed to assess Watts et al. (2011) tripartite conceptualization of critical consciousness (Rapa & Geldhof, 2020).
Time Issues	Administration: <5 minutes. Scoring: <5 minutes.
Subscales and Scoring	The CCS-S consists of four subscales: Critical Reflection - Perceived Inequality, Critical Reflection - Egalitarianism, Critical Motivation, and Critical Action - Sociopolitical Participation (Rapa et al., 2020). Critical Reflection – Perceived Inequality consists of items that assess one's knowledge or awareness of the constraints on opportunity across gender, ethnic-racial, and socioeconomic lines. The Critical Reflection – Egalitarianism subscale consists of items that assess the belief that all groups of people should be treated as equals in society. Critical Motivation consists of items that assess one's commitment and agency to make a difference in society and correct racial and economic inequalities. Lastly, the Critical Action subscale consists of items that assess one's participation in activities to promote equality and social justice. Items are rated on a 6-point Likert scale, ranging from 1 (strongly disagree) to 6 (strongly agree). Scores for all four subscales are calculated by averaging all items for a given subscale. Higher scores reflect a higher degree of critical consciousness.
Psychometric Properties	Rapa and colleagues (2020) demonstrated good reliability and validity of the CCS-S. Rapa and colleagues (2020) provide evidence supporting measurement invariance (i.e., that the scales function similarly) across ethnic-racial identification, age, and gender groups.
Norms and any normative data re: diversity for each instrument	The CCS-S was developed and validated with racially diverse non-clinical US-based samples, providing preliminary evidence for the use of this measure with racially diverse US samples, however, given the recent development of this scale, cultural and translation bias of the CSS has not yet been examined internationally.
Translations	N/A
Sensitivity to Change	N/A

Item	Information
Sample references	Rapa, Bolding, C. W., & Jamil, F. M. (2020). Development and initial validation of the short critical consciousness scale (CCS-S). *Journal of Applied Developmental Psychology, 70*, 101164. https://doi.org/10.1016/j.appdev.2020.101164 Diemer, M. A., Rapa, L. J., Park, C. J., & Perry, J. C. (2017). Development and validation of the critical consciousness scale. *Youth & Society, 49*(4), 461–483. https://doi.org/10.1177/0044118X14538289 Diemer, M. A., Mistry, R. S., Wadsworth, M. E., López, I., & Reimers, F. (2012). Best practices in conceptualizing and measuring social class in psychological research. *Analyses of Social Issues and Public Policy, 13*(1), 77–113. https://doi.org/10.1111/asap.12001.
Website Resources	N/A
How to Obtain/Cost	Contact authors to request permission for use.
Administration Types	Paper and Pencil
Analytics	No
Benchmarking	N/A

Group Leadership Outcome Measures

Given that one of the utilities of treatment outcome monitoring is to inform therapist development and improvement, the use of measures to assess effective leadership qualities or clinical effectiveness in group practice may be of interest to practitioners and agencies. Although using traditional outcome measures to routinely monitor patient outcome during treatment can provide invaluable information about patients' progress and alert therapists to intervene when needed, information about why a patient may not be progressing is often not available. Using measures that assess group leadership qualities and behaviors in conjunction with traditional outcome measures will provide group leaders with feedback on best ways to intervene. For example, if the group-as-a-whole is not progressing in group therapy and feedback indicates that the leaders are perceived as cold and distant by group members, then this feedback can provide insight into the leaders' potential contribution to the group's lack of progress. In addition, group leadership outcome measures that assess group leader qualities and behaviors can be used in supervision to help group leaders and as evaluative tools to assess the effectiveness of group training programs. Lastly, group leadership measures can be used by group leaders in supervision to gain insight and awareness of their qualities and behaviors that might inform their professional development. We recommend the following measures to assess group training and group leader outcomes: the Group Leader Self-Assessment (GLSA) Tool (Barnes et al., 2020), the Group Psychotherapy Intervention Rating Scale (GPIRS) (Chapman et al., 2010), and the Multicultural Orientation (MCO) Inventory (Owen et al., 2011; Owen, 2013).

Group Leader Self-Assessment (GLSA; Barnes et al., 2020)

The GLSA was developed to assess the effectiveness of group leader training and can be used to help trainees identify goals for skill development and realize growth in leadership abilities. Group-leader trainees are asked to self-assess their group-leader ability in relation to key leader roles and functions (Barnes et al., 2020). As a result, the GLSA may prove helpful as an evaluative tool for group training programs.

The GLSA is a 29-item self-report measure. Items assess group leadership qualities and are rated on a 6-point Likert scale (1 = strongly disagree to 6 = strongly agree). Initial analyses indicated a four-factor structure for the GLSA indicating four scales: Support and Caring, Meaning Attribution, Executive Functions, and Emotional Activation. The Support and Caring scale consists of items that assess group leaders warmth, acceptance, and support. The Meaning Attribution scale consists of items that assess group leaders' ability to ascribe meaning to group work, such as translating feelings and experiences and providing cognitive framework for change. The Executive Functions scale assesses group leaders' ability to structure the group, including managing time, setting productive norms, and suggesting procedures. Finally, the Emotional Activation scale assesses group leaders' ability to confront, self-disclose, and model risk-taking.

A total score is calculated by summing all items. Total score can range from 29–174 with high scores representing greater group leadership qualities. The GLSA can be administered and scored in approximately 5–8 minutes. In a study by Barnes and colleagues (2020), the GLSA demonstrated good construct validity, good test-retest reliability, and responsiveness to change. However, this measure has not undergone extensive testing and the use and interpretation of data should be done with caution. There are no clinical cut-off scores or reliable change indexes for the GLSA. The GLSA was developed and validated with a majority White US-based sample and given the recent development of this form, additional cross-cultural validation studies have not been conducted to date. See Table 4.12 for more information on the GLSA.

Table 4.12 Group Leader Self-Assessment (GLSA)

Item	Information
Name of Instrument	Group Leader Self-Assessment (GLSA)
Authors	Mary Alicia Barnes, Sharan L. Schwartzberg, Gary Bedell, Eleanor Counselman, and Elizabeth Marfeo
Source	Barnes, M. A., Schwartzberg, S. L., Bedell, G., Counselman, E., & Marfeo, E. (2020). The Group-Leader Self-Assessment (GLSA) Tool: Preliminary Study of Reliability and Validity. *The Journal for Specialists in Group Work, 45*(4), 277–291. https://doi.org/10.1080/01933922.2020.1799466
Brief Description	The GLSA was developed to assess the effectiveness of group leader training and can be used to help trainees identify goals for skill development and realize growth in leadership abilities. Group-leader trainees are asked to self-assess their group-leader ability in relation to key leader roles and functions (Barnes et al., 2020). As a result, the GLSA may prove helpful as an evaluative tool for group training programs. The GLSA is a 29-item self-report measure. Items assess group leadership qualities and are rated on a 6-point Likert scale (1 = strongly disagree to 6 = strongly agree).
Time Issues	Administration: 5–8 minutes. Scoring: 5–8 minutes.
Subscales and Scoring	Initial analyses indicated a four-factor structure for the GLSA indicating four scales: Support and Caring, Meaning Attribution, Executive Functions, and Emotional Activation. The Support and Caring scale consists of items that assess group leaders warmth, acceptance, and support. The Meaning Attribution scale consists of items that assess group leaders' ability to ascribe meaning to group work, such as translating feelings and experiences and providing cognitive framework for change. The Executive Functions scale assesses group leaders' ability to structure the group, including managing time, setting productive norms, and suggesting procedures. Finally, the Emotional Activation scale assesses group leaders' ability to confront, self-disclose, and model risk-taking. A total score is calculated by summing all items. Total score can range from 29–174 with high scores representing greater group leadership qualities.

Item	Information
Psychometric Properties	The GLSA has demonstrated good construct validity, good test-retest reliability, and responsiveness to change. However, this measure has not undergone extensive testing and the use and interpretation of data should be done with caution.
Norms and any normative data re: diversity for each instrument	The GLSA was developed and validated with a majority White US-based sample and given the recent development of this form, additional cross-cultural validation studies have not been conducted to date.
Translations	N/A
Sensitivity to Change	N/A
Sample references	Barnes, M. A., Schwartzberg, S. L., Bedell, G., Counselman, E., & Marfeo, E. (2020). The Group-Leader Self-Assessment (GLSA) Tool: Preliminary Study of Reliability and Validity. *The Journal for Specialists in Group Work, 45*(4), 277–291. https://doi.org/10.1080/01933922.2020.1799466
Website Resources	N/A
How to Obtain/Cost	Contact authors to request permission for use
Administration Types	Paper and Pencil
Analytics	No
Benchmarking	N/A

Group Psychotherapy Intervention Rating Scale (GPIRS) (Chapman et al., 2010)

The GPIRS was developed to assess leaders' ability to perform interventions aimed at enhancing group cohesion (Chapman et al., 2010). Specifically, the GPIRS is based on three dimensions that are shown to have the strongest relationship with group cohesion (Burlingame et al., 2002: group structuring, verbal interaction, and creating and maintaining a therapeutic emotional climate). As a result, the GPIRS can be conceptualized as a pan-theoretical measure of group leadership interventions.

The GPIRS is a 48-item observer-rated measure of group leader interventions. Items are scored on a 5-point Likert-type scale, each item rating therapist interventions qualitatively on the basis of clarity of delivery: poor (1), adequate (2), well done (3), or excellent (4). The GPIRS consists of three subscales: group structuring, verbal interactions, and creating and maintaining a therapeutic emotional climate. Trained raters assess two facets to every item score: a) the clarity of interventions as delivered by the group leader; and b) the quantity of each type of intervention used by the group leader. As a result, the GPIRS is rated strictly on the basis of the observable behaviors of the group leader (Chapman et al., 2010). Chapman and colleagues (2010) demonstrated good internal validity and concurrent validity for the GPIRS. Despite this preliminary evidence, there is limited research to support and further test the psychometric properties of the GPIRS is necessary. Therefore, the use and interpretation of data should be done with caution. There is no clinical cut-off or reliable change index for the GPIRS. The GPIRS was developed and validated with majority US-based White samples, and unfortunately, there is a paucity of research on the cross-cultural validity and use of the GPIRS. See Table 4.13 for more information on the GPIRS.

Table 4.13 Group Psychotherapy Intervention Rating Scale (GPIRS)

Item	Information
Name of Instrument	Group Psychotherapy Intervention Rating Scale (GPIRS)
Authors	Christopher L. Chapman, Elizabeth L. Baker, Greg Porter, Stephen D. Thayer, and Gary M. Burlingame
Source	Chapman, C. L., Baker, E. L., Porter, G., Thayer, S. D., & Burlingame, G. M. (2010). Rating group therapist interventions: The validation of the Group Psychotherapy Intervention Rating Scale. *Group Dynamics: Theory, Research, and Practice, 14*(1), 15. https://doi.org/10.1037/a0016628
Brief Description	The GPIRS was developed to assess leaders' ability to perform interventions aimed at enhancing group cohesion (Chapman et al., 2010). Specifically, the GPIRS is based on three dimensions that are shown to have the strongest relationship with group cohesion (Burlingame et al., 2002: group structuring, verbal interaction, and creating and maintaining a therapeutic emotional climate (Burlingame et al., 2002). As a result, the GPIRS can be conceptualized as a pan-theoretical measure of group leadership interventions.
	The GPIRS is a 48-item observer-rated measure of group leader interventions. Items are scored on a 5-point Likert-type scale, each item rating therapist interventions qualitatively on the basis of clarity of delivery: poor (1), adequate (2), well done (3), or excellent (4).
Time Issues	Administration: Scoring:
Subscales and Scoring	The GPIRS consists of three subscales: group structuring, verbal interactions, and creating and maintaining a therapeutic emotional climate. Trained raters assess two facets to every item score: (a) the clarity of interventions as delivered by the group leader, and (b) the quantity of each type of intervention used by the group leader. As a result, the GPIRS is rated strictly on the basis of the observable behaviors of the group leader (Chapman et al., 2010).
Psychometric Properties	Chapman and colleagues (2010) demonstrated good internal validity and concurrent validity for the GPIRS. Despite this preliminary evidence, there is limited research to support the psychometric properties of the GPIRS. More research on the scale's validity is necessary to strengthen evidence for its clinical use.
Norms and any normative data re: diversity for each instrument	There is no clinical cut-off or reliable change index for the GPIRS. The GPIRS was developed and validated with majority US-based White samples, and unfortunately, there is a paucity of research on the cross-cultural validity and use of the GPIRS.
Translations	N/A
Sensitivity to Change	N/A
Sample references	N/A
Website Resources	N/A
How to Obtain/Cost	Contact authors to request permission for use
Administration Types	Paper and Pencil
Analytics	No
Benchmarking	N/A

Multicultural Orientation (MCO) Inventory

The MCO inventory assesses patients' perceptions of their therapist on the three pillars of the Multicultural Orientation (MCO) Framework: Cultural Humility, Cultural Opportunities, and Cultural Comfort (Owen, 2013; Owen et al., 2011). The MCO framework complements the traditional model of therapist multicultural competencies and represents a way of being with clients (Owen et al., 2011). The MCO inventory consists of the Cultural Humility Scale (CHS) (Hook et al., 2013), the Cultural Opportunities Scale (Owen et al., 2016), and the Therapist Cultural Comfort Scale (TCCS) (Pérez-Rojas et al., 2019).

Cultural Humility Scale (CHS) (Hook et al., 2013). The CHS is a 12-item scale that assesses therapists' cultural humility. Cultural humility is characterized by a therapist's stance of openness and curiosity about their clients' cultural identities and experiences (Hook et al., 2013; Owen et al., 2016). Research has demonstrated a positive relationship between clients' perceptions of their therapist's cultural humility and their ratings of the therapeutic working alliance and treatment outcome (Hook et al., 2013; Owen et al., 2016). In addition, the CHS has been used within a group therapy context to measure both the group's cultural humility and the leaders' cultural humility (Grimes & Kivlighan, 2021).

The CHS is a patient-rated measure of therapist or group leader cultural humility. Clients are instructed as follows: *Please think about your counselor. Using the scale below, please indicate the extent to which you agree or disagree with the following statements about your counselor. Regarding the core aspect(s) of my cultural background, my counselor…* Example items include *is open to explore, assumes they already know a lot* (reverse coded), and *is a know-it-all* (reverse coded). Each item is rated on a 5-point scale, ranging from 1 (strongly disagree) to 5 (strongly agree). A total score is calculated by averaging all items. Higher scores represent higher levels of cultural humility. The CHS has demonstrated good reliability and validity in previous studies (Owen et al., 2016). There is no clinical cut-off or reliable change index available for the CHS.

Cultural Opportunities Scale (Owen et al., 2016)

Cultural opportunities are instances during a therapy session when there is an opening for purposeful and meaningful discussion of a client's cultural identity and experiences (Owen et al., 2011; Owen et al., 2016). These moments might involve direct naming of the cultural identity, or a more indirect exploration of the topic (Owen et al., 2016). Owen and colleagues (2016) found that clients who perceived their therapists to take more opportunities to discuss their most salient cultural identity had more positive treatment outcomes.

The Cultural Opportunities Scale is a 5-item scale that assesses clients' perceptions of their therapist's cultural missed opportunities. Clients are instructed as follows: *There are times where clients wish their therapist would have discussed certain issues more in depth. These opportunities come and go. Sometimes they are important and other times, they are not. Please rate the following items regarding these opportunities.* Example items include *My therapist discussed my cultural background in a way that worked for me* (reverse coded) and *There were many chances to have deeper discussions about my cultural background that never happened.* Each item is rated on a 5-point scale, ranging from 1 (strongly disagree) to 5 (strongly agree). A total score is calculated by averaging all items. Higher scores represent higher levels of missed cultural opportunities. Previous studies have demonstrated good reliability and validity of this measure (Owen et al., 2016). There is no clinical cut-off or reliable change index available for the Cultural Opportunities Scale.

Therapist Cultural Comfort Scale (TCCS) (Pérez-Rojas et al., 2019). Cultural comfort represents therapists' behavioral, physiological, and emotional experiences during discussions of cultural issues, experiences, and topics (Owen et al., 2017). Therapists' cultural comfort is positively related to clients' treatment outcomes (Owen et al., 2017). The TCCS is a 13-item scale that assesses clients' perceptions of their therapist's cultural comfort. Clients are instructed as follows: *When important parts of my culture come up or are discussed, my therapist…* Example items include *…stumbles with words* (reverse scored), *…seems comfortable talking to me, … seems genuine,* and *…seems annoyed* (reverse scored). Items are rated on a 5-point scale, ranging from 1 (strongly disagree) to 5 (strongly agree). A total score is calculated by averaging all items. Higher scores represent higher levels of cultural comfort. The TCCS has demonstrated good validity and reliability (Pérez-Rojas et al., 2019). There is no clinical cut-off or reliable change index available for the TCCS.

The measures within the MCO inventory were largely developed and validated with majority US-based White samples, and currently there is a lack of evidence of cross-cultural use and validity. Further research is needed to examine the validity and reliability of the MCO inventory internationally and with non-English speakers. See Table 4.14 for more information on the MCO inventory.

Table 4.14 Multicultural Orientation Inventory-Cultural Humility Scale; (CHS); Missed Cultural Opportunities Scale (COS); Therapist Cultural Comfort Scale (TCCS)

Item	Information
Name of Instrument	Multicultural Orientation Inventory-Cultural Humility Scale; (CHS); Missed Cultural Opportunities Scale (COS); Therapist Cultural Comfort Scale (TCCS)
Authors	CHS: Joshua Hook, Don E. Davis, Jesse Owen, Everett L. Worthington, and Shawn O. Utsey. COS: Jesse Owen, Karen Tao, Joanna Drinane, and Joshua Hook. TCCS: Andres E. Perez-Rojas, Theodore t. Bartholomew, Allison J. Lockard, and Jazmin M. Gonzalez.
Source	Hook, J.N., Davis, D. E., Owen, J., Worthington, E. L., & Utsey, S. O. (2013). Cultural Humility: Measuring Openness to Culturally Diverse Clients. Journal of Counseling Psychology, 60(3), 353–366. https://doi.org/10.1037/a0032595 Owen, J., Tao, K. W., Drinane, J. M., Hook, J., Davis, D. E., & Kune, N. F. (2016). Client Perceptions of Therapists' Multicultural Orientation: Cultural (Missed) Opportunities and Cultural Humility. Professional Psychology, Research and Practice, 47(1), 30–37. https://doi.org/10.1037/pro0000046 Pérez-Rojas, Bartholomew, T. T., Lockard, A. J., & González, J. M. (2019). Development and Initial Validation of the Therapist Cultural Comfort Scale. Journal of Counseling Psychology, 66(5), 534–549. https://doi.org/10.1037/cou0000344
Brief Description	**CHS:** The CHS is a 12-item scale that assesses therapists' cultural humility. Cultural humility is characterized by a therapist's stance of openness and curiosity about their clients' cultural identities and experiences (Hook et al., 2013; Owen et al., 2016). The CHS is a patient-rated measure of therapist or group leader cultural humility. Each item is rated on a 5-point scale, ranging from 1 (strongly disagree) to 5 (strongly agree). COS: The Cultural Opportunities Scale is a 5-item scale that assesses clients' perceptions of their therapist's cultural missed opportunities. Each item is rated on a 5-point scale, ranging from 1 (strongly disagree) to 5 (strongly agree). **TCCS:** The TCCS is a 13-item scale that assesses clients' perceptions of their therapist's cultural comfort. Items are rated on a 5-point scale, ranging from 1 (strongly disagree) to 5 (strongly agree) (Pérez-Rojas et al., 2019).
Time Issues	Administration: 10 minutes. Scoring: 10 minutes.

Item	Information
Subscales and Scoring	CHS: A total score is calculated by averaging all items. Higher scores represent higher levels of cultural humility. COS: A total score is calculated by averaging all items. Higher scores represent higher levels of missed cultural opportunities. TCCS: A total score is calculated by averaging all items. Higher scores represent higher levels of cultural comfort.
Psychometric Properties	CHS: The CHS has demonstrated good reliability and validity in previous studies (Owen et al., 2016). COS: Previous studies have demonstrated good reliability and validity of this measure (Owen et al., 2016). TCCS: The TCCS has demonstrated good validity and reliability (Pérez-Rojas et al., 2019).
Norms and any normative data re: diversity for each instrument	The measures within the MCO inventory were largely developed and validated with majority US-based White samples, and currently there is a lack of evidence of cross-cultural use and validity.
Translations	N/A
Sensitivity to Change	N/A
Sample references	Hook, J.N., Davis, D. E., Owen, J., Worthington, E. L., & Utsey, S. O. (2013). Cultural Humility: Measuring Openness to Culturally Diverse Clients. Journal of Counseling Psychology, 60(3), 353–366. https://doi.org/10.1037/a0032595 Owen, J., Tao, K. W., Drinane, J. M., Hook, J., Davis, D. E., & Kune, N. F. (2016). Client Perceptions of Therapists' Multicultural Orientation: Cultural (Missed) Opportunities and Cultural Humility. Professional Psychology, Research and Practice, 47(1), 30–37. https://doi.org/10.1037/pro0000046 Pérez-Rojas, Bartholomew, T. T., Lockard, A. J., & González, J. M. (2019). Development and Initial Validation of the Therapist Cultural Comfort Scale. Journal of Counseling Psychology, 66(5), 534–549. https://doi.org/10.1037/cou0000344
Website Resources	N/A
How to Obtain/Cost	Contact authors to obtain permission for use.
Administration Types	Paper and Pencil
Analytics	No
Benchmarking	N/A

Case Example #1

Dr. Nguyen is an early career psychologist who was hired five years ago by a mental health agency that provides services to adults in a medium sized urban center. She was hired in part to develop a group treatment program for the agency. The agency had few groups running at the time of Dr. Nguyen's hire, but wished to expand this service. The groups she developed or added included time-limited interpersonal process groups for depression and relationship problems. Dr. Nguyen also developed new psychoeducation groups for clients and their families. The groups were led by herself, social workers, and counselors. From the beginning, she established that client outcomes in the process and psychoeducation groups must be assessed at pre- mid- and post-treatment by giving a few brief scales related to the theme or goals of the groups. She convinced the agency to devote a modest number of resources to collect the data from clients systematically and to enter the data in a database. She used the PHQ-9 for the groups on depression, the IIP-32 (Barkham et al., 1996) for the relationship problems groups, and the GAD-7 (Spitzer et al., 2006) and the WHOQOL-BREF (World Health Organization, 2012) to members of all groups. She also asked the agency and therapists to keep track of the number of client dropouts (clients who unilaterally left therapy prior to completing treatment) and attendance. Fictional illustrative data from the groups set up by Dr. Nguyen is provided in Table 4.15.

Recently the mental health agency announced a restructuring process by which they were evaluating their entire programming to determine which aspects to keep, change, or discontinue. The agency was also considering which programs to add. Unlike other programs within the agency, Dr. Nguyen's group program had outcome data to help make these decisions. For example, she found that on average, clients in the depression groups improved reliably from pre- to post-treatment on the PHQ-9, and members in the Interpersonal Problems groups improved on the IIP-32. Members in both process groups also showed moderate positive improvements in their quality-of-life scores. However, she noticed that clients in these groups whose initial presenting problems included significant symptoms of anxiety showed only very modest improvement on the GAD-7. The results for the psychoeducation groups showed similar findings for depression and interpersonal problems. However, Quality of Life scores did not improve in the psychoeducation groups, and GAD-7 scores were unchanged at post-treatment for those clients with anxiety symptoms at the start of psychoeducation. She also noted that the rate of client dropout was higher and session attendance was lower in the psychoeducation versus the process groups. On average, the rate of dropping out is approximately 19 percent in randomized controlled trials and 38 percent in community practices (Swift & Greenberg, 2012). Finally, she found that about 15 percent of clients in all treatment groups were reliably worse at the end of treatment, and this troubled her. Average rates of deterioration in community practices tend to be somewhere between 5 percent and 10 percent (Shimokawa et al., 2010).

Dr. Nguyen was able to use the information from her outcome monitoring to suggest some alterations to the group program. First, she suggested no changes to the content of the process groups for depression and interpersonal problems, but she did suggest redirecting those clients with significant symptoms of generalized anxiety to a new group specifically to treat generalized anxiety symptoms. She began investigating evidence-based alternatives for these clients, as no group for generalized anxiety disorder were offered previously at the agency. Second, she felt that more significant changes should be made to the psychoeducation groups, including changing the content of the groups to focus more on quality-of-life issues, adding more activities to reduce dropping out, and adding a separate psychoeducation group for those with significant symptoms of anxiety. Third, she convened a meeting with the therapists in the psychoeducation groups and a focus group of former clients to brainstorm on how to reduce dropout rates and increase attendance. Fourth, Dr. Nguyen wanted a better system to identify early those clients who deteriorated so that they could be supported by therapists and the groups. She proposed to the agency that they engage in progress monitoring of clients; each client would complete a brief measure of distress

Table 4.15 Fictional Illustrative Group Outcome Data

	Process Groups (k = 8 groups, n = 64 clients)		Psychoeducation Groups (k = 10 groups, n = 80 clients)	
	PHQ-9	WHQOL	PHQ-9	WHQOL
Pre mean (SD)	16.20 (6.42)	75.01 (21.50)	15.70 (5.71)	78.87 (24.20)
Post mean (SD)	9.75 (5.59)	66.50 (20.03)	13.33 (7.25)	77.80 (20.00)
Improved	51%	44%	40%	12%
Recovered	36%	21%	19%	6%
Dropped out	29%		45%	

Note: Pre- and post-treatment means (M) and standard deviations (SD), percent reliably improved and percent reliably recovered at post-treatment of the Patient Health Questionnaire (PHQ-9) and the Brief World Health Organization Quality of Life scale (WHQOL).
Note: These data are fictional and for illustrative purposes only.

such as the OQ-45 or the ORS after each group session and that this information be fed back to the therapists. Dr. Nguyen presented the agency with compelling research evidence on the efficacy of progress monitoring (e.g., Lambert et al., 2018). She proposed that the agency give therapists sufficient time to engage in this activity and to attend in-service education sessions on how best to use progress monitoring. For example, progress monitoring might be used to identify clients at risk of deteriorating or dropping out which would alert the therapist to intervene differently with these clients such as revisiting the collaborative agreement on the tasks and goals of therapy or phone calls between sessions.

Case Example #2

Naomi identifies as a 21-year-old white Jewish American cisgender woman who will participate in a six-month intergroup dialogue group on race at her Midwestern university. Half of the group membership will consist of white members and half of Black members. The goal of the group is to promote cross-cultural understanding for individuals from different races and allow opportunities for students to gain awareness of their own racial identity and experiences of privilege and oppression. The leaders of her group plan to track diversity-related outcomes by assessing each group member prior to the start of the group, periodically (e.g., monthly or quarterly), and at the end of the intergroup dialogue.

Naomi met with the group leaders for a group preparation session wherein the leaders explained the goals of the group, group norms, and how the group will function, and to administer baseline assessments. The group leaders explained the purpose of the measures and then asked Naomi to complete two questionnaires—the SEE and the CCS-S. It took Naomi approximately 5–10 minutes to complete the measures and the group leaders were available to answer any questions about the measures, but Naomi had no questions. The group leaders reviewed the measures to make sure Naomi filled them out completely. They then discussed her specific goals for the group (what she hoped to gain from participating in the group). Naomi identified her goals as follows: "I hope to learn about others' lived experiences and learn about myself and any potential blind spots I have." She added to this, "I sometimes get nervous talking about race or I worry that I might say the wrong thing. So, I am often quiet during conversations of race, but I want to feel more comfortable to speak about race issues." Before the group started, the leaders reviewed Naomi's results from the questionnaires. The group leaders noted that Naomi's scores were notably high on the critical reflection- perceived inequality ($M = 4.55$) and the critical reflection − egalitarianism ($M = 4.76$) subscales compared to her scores on the critical motivation ($M = 3.01$) and the critical action - sociopolitical participation ($M = 2.25$) subscales. This might indicate that although Naomi endorsed moderate to high levels of critical reflection, she reported low levels of motivation and participation. This may indicate that Naomi is cognizant of racial injustices and endorsing equalitarian beliefs, but she may not be committed to social justice action or change in her daily life. Similarly, Naomi endorsed moderate levels on the empathic perspective taking, acceptance of cultural differences, and empathic awareness subscales ($M = 4.0, 4.2, 4.15$, respectively), but low levels on the empathic feeling and expression subscales ($M = 2.30$). Again, these scores indicate that Naomi had some insight about systems of oppression that many members of marginalized groups experience, but she may be uncomfortable or unaware of how to engage in social justice and equitable action.

After the second month of the group, the leaders again ask Naomi and the other members to fill out the questionnaires. The leaders then learned that Naomi's answers revealed only minor changes. Naomi's scores on the critical motivation ($M = 3.01$) and critical action - sociopolitical participation ($M = 2.25$) subscales of the CCS-S and the empathic feeling and expression subscale ($M = 2.30$) of the SEE only marginally increased over the past two months. This indicated little change in Naomi's motivation and participation related to social justice action. Upon reviewing

Naomi's scores, the group leaders planned to explore barriers to her participation in social justice activities more explicitly with Naomi, as well as explore these behaviors more in depth with the group-as-a-whole to promote social learning and mutual influence across members. The group leaders hoped these interventions at the individual and group level will help Naomi develop greater critical motivation and action.

At the end of the intergroup dialogue, Naomi completed the questionnaires again. Upon review of the post-group results, the leaders noted that Naomi made considerable progress as measured by the CCS-S and SEE. Naomi's scores on the critical motivation ($M = 5.01$) and critical action - sociopolitical participation ($M = 4.85$) subscales of the CCS-S and the empathic feeling and expression subscale ($M = 5.24$) of the SEE were moderate to high. Toward the end of the group, Naomi noted, "I always recognized injustice and inequitable treatment of others in the world, but I was uncomfortable talking about these and I did not know what to do to be a part of the solution. This group allowed me to realize these aspects of myself and challenged me to be more active in creating a more just and equitable world." She continued, "I have joined several student organizations to promote racial and gender equality, and I feel motivated to continue this work in the future."

In addition to quantitative outcome data, these qualitative reports can also serve to inform the group leaders' assessment of Naomi's change over the course of the group. These qualitative reports can serve to further support quantitative data collected or add more richness to quantitative reporting. Combining both qualitative reports and quantitative data may prove beneficial for group leaders.

Conclusion

We outlined in this chapter numerous reasons to engage in progress and outcome monitoring of participants who engage in group therapy. We also provided several resources about how to evaluate if a measure is valid and reliable, how to obtain such measures, and which measures we recommend. Two case examples show how measures can be used in different contexts to assess client outcomes, modify programming, and argue for additional resources. Group therapists have an obligation to their clients, the profession, and to funding sources to provide treatment according to best practices. Assessing outcomes is a means of fulfilling this obligation. But more than that, progress and outcome monitoring provide the group therapist with important, reliable, and valid information about the current state of the group and clients, and of the effectiveness of their interventions. Assessing outcomes and client progress are a means by which clinical judgement can be supplemented so that group therapists can make unbiased decisions about continuing with a current group therapy as is or making adjustments to improve client outcomes. Further, outcome monitoring may allow a therapist to gain insights into areas of clinical effectiveness and growth. Being a psychotherapist, including a group therapist, means a commitment to service and to lifelong learning. Progress and outcome monitoring are a means by which group therapists can be informed about what learning and development they may need to undertake. They are also a means by which clients may know if a service they are considering is effective so that they can make informed decisions about their care.

References

Albar, M. J., García-Ramírez, M., Perez Moreno, P., Luque-Ribelles, V., Garrido, R., & Bocchino, A. (2015). Adaptation to Spanish of an ethnocultural empathy scale. *Texto & Contexto-Enfermagem*, 24, 621–628.

Albiero, P. & Matricardi, G. (2013). Empathy towards people of different race and ethnicity: Further empirical evidence for the Scale of Ethnocultural Empathy. *International Journal of Intercultural Relations*, 37(5), 648–655. doi:10.1016/j.ijintrel.2013.05.003.

Alldredge, C. T., Burlingame, G. M., Yang, C., & Rosendahl, J. (2021). Alliance in group therapy: A meta-analysis. *Group Dynamics: Theory, Research, and Practice*, 25(1), 13–28. doi:10.1037/gdn0000135.

American Psychological Association. (2017). *Ethical principles of psychologists and code of conduct*. Washington, DC: Author.

Bardeen, J. R., Fergus, T. A., & Orcutt, H. K. (2012). An examination of the latent structure of the Difficulties in Emotion Regulation Scale. *Journal of Psychopathology and Behavioral Assessment*, 34(3), 382–392. doi:10.1007/s10862-012-9280-y.

Barkham, M., Hardy, G. E., & Startup, M. (1996). The IIP-32: A short version of the Inventory of Interpersonal Problems. *British Journal of Clinical Psychology*, 35(1), 21–35. doi:10.1111/j.2044-8260.1996.tb01159.x.

Barnes, M. A., Schwartzberg, S. L., Bedell, G., Counselman, E., & Marfeo, E. (2020). The Group-Leader Self-Assessment (GLSA) Tool: Preliminary Study of Reliability and Validity. *The Journal for Specialists in Group Work*, 45(4), 277–291. doi:10.1080/01933922.2020.1799466.

Beidas, R. S. et al. (2015). Free, brief, and validated: Standardized instruments for low-resource mental health settings. *Cognitive and Behavioral Practice*, 22, 5–19. doi:10.1016/j.cbpra.2014.02.002.

Bjureberg, J. et al. (2016). Development and validation of a brief version of the difficulties in emotion regulation scale: the DERS-16. *Journal of psychopathology and behavioral assessment*, 38(2), 284–296. doi:10.1007/s10862-015-9514-x.

Burlingame, G. M., Dunn, T., Hill, M., Cox, J., Wells, M. G., Lambert, M. J., & Brown, G.S. (2004). *Administration and Scoring Manual for the YOQ-30.2 (Youth Outcome Questionnaire-30 Version 2.0)*. Salt Lake City, UT: American Professional Credentialing Services.

Burlingame, G. M., Fuhriman, A., & Johnson, J. E. (2002). Cohesion in group psychotherapy. In J. C. Norcross (Ed.), *Psychotherapy relationships that work: Therapist contributions and responsiveness to patients* (pp. 71–87). New York: Oxford University Press.

Burlingame, G. M., Seebeck, J. D., Janis, R. A., Whitcomb, K. E., Barkowski, S., Rosendahl, J., & Strauss, B. (2016). Outcome differences between individual and group formats when identical and nonidentical treatments, patients, and doses are compared: A 25-year meta-analytic perspective. *Psychotherapy*, 53(4), 446–461. doi:10.1037/pst0000090.

Burnes, T. R. & Ross, K. L. (2010). Applying social justice to oppression and marginalization in group process: Interventions and strategies for group counselors. *The Journal for Specialists in Group Work*, 35 (2), 169–176. doi:10.1080/01933921003706014.

Canadian Psychological Association. (2017). *Canadian code of ethics for psychologists* (4th ed.). Ottawa, ON: Author.

Chapman, C. L., Baker, E. L., Porter, G., Thayer, S. D., & Burlingame, G. M. (2010). Rating group therapist interventions: The validation of the Group Psychotherapy Intervention Rating Scale. *Group Dynamics: Theory, Research, and Practice*, 14(1), 15. doi:10.1037/a0016628.

Chen, E. C., Kakkad, D., & Balzano, J. (2008). Multicultural competence and evidence-based practice in group therapy. *Journal of Clinical Psychology*, 64(11), 1261–1278. doi:10.1002/jclp.20533.

Clark, L. A. & Watson, D. (2019). Constructing validity: New developments in creating objective measuring instruments. *Psychological Assessment*, 31(12), 1412–1427. doi:10.1037/pas0000626.

Constantino, M. J., Boswell, J. F., Coyne, A. E., Swales, T. P., & Kraus, D. R. (2021). Effect of matching therapists to patients vs assignment as usual on adult psychotherapy outcomes: A randomized clinical trial. *JAMA Psychiatry*. doi:10:1001/jamapsychiatry.2021.1221.

Coutinho, J., Ribeiro, E., Ferreirinha, R., & Dias, P. (2010). The Portuguese version of the Difficulties in Emotion Regulation Scale and its relationship with psychopathological symptoms. *Archives of Clinical Psychiatry (São Paulo)*, 37, 145–151.

De Francisco Carvalho, L. & Rocha, G. (2009). Translation and cultural adaptation of Outcome Questionnaire (OQ-45) to Brazil. *Psico-USF*, 14, 309–316. doi:10.1590/S1413-82712009000300007.

de Jong, K., Nugter, M. A., Polak, M. G., Wagenborg, J. E., Spinhoven, P., & Heiser, W. J. (2007). The Outcome Questionnaire (OQ-45) in a Dutch population: A cross-cultural validation. *Clinical Psychology & Psychotherapy: An International Journal of Theory & Practice*, 14(4), 288–301.

Dessel, A., Rogge, M. E., & Garlington, S. B. (2006). Using intergroup dialogue to promote social justice and change. *Social work*, 51(4), 303–315. doi:10.1093/sw/51.4.303.

Diemer, M. A. & Blustein, D. L. (2006). Critical consciousness and career developmentamong urban youth. *Journal of Vocational Behavior*, 68, 220–232. doi:10.1016/j.jvb.2005.07.001.

Dozois, D. J. A. et al. (2014). The CPA PresidenNaomil Task Force on Evidence-based Practice of Psychological Treatments. *Canadian Psychology/Psychologie canadienne*, 55, 153–160. doi:10.1037/a0035767.

Duncan, B. L. (2012). The Partners for Change Outcome Management System (PCOMS): The Heart and Soul of Change Project. *Canadian Psychology/Psychologie canadienne*, 53(2), 93.

Duncan, B. L. & Reese, R. J. (2015). The Partners for Change Outcome Management System (PCOMS) revisiting the client's frame of reference. *Psychotherapy*, 52(4), 391. doi:10.1037/pst0000026.

Faustino, B. & Vasco, A. B. (2020). Factor Structure and Convergent Validity of the Portuguese version of the Inventory of Interpersonal Problems–32. *Journal of Relationships Research*, 11.

Flückiger, C., Del Re, A. C., Wampold, B. E., & Horvath, A. O. (2018). The alliance in adult psychotherapy: A meta-analytic synthesis. *Psychotherapy*, 55(4), 316–340. doi:10.1037/pst0000172.

Giromini, L., Velotti, P., De Campora, G., Bonalume, L., & Cesare Zavattini, G. (2012). Cultural adaptation of the difficulties in emotion regulation scale: Reliability and validity of an Italian version. *Journal of clinical psychology*, 68(9), 989–1007.

Gratz, K. L. & Roemer, L. (2004). Multidimensional assessment of emotion regulation and dysregulation: Development, factor structure, and validation of the difficulties in emotion regulation scale. *Journal of psychopathology and behavioral assessment*, 26(1), 41–54. doi:10.1023/B:JOBA.0000007455.08539.94.

Grenon, R., Schwartze, D., Hammond, N., Ivanova, I., Mcquaid, N., Proulx, G., & Tasca, G. A. (2017). Group psychotherapy for eating disorders: A meta-analysis. *International Journal of Eating Disorders*, 50(9), 997–1013. doi:10.1002/eat.22744.

Grimes, J. L. & Kivlighan, D. M., III. (2022). Whose multicultural orientation matters most? Examining additive and compensatory effects of the group's and leader's multicultural orientation in group therapy. *Group Dynamics: Theory, Research, and Practice*, 26(1), 58–70. doi:10.1037/gdn0000153.

Gurin, P., Nagda, B. R. A., & Zúñiga, X. (2013). *Dialogue across difference: Practice, theory, and research on intergroup dialogue*. Russell Sage Foundation.

Gyani, A., Shafran, R., Rose, S., & Lee, M. J. (2015). A qualitative investigation of therapists' attitudes towards research: Horses for courses? *Behavioural and Cognitive Psychotherapy*, 43, 436–448. doi:10.1017/S1352465813001069.

Hafkenscheid, A., Duncan, B. L., & Miller, S. D. (2010). The Outcome and Session Rating Scales: A cross-cultural examination of the psychometric properties of the Dutch translation. *Journal of Brief Therapy*, 7(1), 1–12.

Harry, M. L., Coley, R. Y., Waring, S. C., & Simon, G. E. (2021). Evaluating the cross-cultural measurement invariance of the PHQ-9 between American Indian/Alaska Native adults and diverse racial and ethnic groups. *Journal of affective disorders reports*, 4, 100121.

He, X. Y., Li, C. B., Qian, J., Cui, H. S., & Wu, W. Y. (2010). Reliability and validity of a generalized anxiety disorder scale in general hospital outpatients. *Shanghai Arch Psychiatry*, 22(4), 200–203.

Hook, J. N., Davis, D. E., Owen, J., Worthington Jr, E. L., & Utsey, S. O. (2013). Cultural humility: Measuring openness to culturally diverse clients. *Journal of counseling psychology*, 60(3), 353. doi:10.1037/a0032595.

Horowitz, L. M., Alden, L. E., Wiggins, J. S. et al. (2000). *IIP – Inventory of Interpersonal Problems Manual*. San Antonio, TX: The Psychological Corporation.

Horowitz, L. M., Rosenberg, S. E., & Bartholomew, K. (1993). Interpersonal problems, attachment styles, and outcome in brief dynamic psychotherapy. *Journal of Consulting and Clinical Psychology*, 61(4), 549–560. doi:10.1037/0022-006X.61.4.549.

Horowitz, L. M., Alden, L. E., Kordy, H., & Strauß, B. (2000). *Inventar zur Erfassung interpersonaler Probleme: deutsche Version; IIP-D*. Beltz-Test.

Hunsley, J. & Lee, C. M. (2007). Research-informed benchmarks for psychological treatments: Efficacy studies, effectiveness studies, and beyond. *Professional Psychology: Research and Practice*, 38, 21–33. doi:10.1037/0735-7028.38.1.21,

Hunsley, J. & Mash, E. J. (Eds). (2018). *A guide to assessments that work* (2nd ed.). New York, NY: Oxford University Press. doi:10.1093/medpsych/9780190492243.001.0001.

Ionita, G. & Fitzpatrick, M. (2014). Bringing science to clinical practice: A Canadian survey of psychological practice and usage of progress monitoring measures. *Canadian Psychology*, 55, 187–196. doi:10.1037/a0037355.

Iraurgi, I. & Penas, P. (2021). Outcomes Assessment in Psychological Treatment: Spanish adaptation of OQ-45 (Outcome Questionnaire). *Revista Latinoamericana de Psicología*, 53, 56–63.

Jacobson, N. S. & Truax, P. (1991). Clinical significance: A statistical approach to defining meaningful change in psychotherapy research. *Journal of Consulting and Clinical Psychology*, 59(1), 12–19. doi:10.1037/0022-006X.59.1.12.

Janis, R. A., Burlingame, G. M., Svien, H., Jensen, J., & Lundgreen, R. (2020). Group therapy for mood disorders: A meta-analysis. *Psychotherapy Research*. Advance online publication. https://doi.org/10.1080/10503307.2020.1817603.

Kiesler, D. J. (1996). *Contemporary interpersonal theory and research: Personality, psychopathology, and psychotherapy*. Wiley.

Kivlighan III, D. M. & Chapman, N. A. (2018). Extending the multicultural orientation (MCO) framework to group psychotherapy: A clinical illustration. *Psychotherapy*, 55(1), 39. doi:10.1037/pst0000142.

Knoll, M., Ionita, G., Tomaro, J., Chen, V., & Fitzpatrick, M. (2016). Progress monitoring measures: The interaction of clinician initial motivation with selection and maintenance issues. *Psychology*, 7, 444–458. doi:10.4236/psych.2016.73046.

Kroenke K, Spitzer R. L., Williams, J. B., Lowe B. (2010). The patient health questionnaire somatic, anxiety, and depressive symptom scales: a systematic review. *General Hospital Psychiatry*, 32(4), 345–359. doi:10.1016/j.genhosppsych.2010.03.006.

Lafontaine, M.-F., Brassard, A., Lussier, Y., Valois, P., Shaver, P. R., & Johnson, S. M. (2015). Selecting the best items for a short-form of the Experiences in Close Relationships Questionnaire. *European Journal of Psychological Assessment*, 32(2). doi:10.1027/1015-5759/a000243.

Lambert, M. J. (2017). Maximizing psychotherapy outcome beyond evidence-based medicine. *Psychotherapy and Psychosomatics*, 86, 80–89. doi:10.1159/000455170.

Lambert, M. J. et al. (2004). *Administration and scoring manual for the Outcome Questionnaire-45*. Salt Lake City, UT: OQ Measures.

Lambert, M. J., Smart, D. W., Campbell, M. P., Hawkins, E. J., Harmon, C., & Slade, K. L. (2006). Psychotherapy outcome, as measured by the OQ-45, in African American, Asian/Pacific Islander, Latino/a, and Native American clients compared with matched Caucasian clients. *Journal of College Student Psychotherapy*, 20(4), 17–29.

Lambert, M. J., Whipple, J. L., & Kleinstäuber, M. (2018). Collecting and delivering progress feedback: A meta-analysis of routine outcome monitoring. *Psychotherapy*, 55(4), 520–537. https://doi.org/10.1037/pst0000167.

Leary, T. (1957). *Interpersonal diagnosis of personality: A functional theory and methodology for personality evaluation*. Ronald Press.

Li, J., Han, Z. R., Gao, M. M., Sun, X., & Ahemaitijiang, N. (2018). Psychometric properties of the Chinese version of the Difficulties in Emotion Regulation Scale (DERS): Factor structure, reliability, and validity. *Psychological assessment*, 30(5), e1.

Lo Coco, G., Gullo, S., Albano, G., Brugnera, A., Flückiger, C., & Tasca, G. A. (2022). The alliance-outcome association in group interventions: A multilevel meta-analysis. *Journal of Consulting and Clinical Psychology*. Advance online publication. doi:10.1037/ccp0000735.

Lo Coco, G., Mannino, G., Salerno, L., Oieni, V., Di Fratello, C., Profita, G., & Gullo, S. (2018). The Italian version of the inventory of interpersonal problems (IIP-32): psychometric properties and factor structure in clinical and non-clinical groups. *Frontiers in psychology*, 9, 341.

Mallinckrodt, B. & Wang, C. C. (2004). Quantitative methods for verifying semantic equivalence of translated research instruments: a Chinese version of the experiences in close relationships scale. *Journal of Counseling Psychology*, 51(3), 368.

Merta, R. J. (1995). *Group work: Multicultural perspectives*.

Miller, S. D., Duncan, B. L., Brown, J., Sparks, J. A., & Claud, D. A. (2003). The outcome rating scale: A preliminary study of the reliability, validity, and feasibility of a brief visual analog measure. *Journal of brief Therapy*, 2(2), 91–100.

Miller, S. D., Duncan, B. L., Sorrell, R., & Brown, G. S. (2005). The Partners for Change Outcome Management System. *Journal of Clinical Psychology*, 61(2), 199–208. doi:10.1002/jclp.20111.

Moriarty, A. S., Gilbody, S., McMillan, D., & Manea, L. (2015). Screening and case finding for major depressive disorder using the Patient Health Questionnaire (PHQ-9): a meta-analysis. *General hospital psychiatry*, 37(6), 567–576.

Muir, H. J., Coyne, A. E., Morrison, N. R., Boswell, J. F., & Constantino, M. J. (2019). Ethical implications of routine outcomes monitoring for patients, psychotherapists, and mental health care systems. *Psychotherapy*, 56(4), 459. https://doi.org/10.1037/pst0000246.

Owen, J. (2013). Early career perspectives on psychotherapy research and practice: Psychotherapist effects, multicultural orientation, and couple interventions. *Psychotherapy*, 50, 496–502. doi:10.1037/ a0034617.

Owen, J., Tao, K. W., Drinane, J. M., Hook, J., Davis, D. E., & Kune, N. F. (2016). Client perceptions of therapists' multicultural orientation: Cultural (missed) opportunities and cultural humility. *Professional Psychology: Research and Practice*, 47(1), 30–37. https://doi.org/10.1037/pro0000046.

Owen, J. J., Tao, K., Leach, M. M., & Rodolfa, E. (2011). Clients' perceptions of their psychotherapists' multicultural orientation. *Psychotherapy*, 48, 274–282. doi:10.1037/a0022065.

Özdikmenli-Demir, G. & Demir, S. (2014). Testing the psychometric properties of the Scale of Ethnocultural Empathy in Turkey. *Measurement and Evaluation in Counseling and Development*, 47(1), 27–42.

Parkerson, H. A., Thibodeau, M. A., Brandt, C. P., Zvolensky, M. J., & Asmundson, G. J. (2015). Cultural-based biases of the GAD-7. *Journal of Anxiety Disorders*, 31, 38–42.

Pérez-Rojas, A. E., Bartholomew, T. T., Lockard, A. J., & González, J. M. (2019). Development and iniNaomil validation of the Therapist Cultural Comfort Scale. *Journal of counseling psychology*, 66(5), 534–549. doi:10.1037/cou0000344.

Persons, J. B., Koerner, K., Eidelman, P., Thomas, C., & Liu, H. (2016). Increasing psychotherapists' adoption and implementation of the evidence-based practice of progress monitoring. *Behaviour Research and Therapy*, 76, 24–31. doi:10.1016/j.brat.2015.11.004.

Pinner, D. H. & Kivlighan, D. M., III. (2018). The ethical implications and utility of routine outcome monitoring in determining boundaries of competence in practice. *Professional Psychology: Research and Practice*, 49, 247–254. doi:10.1037/pro0000203.

Puschner, B., Kraft, S., & Bauer, S. (2004). Interpersonal problems and outcome in outpatient psychotherapy: Findings from a long-term longitudinal study in Germany. *Journal of Personality Assessment*, 83(3), 223–234.

Rapa, L. J., Bolding, C. W., & Jamil, F. M. (2020). Development and iniNaomil validation of the short critical consciousness scale (CCS-S). *Journal of Applied Developmental Psychology*, 70, 101164. doi:10.1016/j.appdev.2020.101164.

Rapa, L. J. & Geldhof, G. J. (2020). Critical consciousness: New directions for understanding its development during adolescence. *Journal of applied developmental psychology*, 70, 101187. 10. 1016/j. appdev.2020. 101187.

Rasoal, C., Jungert, T., Hau, S., & Andersson, G. (2011). Development of a Swedish version of the scale of ethnocultural empathy. *Psychology*, 2(6), 568–573.

Raz Gross, M. D., Glasser, S., Jacobson, D. M., Levitan, G., & Ponizovsky, A. M. (2015). Validation of the Hebrew and Arabic versions of the Outcome Questionnaire (OQ-45). *Israel Journal of Psychiatry*, 52(1), 33.

Ribeiro, M. D. (Ed.) (2020). *Examining social identities and diversity issues in group therapy: Knocking at the boundaries*. Routledge.

Ridley, C. R. & Lingle, D. W. (1996). Cultural empathy in multicultural counseling: A multidimensional process model. In P. B. Pedersen, J. G. Draguns, W. J. Lonner, & J. E. Trimble (Eds), *Counseling across cultures* (pp. 21–46). Sage Publications, Inc.

Rugancı, R. N. & Gençöz, T. (2010). Psychometric properties of a Turkish version of the Difficulties in Emotion Regulation Scale. *Journal of Clinical Psychology*, 66(4), 442–455.

Salazar, J., Martí, V., Soriano, S., Beltran, M., & Adam, A. (2010). Validity of the Spanish version of the Inventory of Interpersonal Problems and its use for screening personality disorders in clinical practice. *Journal of personality disorders*, 24(4), 499–515.

Schuman, D. L., Slone, N. C., Reese, R. J., & Duncan, B. (2015) *Efficacy of client feedback in group psychotherapy with soldiers referred for substance abuse treatment*, Psychotherapy Research, 25:4, 396–407. doi:10.1080/10503307.2014.900875.

She, Z. et al. (2018). Client feedback in China: A randomized clinical trial in a college counseling center. *Journal of Counseling Psychology*, 65(6), 727.

She, Z., Sun, Q. W., & Jiang, G. R. (2017). Reliability and validity of Chinese version of Outcome rating scale. *Chinese Journal of Clinical Psychology*, 25(2), 272-275.

Shimokawa, K., Lambert, M. J., & Smart, D. W. (2010). Enhancing treatment outcome of patients at risk of treatment failure: Meta-analytic and mega-analytic review of a psychotherapy quality assurance system. *Journal of Consulting and Clinical Psychology*, 78, 298–311. doi:10.1037/a0019247.

Sighinolfi, C., Norcini Pala, A., Chiri, L. R., Marchetti, I., & Sica, C. (2010). Difficulties in emotion regulation scale (DERS): the Italian translation and adaptation. *Psicoterapia Cognitiva Comportamentale*, 16(2), 141–170.

Skevington, S. M., Lotfy, M., & O'Connell, K. A. (2004). The World Health Organization's WHOQOL-BREF quality of life assessment: psychometric properties and results of the international field trial. A report from the WHOQOL group. *Quality of life Research*, 13(2), 299–310.

Slone, N. C., Reese, R. J., Mathews-Duvall, S., & Kodet, J. (2015). Evaluating the efficacy of client feedback in group psychotherapy. *Group Dynamics: Theory, Research, and Practice*, 19(2), 122–136. doi:10.1037/gdn0000026.

Solstad, S. M., Castonguay, L. G., & Moltu, C. (2017). Patients' experiences with routine outcome monitoring and clinical feedback systems: A systematic review and synthesis of qualitative empirical literature. *Psychotherapy Research*, 29, 157–170. doi:10.1080/10503307.2017.1326645.

Spitzer R. L., Kroenke, K, Williams, J. B. W., Löwe, B. (2006). A Brief Measure for Assessing Generalized Anxiety Disorder: The GAD-7. *Archives of Internal Medicine*, 166 (10), 1092–1097. doi:10.1001/archinte.166.10.1092.

Strauss, B. & Burgmeier-Lohse, M. (1994). Evaluation einer stationären Langzeitgruppenpsychotherapie—Ein Beitrag zur differentiellen Psychotherapieforschung im stationären Feld [Evaluation of inpatient long term group psychotherapy–a contribution to differential psychotherapy research on inpatient settings]. *Psychotherapie, Psychosomatik, medizinische Psychologie*, 44(6), 184–192.

Strupp, H. H., Horowitz, L. M., & Lambert, M. J. (1997). *Measuring patient changes in mood, anxiety, and personality disorders: Toward a core battery*. American Psychological Association.

Sullivan, H. S. (1953). *The interpersonal theory of psychiatry*. Norton.

Swift, J. K. & Greenberg, R. P. (2012). Premature discontinuation in adult psychotherapy: A meta-analysis. *Journal of Consulting and Clinical Psychology*, 80(4), 547–559. doi:10.1037/a0028226.

Tasca, G. A., Brugnera, A., Baldwin, D., Carlucci, S., Compare, A., Balfour, L., … & Lafontaine, M. F. (2018). Reliability and validity of the Experiences in Close Relationships Scale-12: Attachment dimensions in a clinical sample with eating disorders. *International Journal of Eating Disorders*, 51(1), 18–27. doi:10.1002/eat.22807.

Tasca, G. A., Angus, L., Bonli, R., Drapeau, M., Fitzpatrick, M., Hunsley, J., & Knoll, M. (2019). Outcome and progress monitoring in psychotherapy: Report of a Canadian Psychological Association Task Force. *Canadian Psychology/Psychologie canadienne*, 60(3), 165 177. doi:10.1037/cap0000181.

Vanheule, S., Desmet, M., & Rosseel, Y. (2006). The factorial structure of the Dutch translation of the inventory of interpersonal problems: a test of the long and short versions. *Psychological assessment*, 18(1), 112.

Walfish, S., McAlister, B., O'Donnell, P., & Lambert, M. J. (2012). An investigation of self-assessment bias in mental health providers. *Psychological Reports*, 110, 639–644. doi:10.2466/02.07.17.PR0.110.2.639-644.

Wang, Y. W., Davidson, M. M., Yakushko, O. F., Savoy, H. B., Tan, J. A., & Bleier, J. K. (2003). The scale of ethnocultural empathy: development, validation, and reliability. *Journal of counseling psychology*, 50(2), 221–234. https://doi.org/10.1037/0022-0167.50.2.221.

Watts, R. J., Griffith, D. M., & Abdul-Adil, J. (1999). Sociopolitical development as an antidote for oppression—Theory and action. *American Journal of Community Psychology*, 27, 255–271. doi:10.1023/A:1022839818873.

White, B. A., Miles, J. R., Frantell, K. A., Muller, J. T., Paiko, L., & LeFan, J. (2019). Intergroup dialogue facilitation in psychology training: Building social justice competencies and group work skills. *Journal of Diversity in Higher Education*, 12(2), 180–190. doi:10.1037/dhe0000089.

Wiseman, H, Mayseless, O, & Sharabany, R. (2006). Why are they lonely? Perceived quality of early relationships with parents, attachment, personality predispositions and loneliness in first-year university students. *Personality and Individual Differences*. 40, 237–248.

World Health Organization. (1996). WHOQOL-BREF: introduction, administration, scoring and generic version of the assessment: field trial version, December 1996 (No. WHOQOL-BREF). World Health Organization.

World Health Organization. (2012). WHOQOL User Manual. Retrieved from www.who.int/toolkits/whoqol.

5   Enhancing Group Therapy Outcomes with Measurement-Based Care

Paul L. Hewitt and Shi Min Liew

In this chapter we will use two examples illustrating various elements of measurement-based care (MBC) as well as procedures and issues discussed in previous chapters to enhance the effectiveness of group therapy whether it is used for clinical purposes, research, or program evaluation, or a combination of all three. There are several overarching principles in these examples that we believe are crucial in conducting effective group psychotherapy for patients that are embraced in the MBC perspective. These include the importance of a focus on not just symptoms (or groups of symptoms defined as disorders) but on transdiagnostic issues in the assessment, formulation, and group treatment of difficulties. Secondly, we underscore the importance of establishing, from the beginning, a collaborative atmosphere that includes the patient in the process of assessment and group treatment and enhances patients' benefit from that treatment. Thirdly, we underscore the importance of high-quality clinical decision making in conducting the treatment that is based upon empirically demonstrated approaches that pay attention to scientific principles and evidence. We owe it to patients to be thoughtful, careful, and effective in the clinical work we do.

We will be describing two separate group treatments that involved elements of MBC as described in Chapter 1 from two different healthcare sites using two different group therapy approaches. Thus, the chapter is broken into two sections to illustrate different elements of MBC from the perspective of two different clinicians considering somewhat different issues and making decisions in the design, implementation, evaluation and reporting on effectiveness of each of their treatments. The first example, from an outpatient clinic in a public hospital setting in Singapore, demonstrates a group treatment program emphasizing interpersonal styles and problems that have been viewed as transdiagnostic factors underlying a large number of symptoms and disorders. The second example, from a university clinical treatment and research setting in Vancouver, Canada, focuses on the assessment and treatment of perfectionism, which is a core multidimensional personality vulnerability or transdiagnostic factor associated with the experience of myriad symptoms, syndromes, and disorders (see Bieling et al., 2004; Hewitt et al., 2017). The two examples provide an illustration of some of the considerations that clinicians had in preparing and conducting MBC group psychotherapy. The examples also provide an opportunity to consider some of the assessment issues germane to group psychotherapy treatment in different cultures, using different treatment orientations, and with different health care systems. Moreover, the examples are illustrative of evidence-gathering that can be used not only to evaluate the effectiveness and direct the refinement of the treatment for patients but also for the demonstration of the utility and appropriateness of such treatment for managers and others providing resources for patient care. In these examples, there is great emphasis placed on the evaluation and quality of measures used both in terms of the reliability and validity of instruments (which is crucial to make accurate and important claims of benefit, refinements

DOI: 10.4324/9781003255482-5

to treatment, and effectiveness of the group treatment program to agencies), but also on the utility of the measurements in terms of time commitment and potential fatigue of patients in the process of obtaining treatment. We believe, as has been demonstrated extensively in the research literature (see Wampold & Imel, 2015), that recruiting and maintaining a collaborative and supportive therapeutic alliance from the start can be extremely beneficial in optimizing treatment effects. The three attributes of therapeutic alliance are 1) the bond between the patient and therapist; 2) therapist's empathic understanding; and 3) a level of agreement between patient and therapist with regards to the goals and task of treatment (Bordin, 1979). It should be noted that in the group psychotherapy alliance can occur between a particular member and another member, a subgroup, the whole group, or the therapists. It is important that patients feel that they are heard and are not simply passive recipients of an assessment and treatment protocol; that their own unique issues and concerns are articulated and understood by clinicians and that the issues and concerns are dealt with and evaluated within the group treatment context. Thus, clinicians can choose to engage patients in MBC from the start which we believe can provide an optimum treatment experience, mitigate dropouts and noninvolvement in the process, and, indeed, influence positive treatment outcomes (see Hewitt et al. 2020; McLeod et al., 2021).

We discuss personality pathology and interpersonal/relational difficulties as the core underlying processes that require specific attention in terms of treatment. Group treatment goals that extend beyond symptom or episode reduction, from our perspective, are crucial; despite the fact that numerous group therapy approaches focus solely on symptom reduction. Personality and relational styles and problems have long been implicated in the etiology of many disorders and dysfunctions (see Blatt, 2004; Bornstein, 2005; Tasca et al. 2021) and both clinicians and researchers have been encouraged to focus on "patient characteristics and personality vulnerabilities that bear directly and indirectly on the psychopathology the patient exhibits rather than on the symptoms of the clinical syndrome per se" (Hewitt et al., 2008). Based on this approach, the clinicians in the following case examples reasoned that simply focusing on reducing symptoms of a disorder and allowing patients to continue carrying predispositions for those symptoms or disorder with them into the future seems of limited service for those individuals. This perspective is often of great appeal to front-line clinicians working in various clinical agencies who see patients who appear to experience only temporary relief of the distress and symptoms and express concern over relapse and the reappearance of symptoms or who continue to need subsequent treatment. A more practical consideration is that agencies can support treatments that focus on transdiagnostic factors that underly and maintain numerous disorders rather than have separate treatments for separate disorders.

Why Group Treatment?

Group psychotherapy can be particularly potent in treating transdiagnostic personality vulnerability factors (e.g., Marmarosh & Tasca, 2013; Tasca et al., 2021), especially for those that have relational elements that influence maladaptive outcomes and present challenges for both patients and therapists (e.g., Hewitt et al., 2017; Kramer, 2019). Although all forms of therapy require a willingness to reveal one's self and vulnerability, group therapy may, at first, present a daunting and frightening prospect for patients; thus, working with patients from the start to mitigate the fears of revealing the self is important.

There are numerous characteristics of group psychotherapy that make it challenging for participants who need to have reasonable goals and expectations and need to be motivated, cooperative with others, and capable of forming connections with others (Dies & Dies, 1993; Marmarosh & Sproul, 2021). Many of these hurdles can be addressed by knowledgeable clinicians employing appropriate assessment and treatment techniques and interventions. Navigating these hurdles can provide excellent opportunities for therapeutic benefit (Bernard et al., 2008; Garceau et al., 2021; Yalom & Leszcz, 2020). Furthermore, appropriate measurement and assessment procedures, individualized assessment feedback, and pre-group preparation, can be used to facilitate participation and engagement, potentially mitigate dropout, and, ultimately, enhance the treatment benefits (see Burlingame et al., 2006; Constantino et al., 2018; Tasca et al., 2021). Moreover, the initial assessment and ongoing data gathering, the results of which are shared directly with the patient over the course of the group treatment, can provide an excellent basis for establishment and maintenance of the therapeutic alliance and group cohesion factors extremely important in therapeutic benefit (Hilsenroth & Cromer, 2007).

The initial measurement-based assessment process provides an excellent starting point for 1) establishment of a caring environment for patients; 2) demonstration for patients that there is concern for the uniqueness of the individual even though it is a group context; 3) inclusion of a collaborative enterprise where patients' unique context and concerns are acknowledged and understood; and 4) engagement of the patients to be a collaborator in their treatment, which can ease the sometimes difficult demand to be deeply forthcoming throughout the process of assessment and treatment. As well, by building in measures of functioning at various points in the treatment and providing feedback to group therapy patients the process can facilitate their engagement in that treatment and affect treatment outcome (Lambert & Shimokawa, 2011).

Example One: Group Treatment of Interpersonal Problems

This section illustrates a case study of a transdiagnostic group psychotherapy program in a hospital outpatient clinic. Specifically, it brings the readers through some important considerations and practical decisions made regarding an MBC approach in this clinical context. The case also highlights how the clinician had addressed common concerns, such as assessment fatigue and dropouts.

Description of Location and Context

The following case example took place in Singapore, a sovereign island country and city-state in South East Asia, founded in 1965. Besides having the busiest cargo seaport, this cosmopolitan nation is also a finance and tourism hub. The population consists of residents from four main ethnic categories: Chinese, Malays, Indians and other races. Singapore's primary language is English while other official languages include Mandarin, Malay and Tamil. The average years of education in Singapore is 11.2, and 32.4 percent of its population that are above 25 years old graduated with degrees. Singapore is home to 10 religions and Singaporeans have the constitutional right to practice any religion. Despite the common belief that all Asian countries possess a strong collectivistic culture, Singapore has a unique mix of Asian and Western cultural influences with the younger generation more aligned with individualistic traits and values of the West.

Singapore's mental health statistics are comparable to those in the United States, with the lifetime prevalence of mental disorders at 14.2 percent with suicide being the leading cause of death among its youths (10 to 29 years old; Samaritans of Singapore, 2021). The three most common mental health conditions are Major Depressive Disorder, Alcohol Abuse and, Obsessive Compulsive Disorder (Subramaniam et al., 2020).

The following case example of a group intervention was conducted in an outpatient clinic setting within a general medical hospital based in northern Singapore. This clinic predominately treats individuals with mild to moderate mood and anxiety disorders. The clinician who led the group interventions in this case study is a Masters-level trained clinical psychologist and a Certified Group Psychotherapist conferred by the American Group Psychotherapy Association (AGPA). She is also the second author of this chapter. Her theoretical approach for group treatment is based on interpersonal and psychodynamic perspectives. More specifically, the group treatment focus was on transdiagnostic issues, meaning that the work focused on underlying constructs that are thought to give rise to symptoms; this orientation is in contrast to the majority of groups in Singapore which follow group protocols that are typically focused on a disorder or topic (e.g., Depression, Panic Disorder, Insomnia, Anger Management, Chronic Pain; Ooi et al., 2016). But focusing on a disorder or topic as the basis of group composition poses several recruitment challenges, such as slow and inconsistent flow of referrals, heightened potential of group members dropping out prematurely, and relatively few group offerings every year. Furthermore, group programs narrowly targeting specific disorders or topics tend to be piecemeal as they use circumscribed interventions for distinct symptoms or disorders and, thus require patients potentially to engage in multiple treatments. Given the premise that it is more resource- and time-efficient to provide integrative treatments focusing on an array of variables common across multiple diagnoses, the clinician explored models with transdiagnostic application.

In Singapore, hospital administrators are more likely to approve of structured group programs (i.e. psychoeducation and skills-based groups) and provide funds for its employees to be trained in them (Liew & Whittingham, 2020). Few local group leaders are trained in groups targeting group processes and interpersonal dynamics which affect emotional well-being and underlie the maintenance of psychopathology. Considering the various systemic factors and treatment needs, the present clinician was inclined towards a transdiagnostic treatment approach specifically targeting interpersonal difficulties as the main focus of group intervention, despite the fact that this approach was an exception to the general trend in the present clinical setting.

Group Treatment of Transdiagnostic Interpersonal Problems

Focused Brief Group Therapy (FBGT) is a semi-structured, integrative, interpersonal group therapy approach designed to accurately and reliably target reductions in interpersonal distress in eight sessions (Whittingham, 2015). A primary aim of FBGT group leaders is to facilitate the activation of adaptive interpersonal behaviors among group members in the here-and-now. The approach uses an assessment tool—the IIP-32—to focus treatment around specific interpersonal areas of distress. Members then enact behavioral goals during the here-and-now of the group. As a result, group members act on the here-and-now of the group and are invited to provide and request feedback from the group regarding each other's behavioral goal attempts in order to shape or reinforce their group behaviors and create new, adaptive schemas (Whittingham, 2015; Whittingham, 2018). In addition to its roots to interpersonal theory to address interpersonal behaviors, FBGT also sheds light on the intentions of these behaviors through group members' attachment styles (Whittingham, 2017). It is also non-shaming, person-centered and strengths-focused. A unique feature of this approach is the collaborative process of using assessment tools and exploring their results in real time with the group members both individually and collectively (Whittingham, 2018). The following sections will detail considerations in implementing FBGT and employing group assessment measures as well as elucidating the adaptations needed to tailor psychotherapy approaches for clinical populations in non-Western countries.

Culturally responsive interventions involve adapting evidence-based psychotherapy to incorporate components that are contextually relevant and culturally meaningful. The primary aim is to maintain fidelity to the core features of the psychotherapy approach while integrating certain cultural elements to make the approach meaningful to the particular treated population. Delivering culturally informed treatment is essential to increase treatment acceptability, patient satisfaction and effectiveness (Chowdhary et al., 2014; Hall et al., 2016).

Group members gather with different intersecting identities, such as race, sexual orientation, gender, age, ethnicity and religion (Ribeiro, 2020). As a result, pre-group interviews should explore members' identifications with differing cultural groupings and how these identifications shape their perception and experiences of their presenting problems, their expectations of therapy, and their understanding of the therapist's and members' roles. In the present example, the group therapist had selected certain questions from the Group Therapy Questionnaire-Short Form (GTQ-S); MacNair & Corazzini, 1994; MacNair-Semands, 2002) as recommended in the FBGT model. Some of the specific items selected from the GTQ-S included the checklist of interpersonal problems, identification of roles held in one's current family or intimate relationships that contribute to interpersonal difficulties, fears about group therapy, and potential obstacles which might prevent or limit attainment of goals. While it would be ideal to administer a standalone questionnaire which specifically delves into assessing group member's cultural affiliations and their impacts on interpersonal functioning and mood, this would necessitate additional time and effort on the group members to complete them during the pre-group meeting. Consequently, the local group therapist sought to gather relevant cultural information with several specific questions regarding cultural influences to avoid fatigue. For example, questions such as "were there any remarkable cultural influences in your current interpersonal struggles" and "are there any group-related nuances specific to your culture that we should be aware of" were included in the clinical interview segment of the pre-group screening session. Parenthetically, it was also necessary for the group therapist herself to develop awareness of the various racial identities in order to develop deeper sensitivity and connection with group members (Bemak & Chung, 2019). For example, discussion of sexual topics and expression with individuals of differing gender (apart from their spouses) is generally forbidden among Muslims.

Screening and Assessment

As suggested by Chen and colleagues (2008), the "local clinical scientist" method is especially important when there is limited research guidance regarding how to adapt interventions a group different from the group the approach was developed on. In the present case study, the group therapist attempted to select culturally appropriate and sensitive measures to monitor group processes and outcomes (Liew & Whittingham, 2020; Whittingham, 2018). Findings from the measures administered and gathered at various junctures of the group program facilitates elaboration of the individual group members' clinical formulations and allows a more comprehensive understanding of individual members' and the entire group's emotional functioning. The use of measures to achieve these overarching objectives was clearly communicated to the group members during the pre-group meeting and reiterated throughout the group sessions. During the individual pre-group sessions, each group member completed the measures in-person with ongoing opportunities provided by the group leader to clarify any item(s) that were not understood.

The use of measures in psychotherapy does raise the concern of assessment fatigue. In the present study, this concern was mitigated by 1) encouraging collaborative engagement of the patients on their outcomes and group process; 2) appropriate time allocation to complete the self-reported measures; and 3) familiarity of some of the questionnaires. And of particular importance, the group therapist had prepared the group members during the pre-group sessions regarding the frequency of measures administration consistent with Liew and Whittingham (2020) contributing to the engagement of the group members in this process. Fortunately, complaints regarding effort and time taken to complete the measures were rare. Whenever that occurred, the group therapist provided some reinforcement of the rationale of the routine outcome monitoring (i.e., informing their treatment progress and allowing group therapist to provide better care in subsequent sessions). Furthermore, one of the assessment measures was an outcome measure, the Depression Anxiety and Stress Scale (DASS-21) (Lovibond & Lovibond, 1995) which local clinicians and patients were familiar with, as it has been commonly administered in Singapore. This sense of familiarity provided group members with a degree of comfort in the assessments based on anecdotal reports.

Despite the frequent and lengthy outcome and process questionnaires (see Table 5.1), the therapist found a high degree of cooperation of most of group members across the eight group sessions, assessed as 93.3 percent completion rate. Several of the members verbally shared that they were keen to closely track their treatment progress and hence, appreciated the administration of assessment measures at various points of their treatment.

In the present case example, two mood symptoms outcome measures—the DASS-21 (Lovibond & Lovibond, 1995) and OQ30.2 (Lambert et al., 2004)—were used. With the intention to evaluate group engagement and prevent dropout in a timely manner, process measures were also incorporated. The primary process measure administered was the Group Climate Questionnaire (GCQ) (MacKenzie, 1981), supplemented with a brief 4-item process measure (i.e., Group Session Rating Scale; GSRS) (Quirk et al., 2013), both described earlier in this volume. The purpose of this additional process measure was to quickly collect feedback from group members for every session to identify intricate developments of the group process which might not have been captured by the GCQ, since it was administered in only three of the eight group sessions as per the FBGT model. Clarification and confirmation regarding their individual or group needs could also be promptly performed upon reviewing the ratings of the four items on the GSRS (i.e. relationship, goals and topics, approach or method, overall) after each group session. For future groups, it could be helpful to track functional measures such as hospital admissions, relapses, and both work and social functioning (e.g., Work and Social Adjustment Scale; Mundt & Marks, 2002).

Table 5.1 Outcome and Process Measures Administered in Case Study 1

Category	Questionnaire(s)	Administration
Outcome Measures		
Mood	Depression, Anxiety and Stress Scales (DASS- 21; Lovibond & Lovibond, 1995), OQ30.2* (Lambert et al., 2004)	Pre-group, after Session 8
Interpersonal distress	Inventory of Interpersonal Problems* (IIP-32; Horowitz, Alden, Wiggins & Pincus, 2000).	Pre-group, after Session 8
Process Measures		
Group dynamics	Group Session Rating Scale (Quirk, Miller, Duncan & Miller, 2013)	End of each group session
	Group Climate Questionnaire* (MacKenzie, 1983)	After Session 2, 5 and 8
	Session Logs (Liew & Whittingham, 2020)	End of each group session

Note. * denotes measures described in CORE-R.

The defining and transdiagnostic component of FBGT's model (Whittingham, 2015) is its utilization of the interpersonal circumplex which was first developed by Leary (1957). The interpersonal circumplex is an empirically validated conceptualization considered to be the gold standard of analytic tools to understand interpersonal functioning (Horowitz & Strack, 2010). As described earlier in the volume, the Inventory of Interpersonal Problems (IIP-32) measures interpersonal distress along eight scales (i.e., dominant, unassertive, warm, cold, inhibited, disinhibited, focused on self and focused on others). The IIP-32 was the main inventory of this study and was administered during the individual pre-group sessions to facilitate the development of a person-centered clinical formulation. This clinical formulation sought to integrate the IIP-32 ratings with the patient's interpersonal and mood history (obtained via the mood outcome measures and clinical interview responses), and interactional dynamics observed by the group therapist during the pre-group session. Subsequently, the clinical formulation was shared and verified with the patient to refine or confirm it.

To illustrate, let us consider a local case example of Jamie - her ratings for the outcome measures administered at pre-group meeting are detailed in the table below (see Table 5.2). Jamie's clinical formulation was a careful amalgamation of her self-reported ratings, clinical diagnosis (i.e., General Anxiety Disorder), clinical history (including childhood attachment trauma) and interpersonal tendencies (i.e., likes to lead conversation to feel sense of control, difficulties with rejecting and disagreeing with others, fear of offending authority figures). Foremost, her DASS-21 Anxiety score was classified as extremely severe, consistent with her clinical diagnosis and presentation during the pre-group interview. The item analysis on her OQ30.2 revealed that Jamie was unsatisfied with her life and relationships and had concerns about family troubles. This was also reflected in her clinical interview during which she had shared the significant mood disturbances that were a result of conflicts with her siblings and her in-laws' financial and legal woes. Her IIP-32 findings revealed significant

Table 5.2 Jamie's Self-reported Ratings of Outcome Measures at Pre-group Meeting

Category	Questionnaire	Pre-group ratings		
		Subscale	Score	Classification
Mood	Depression, Anxiety and Stress Scales (DASS- 21; Lovibond & Lovibond, 1995)	Depression	8/21	Moderate
		Anxiety	10/21	Extremely severe
		Stress	12/21	Moderate
	OQ30.2* (Lambert et al., 2004)		62	
Interpersonal distress	Inventory of Interpersonal Problems* (IIP-32; Horowitz, Alden, Wiggins, & Pincus, 2000)	Highly assertive	64	Above average
		Focused on own needs	50	Normative
		Cold/Distant	57	Normative
		Socially inhibited	47	Normative
		Non-assertive	63	Above average
		Focused on others' needs	77	Significant difficulty
		Self-sacrificing/ Warm	77	Significant difficulty
		Uninhibited	74	Significant difficulty

Note. IIP-32 scores are T-scores.

distress in her interpersonal responses, such as focusing on others' needs[1], self-sacrificing/warm[2] and uninhibited[3]. In brief, Jamie's psychopathology presented as an array of anxiety and physiological symptoms which she identified as stemming from her interpersonal struggles with her family members and the circumstances of her family environment.

There are a few interpersonal profiles on the IIP-32 which are likely to influence outcomes, leading to group failures, decompensation, or premature dropouts. Specifically, group members with high interpersonal distress scores for the Assertive, Uninhibited, and Focused on Own Needs scales were predicted to present with self-sabotaging behaviors which would counteract their group goals. In the FBGT model, the group leaders inoculate against the self-sabotaging during the pre-group meeting by bringing this issue to light and suggesting behavioral goals to prevent these undesirable consequences (Whittingham, 2015; Whittingham, 2018). For example, Jamie had a score of 74 for the Uninhibited for her IIP-32 during pre-group assessment. It was also observed that few other group members commonly possess significant high scores (cut-off score 70 and above) for struggling with Focused on Others' Needs. Therefore, it was important for the group therapist to give Jamie an inoculation of her potential self-sabotaging and destructive group behavioral tendencies (i.e., inappropriately interrupting others and controlling conversations). Inoculation is a technique developed within FBGT that predicts into possible self-sabotage and collaboratively develops goals with the client to prevent this occurring. Given the make-up of IIP-32 profiles in the group, the other group members were likely to give Jamie space whenever she interrupted and allow her to dominate group conversations. On that account, the group therapist coached Jamie to moderate her sharing to be more consistent with other group members' and to gradually deepen her sharing only after observing that the group members seemed ready for intense emotional content and disclosure.

Group leaders should ideally consider each group member's clinical formulation and how their interpersonal dynamics might impact on the group dynamics. Based on these clinical formulations developed in the pre-group sessions, the group leader and members then collaboratively can form clear, focused, realistic and relevant goals with the intention to progress towards interpersonal flexibility (refer to Jamie's goals in Table 5.3). These goals take the form of interpersonal behaviors through behavioral activation and they are facilitated by the leader during the here-and-now of the group sessions (Whittingham, 2017, 2018). The IIP-32 was also administered at the end of the final group session to assess change in levels of interpersonal distress and the findings were interpreted and discussed with the group members at their individual post-group sessions.

In the first of three trials of the Singapore FBGT groups, there were a few comments during the group about difficulties recalling session progress the following week, as there had been "too many memorable group interactions" and members reported they often struggled to track their own behavioral goals, reflections and progress. In the subsequent two trials, the group therapist added a session log with the purpose of facilitating group members' reflection of their hard work and the group supporting their efforts for that session. At the end of each group session, the group therapist distributed a customized handout for each group member to log their perceived progress and remarkable moments or efforts during the session in an open-ended manner. These session logs were collected and referenced along with the process measure(s) administered for each group session. This was a Singapore adaptation and an off-model feature for FBGT. In addition, this personal log consisted of their individual goals which prompted them to stay on task.

The group therapist distributed these handouts to the group members when they arrived for the group sessions for perusal of their individual goals and previous entries prior to the commencement of each group session. In trials two and three, the group therapist checked in with the group members about their opinion of this session log and it was noted that most appreciated it as a personal reminder of their attempts at working on their behavioral goals session by session. In addition, the group leader's observations of the group members behaviour (i.e. attempts at group tasks and session experience) were generally consistent with the patients' self-report entries in the session logs (see Table 5.3 below for case example of Jamie 's session log). Therefore, it seemed that this added feature was helpful in meeting the needs of the group members and thus, the session log feature was kept and continued in the third trial. Furthermore, the qualitative information written by the group members was analyzed along with the GSRS ratings to connect the ratings on the GSRS items to the rich descriptions in the session logs (Liew & Whittingham, 2020). Moreover, these self-reports (e.g., group experience, tendencies, feedback received) were also taken into account for the group members' individual clinical formulation which was periodically updated by the group leader. Finally, for the patients to be adequately heard, motivated, and engaged to work in the group sessions, the use of all outcome and process measures were presented in a collaborative fashion with the patients during the post-group individual debriefing.

In this example, the group leader had intended to recruit a mix of patients with a variety of sexual and gender identities, age ranges, racial identities, mood diagnoses, and interpersonal tendencies, in order to ensure some heterogeneity in the group composition. This selection process was facilitated by the use of patient responses on the IIP-32 and mood measures, as well as the derived clinical formulation and observations gleaned from the clinical interview. For example, the group leader limited the number of group members who scored high in Dominance or Disinhibited scales in order to prevent these group members from dominating the group's time. In general, the group leader aimed for a

Table 5.3 Sample of Group Session Log

Session	Participant Notes
Jamie 's Goals	1 Share my disagreements and anger (Once per session) 2 To provide and ask for feedback (Once per session) 3 To share my urges to shape conversations
Session 1	Shared my frustrations, became more aware of the urge to shape conversations and made space for the urge
Session 2	It was a very productive session, managed to share my disagreement even thought it was slightly uncomfortable but my anger not so much, but I do realize a lot of anger is self-directed.
Session 3	Shared my disagreement! Still anxiety inducing. Started off today's session with some jitters but it got better. Did not get to share my panic episode because it was brief during session. Not so much anger compared to last week.
Session 4	Shared my personal anger situation. Uncomfortable emotions were dealt with and feedback were received, both positive and constructive ones.
Session 5	Resolved (or I feel) last week's issue. Shared my disagreement while knowing the boundaries. Know what I'm apologizing for and not apologizing for (being specific in what I am sorry about).
Session 6	Shared about my struggles in the past with self-harm. Gave and asked for feedback even though it was uncomfortable to ask for feedback directly.
Session 7	Gave feedback. It was nice to be able to relate with Asher (pseudo name). It was a pretty productive session for me to be able to balance my own needs and support the group – to hear and to be heard.
Session 8	Good closure and understanding of where I stand and am right now interpersonally.

balance of interpersonal styles in an attempt to keep the group balanced and heterogenous across the various interpersonal domains.

Apart from the qualitative data provided by the session logs, none of the formal outcome and process measures had been constructed locally and their normative data were not based on a Singapore population. This is a common problem when assessing treatment effects in Singapore; consequently, we attempted to choose outcome and group process measures that seemed culturally relevant and sensitive. The group leader in this case study decided to "make do" by selecting the most suitable measures while carefully considering the validity of these measures for the current clinical sample. An examination of the IIP-32 scores of the Singapore sample seemed in line with normative samples, contrary to the initial hypothesis that the Singapore sample might yield different patterns of interpersonal distress. Still, the group leader interpreted the findings for each group member with caution. Instead of relying solely on established norms and cut-off scores, the local group leader conscientiously looked out for trends within and between domains and performed item analysis when necessary (Liew & Whittingham, 2020) in an attempt to ensure that instruments developed in different cultures were working in similar ways in Singapore. While aspiring to utilize the instrument in similar ways in Singapore, the item-analysis approach enabled the group leader not to miss any important trends or findings that might be left out due to the likely differences in normative data. Finally, the changes in scores on the measures of outcomes and process were explored in detail with each group member during their individual post-group session with the aim of making meaning among the various sources of data, namely the objective measures, the open-ended session logs, and in-group behavior and subjective experiences (Liew & Whittingham, 2020).

Drop-out Rates

Drop-out in group psychotherapy remains a prominent clinical issue and in this case example, the group therapist was unsure of the dropout rate to expect, given both that it was her first attempt implementing FBGT in an outpatient clinic with adult group members and that the model was established in a very different setting, namely a university counselling center in the United States. A review of the literature revealed that drop-out rates in group therapy varied considerably: Batch (2018), for example, found that it ranged from 10–60 percent for group therapy in the United States while a study from Denmark reported a 20.6 percent dropout rate (Jensen et al., 2014). It was decided that this Singapore case study should be benchmarked against a similar Singapore group to appreciate and mitigate factors that might contribute to drop-outs. Using another Singapore clinical population, Wong (2018) found a 17% drop-out rate in an 8-session cognitive behavioral therapy group program in a Singaporean psychiatric institution outpatient clinic. As we assessed, the drop-out rate for the present case study was lower at 7 percent, consistent with the goals of FBGT (Whittingham, 2018).

Of relevance to the issue of drop-out, a recent Singapore survey revealed that Singaporeans' attitudes towards seeking counselling were dependent on trust towards their counselor and a view of the counselor as one who could understand their issues and empathize significantly (Goh, 2020). This finding, in turn, reinforces the importance of the group leader's emphasis on establishing therapeutic alliance and a collaborative approach to clinical formulation during the pre-group sessions. Hence, with hopes to recruit group members who were motivated and committed, the group leader attempted to enhance participation during the pre-group meeting with provision of a clear description of 1) the work of the group; 2) clinical examples; 3) brief role-plays of the here-and-now approach; 4) activation of adaptive interpersonal behaviors; and 5) interpersonal feedback as the change mechanisms for every patient. In particular, adaptive interpersonal behaviors were collaboratively identified as individual goals in the pre-group meeting and actively examined in the here-and-now, with the help of the other members' feedback. Some examples of these adaptive interpersonal behaviors include verbally expressing both disagreements and negative emotions. Given the rarity of a process group as a form of treatment in Singapore, emphasis on trusting the group process and accountability of group attendance were also made by the group leader. Moreover, the group leader noticed the FBGT model had similar elements matching those postulated for a brief psychoanalytic group, namely rapid cohesion promotion, rapid conceptualizations, broad selection of patients, a clear and specific focus, time limit awareness, active therapists, emphasis on the here-and-now and an interpersonal orientation (Weiss, 2010). Furthermore, favorable outcomes were associated with strong patient commitment and consensus on the group task in time limited group therapy (Lenzo et al., 2014).

Mid-Treatment Assessment

A brief mid-treatment assessment was performed after the fifth session with one of the process measures, the GCQ, which was also administered upon the second and last group session, thus allowing the group leader to observe the overall group and individual trends on engagement, avoidance and conflict. It was observed, for example, that the group tended to peak on engagement and conflict at the midpoint of the group program, consistent with clinical observations that the group was actively working on disagreements and differences in the here-and-now during that period. And in an ongoing way, the group leader routinely monitored the weekly GSRS ratings and the group members' entries in their session logs and provided informal feedback throughout the group sessions.

Post-Treatment Assessment

In the present study, the Reliable Change Index (RCI) (see Chapter 4; Hawley, 1995; Jacobson & Truax, 1991) was calculated for each group member to evaluate whether any pre-post reductions in interpersonal distress and mood symptoms were clinically reliable. In addition, treatment outcomes for the group-as-a-whole were analyzed, in part to make a case to the hospital administration that the group program was worth the resources. The efficacy of the treatment mode has been commonly evaluated by statistical analyses involving comparisons of group means. In the typical case of group research where group sizes are small and various assumptions underlying parametric tests such as the independence of observation are violated, we used non-parametric statistical analyses, specifically the Wilcoxon Signed Ranked Test analysis, which uses the median to evaluate the whole group's change as a whole, to meaningfully evaluate the group intervention. As a core part of accountability, both individual and group treatment effects were presented to the hospital administrators to justify continuation of this group program as part of the hospital's clinical service (explained further in later section).

Consistent with the Focused Brief Group Therapy model (Whittingham, 2015), feedback was provided to each group member individually during post-group sessions. The general format of this session entailed exploration of therapeutic progress on group goals, as perceived both by the patient and the leader, review of attempts of adaptive interpersonal behaviors, and the study of changes in pre- and post-outcome and process measures. Given that there were multiple constructs analyzed and questionnaires administered at various time points of the group program, the leader had prepared a simplified reference document for the patients to provide the feedback. The leader summarized the psychometric findings in a single page handout for the feedback session (refer to Table 5.4 for a sample of the

Table 5.4 Example of Reference Document with Outcome Measures for Jamie's Post-group Meeting

Feedback to each Group Member

Measures	Pre-group score		Post-group score	Comments	Recommendations
DASS					
Depression	8/21	Moderate	7/21 Moderate	• More psycho-somatic features of anxiety (dryness of mouth, trembling)	• Dialectical thinking
Anxiety	10/21	Extremely severe	8/21 Severe		
Stress	12/21	Moderate	6/21 Normal		
OQ-30.2				• Post-group: Satisfied with life and relationships	• Take risks
Mood symptoms Functioning	62		51	• Continues to be concerned about family troubles	
				• Something is wrong with my mind	
IIP-32				• Improved insight and actively trying out new interpersonal behaviors	• Emotional needs: to attend to self (cut back from overly attending to others)
Interpersonal distress	Focusing on others' need Warm/self-sacrificial Uninhibited		All within normative range now		
				• Interpersonal more flexible	

simplified reference document). Moreover, the group leader and patients also discussed and generated some ideas on how to sustain treatment gains from the group intervention (Liew & Whittingham, 2020).

The Table 5.4 handout with summarized psychometric findings, interpersonal behavioral progress and suggestions were also documented in every patient's electronic medical record. This effort was designed to link to patients' respective individual psychotherapists and referring clinicians who worked in the same hospital. To further integrate the group treatment with other treatment interventions, the group leader also had informal check-ins with the group members' individual therapists to inquire about any significant concerns raised about the group experience during their individual psychotherapy sessions. Referencing Jaime's progress in Table 5.4, the group leader briefed Jaime on her observable improvement in stress self-rating and the pattern of Jamie's anxiety features reflected as psychosomatic presentation as elucidated through item analysis of her DASS-21 ratings. Similarly, her overall mood functioning showed a positive change based on her OQ30.2 while items endorsed in the post-group questionnaire revealed that she was satisfied with life and relationships but continued to be concerned about family troubles (this was consistent with Jamie's sharing in the group sessions). Jamie's interpersonal distress on the various scales were in the normative score range after the group program and the group leader had observed that she had demonstrated improved insight and actively attempted appropriate interpersonal behaviors to meet her needs.

During the yearly review of the ongoing clinical services, a brief presentation was given by the group leader to the hospital management to inform them about the treatment effectiveness and provide an accounting for the hospital resources dedicated for this group program. The main findings presented were first, the overview of the reliable changes to IIP-32 behavioral goals selected by group members to be worked on as in Table 5.5, and second, the outcomes sorted according to the breakdown of the IIP-32 scales which the group members had selected to work as in Table 5.6, and third, the treatment effect of the local FBGT for mood outcomes as a group (see Table 5.7). Foremost, more than half of the patients showed reliable improvement on interpersonal scales that were intervention targets whereas no patients showed reliable deterioration (Table 5.5). Furthermore, the group leader observed that patients tended to show greater improvements on Socially Inhibited and Uninhibited scales than on the other six interpersonal scales (Table 5.6). The number of

Table 5.5 Reliable Changes to IIP-32 Goals Selected by Group Members

	No. of reliable improvements (%)	*No. of uncertain change (%)*			*No. of reliable deterioration (%)*
		Improvement	*Deterioration*	*Same*	
Goals selected by group members	15 (53.6%)	7 (25%)	2 (7.1%)	4 (14.3%)	0 (0%)

Table 5.6 Breakdown of IIP-32 Scales and Their Reliable Changes

Selected scales as goals	*No. of reliable improvement (%)*	*No. of uncertain change (%)*			*No. of reliable deterioration (%)*
		Improvement	*Deterioration*	*Same*	
Assertive	2 (67%)	1 (33%)	0 (0%)	0 (0%)	0 (0%)
Focused on Own Needs	1 (50%)	1 (50%)	0 (0%)	0 (0%)	0 (0%)
Cold/Distant	1 (33%)	1 (33%)	0 (0%)	1 (33%)	0 (0%)
Socially Inhibited	3 (50%)	1 (13%)	1 (13%)	1 (13%)	0 (0%)
Non-assertive	0 (0%)	0 (0%)	0 (0%)	0 (0%)	0 (0%)
Focused on Others Needs	2 (40%)	2 (40%)	1 (20%)	0 (0%)	0 (0%)
Warm/Self-sacrifice	2 (50%)	1 (25%)	0 (0%)	1 (25%)	0 (0%)
Uninhibited	4 (80%)	0 (0%)	0 (0%)	1 (20%)	0 (0%)

Table 5.7 Mood Outcomes of Singapore Case Study of FBGT

Variables	*No. of reliable improvements (%)*	*No. of uncertain change (%)*			*No. of reliable deterioration (%)*	*p-value for McNemar Test*
		Improvement	*Deterioration*	*Same*		
DASS						
Depression	7 (50%)	4 (29%)	2 (14%)	0 (0%)	1 (7%)	.008**
Anxiety	2 (14%)	8 (57%)	2 (14%)	1 (7%)	1 (7%)	.25
Stress	5 (36%)	6 (43%)	2 (14%)	1 (7%)	0 (0%)	.063
OQ30.2	9 (64%)	4 (29%)	0 (0%)	0 (0%)	1 (7%)	.004**
IIP-32	8 (57%)	3 (21%)	3 (21%)	0 (0%)	0 (0%)	.008**

*p <.05. ** p <.01. *** p <.001

reliable improvements on Total Interpersonal Distress, measured by overall IIP-32, was greater than number of uncertain or deteriorated change following group treatment (Table 5.7). Similar results were found for mood outcomes including depression and stress as measured by DASS21. On the other hand, reliable improvement rates did not differ from uncertain or deteriorated rates following treatment with 14 percent of the sample showing reliable improvement for anxiety.

Cultural Considerations

As the FBGT was developed in another country and culture and thus required the group leader to adapt some parts of the group program for this clinical sample, it was necessary to evaluate if this group approach was a good match to the local population. As suggested by Soto and colleagues (2018), "one cannot adapt treatments to what one does not know" (p. 1920). Therefore, the group leader sought to understand and regularly assess patients' racial and ethnic backgrounds and their salient worldviews and experiences to explore how they meshed with the group interventions prescribed by the FBGT model. For instance, it had been posited that "Chinese people are not used to expressing their opinions and emotions" (Cheung & Chan, 2002) and that "Chinese people have strong preference toward relation harmony" (Lin, 2002). Similar assumptions were heard among some clinicians in Singapore, all suggesting that a therapy group promoting free exploration of here-and-now dynamics and interpersonal differences might not be effective. However, as the results reveal, these beliefs about cultural influences did not hold in this Singapore case study, as the members (who were majority Chinese) generally discussed their interpersonal and psychological issues freely during group sessions. The group leader credited such forthcoming disclosures and open group explorations to several factors: 1) the consistent reinforcement of desirable and adaptive group behaviors at the initial stage of the group program; 2) the ongoing effort of the therapist to provide a universal safe outlet for emotions and thoughts; 3) to pre-group preparation and orientation aimed at promoting commitment to the group tasks requiring a certain level of tolerance of interpersonal conflicts and tension; and 4) to the comparative youth of the group members who were perhaps more eloquent in the affective language. In addition, the overall success of the group program may also have been due to the shared cultural background of the leader with the majority of group members, in this case Chinese. The common cultures of leader and members could serve to enhance group members' perception of the leader's credibility and therapeutic alliance building (Chen et al., 2008). At the same time, there was some risk that the few non-Chinese group members experienced some sort of exclusion due to this identity variable which is based on cultural similarity. Hence, group leaders should examine and brace themselves for potential challenges due to perceived differences of cultural values and identity, especially so in a culturally diverse country like Singapore.

On the whole, implementation of the FBGT model appears to be promising in the Singapore outpatient setting, with more than three quarters of the participants showing relative improvements and more than half of the participants showing reliable improvement in their interpersonal distress self-report ratings. Moreover, there were also encouraging results for overall distress and depression features among the group members. In comparison to other studies, the low drop-out rate in this case study was also an indication of satisfactory engagement levels among the group members. Notably, the main limitation of this case study is the lack of methodological rigor to rule out the impact of other confounding variables (i.e. ongoing individual psychotherapy and psychiatric medications) that could contribute to the treatment effects. Nonetheless, it was a great start to utilizing the group outcome and process measures to inform and individual's mood states and explore group dynamics in real time, while embracing the time and resource constraints of the hospital setting.

Example Two: Dynamic Relational Group Treatment of Perfectionism

This example provides a description of the MBC approach used with an evidence-based treatment of perfectionism. The example illustrates some of considerations that clinicians have in assessing treatment outcome.

Description of Location and Context

This case example took place in a training clinic in a clinical psychology program in a large university setting in Vancouver, Canada. The clinic provides training for PhD level clinical psychology graduate students who provide assessment and treatment under the direct supervision of a licensed clinical psychologist. The training clinic offers services to the community at large and although students from the university can access the services, the clinic provides services mainly to nonstudent community members. The majority of patients seen in the clinic tend to be treated for anxiety, mood, and personality disorders; however, a large number of patients seek treatment for interpersonal and relational problems. The clinic charges fees on a sliding scale based on patients' income and by far the majority of fees are minimal. The clinic has a focus on training of evidence-based practice that includes concern with effectiveness and efficacy of treatments and clear demonstrations of the effectiveness of the various treatments. The MBC approach fits very well with the clinic mandate both in terms of its emphasis on careful methodology and measurement but also because of the consideration of cultural and diversity issues in measurement-based care. The community that the clinic services is multicultural with mainly European Canadian (47 percent) and Asian Canadian (39 percent) and South Asian Canadian (6 percent) populations.

There were two 5th-year PhD student clinicians providing clinical services in this example. Each clinician was involved in the assessment and treatment process of the group and each conducted initial interviews and psychometric testing pretreatment, mid-treatment, and post-treatment. The two clinicians also acted as co-therapists for the group and provided individual feedback to patients at pre-treatment, mid-treatment and posttreatment. The two clinicians were supervised by a senior clinical psychologist with extensive clinical and supervisory experience who had attended intensive training workshops on the assessment and treatment of core personality vulnerability factors that underlie a variety of clinical syndromes and relational problems often seen in the clinic. The emphasis of the workshop was on perfectionism as a transdiagnostic factor that was presented as not only associated with many disorders but also significant interpersonal and physical health issues (see Hewitt, 2020; Hewitt et al., 2017; Sirois & Molnar, 2016). The workshop focused on the assessment and development of a clinical formulation for each patient that forms the basis for the treatment and the group psychotherapy approach that, based on the research literature, has shown excellent effectiveness in producing clinically significant change (see Hewitt et al., 2015, Hewitt et al., 2020). The dynamic relational approach of the treatment resonated powerfully with the psychologist who had previously focused mainly on symptom reduction group treatments that seemed to deal only temporarily with the patients' difficulties and never seemed to get at core issues for patients. Moreover, the broad clinical problems that the majority of patients in the clinic experienced seemed to fit well with an approach focusing on transdiagnostic personality factors and the psychologist believed that a treatment that focused on these issues would have great utility.

The psychologist had received training in the dynamic relational approach to the treatment of perfectionism in the workshops she attended. The treatment was presented as particularly well-suited to group psychotherapy (see Hewitt et al., 2017) using time-limited groups, with treatment extending for a total of 12 weekly, 90-minute group sessions.

Typically, groups comprised a cohort of eight to ten participants who are selected based on extreme levels of various components of the perfectionistic personality style. Moreover, considerations were given to group composition and, although all patients were selected based on scoring high on at least one element of perfectionism, a mixture of individuals with various elements (e.g., perfectionism traits, perfectionistic self-presentation, and perfectionistic self-relational dialogue) was consistent with the existing treatment research (Hewitt et al., 1991, 2003, 2015). There were two group therapists for each group and, given the time-limited format, groups were closed so that a given cohort began and ended treatment together. Although the workshop presenter indicated that a more open-ended treatment and groups that are open for patients to join at any point are anecdotally effective, the psychologist chose to use the 12-session, closed group approach as this approach had been shown empirically to be effective (Hewitt et al., 2015, Hewitt, Qiu, et al., 2020, Hewitt et al., 2023). Moreover, such a short-term group fit well with the short-term treatment approaches used in the facility and would, potentially, allow a greater number of patients to receive treatment. Finally, with the group beginning and ending the treatment together, allowing the development of group cohesion and the unfolding of relational issues, such as alliance ruptures and both time and opportunity for repairs of those ruptures, among the patients over time. As well, the patients would likely progress through the group developmental stages at a similar rate with similar themes and emotions as group material.

In this treatment, closely following the protocol developed by Hewitt and colleagues (Hewitt et al., 2015, 2017), each participant underwent an extensive initial screening and assessment, and pre-group training session prior to the commencement of the treatment. This included assessment of the various perfectionism components as well as symptoms and work and social functioning to assess the broad effectiveness of the treatment. In addition, assessment of facility with English was assessed as the group treatment was conducted in English and various process-related measures were chosen (e.g., GCQ and GSRS as described above as well as the Therapeutic Factors Inventory; Joyce et al., 2011) were administered throughout the treatment. This was done to provide information that was used to determine the presence of features of treatment that are of particular benefit in outcome and to refine elements of the group treatment in the particular facility. Various measurements at each of the stages were used to guide treatment, evaluate progress, and determine benefit. A crucial component of the treatment, based on years of empirical evidence, was to establish from the start a collaborative and person-centered approach that is maintained throughout the course of treatment.

Screening and Assessment

As the treatment of perfectionism uses a measurement based approach throughout the entire process, the group treatment commenced for each individual with a comprehensive pre-treatment assessment that focused on 1) identifying appropriate participants for group treatment by assessing and considering inclusion and exclusion criteria; 2) identifying the nature and genesis of the various transdiagnostic perfectionism and relational/personality components; 3) identifying the nature and level of the symptoms, distress, and dysfunction the patient was experiencing; and 4) using all the information to derive a working formulation that was used to guide specific treatment goals and road map for both group leaders and patient. The formulation for each patient is an idiographic model of the patient's functioning that offers 1) a depiction of perfectionism elements in terms of their manifestation, development, and maintenance; 2) the purpose perfectionism elements served in the past and serve in the present; and finally 3) how perfectionism features interfere with relations with others and the self and, in turn, creates marked distress for the person and those around them. Using both psychometric and interview data, the initial formulation for each patient was developed by the clinician in consultation with the supervising psychologist. Although a detailed account of the formulation is beyond the scope of this paper, one important element of the formulation that is shared, discussed, and refined with the patient, is the Cyclical Relational Pattern (CRP) (see Hewitt et al. 2020). The CRP has four connected facets that include 1) **Acts of Self**, which involve behaviours, cognitions, affective states, and perceptions; 2) **Expectations of Others** that capture the individual's relational wishes and view of how others will act, feel and think in response to the Acts of Self; 3) **Acts of Others** or the observed reactions of others to the individual's Acts of Self; and 4) **Introject** involving the patient's feelings, thoughts and behaviours toward self that typically are an internalization of the ways in which significant others have treated the individual. For example, based on several measures and interview data, a CRP for one group therapy patient, Roberto, involved his excessive need to always appear absolutely flawless to others (see Hewitt et al., 2003) by closely monitoring his vocabulary, grammar, speech volume and tone, manners, dress, and by letting people know how seemingly 'perfect' he was. By engaging in these Acts of Self, Roberto had an expectation that if he appeared pristine and perfect to others and ensured they knew of his perfection, they would respect, accept and care for him, and not reject, ridicule or abandon him, and be open to an intimate relationship. In reality, his experiences with others' actual behavior was that people were put off by him and seemingly found him distant, not genuine and very difficult to get to know and, as a result, indeed, rejected him. The result of this rejection (or failure as Roberto labelled it) led to him concluding that, once again, there was something wrong with him, that he was deeply flawed, unlovable, and did not matter to others, and that he needed to ensure that he appear even more perfect the next time. Moreover, this pattern was discussed as underlying the significant social anxiety he experienced as well as his marked levels of depression and social hopelessness. The presentation of Roberto's CRP was met, as is often the case, with interest and resonance and he commented that the CRP captured patterns of his behavior in a way he had not considered before but made sense to him. The clinician commented to the supervising psychologist later that the presentation of the feedback and formulation in a collaborative fashion appears to deepen the connection between the patient and the therapist and indicated that this will likely facilitate the patients' participation.

The assessment proper involved two sessions with each individual patient: A data-gathering session and a feedback/goal setting session. The data-gathering session included a fairly standard semi-structured clinical interview and psychometric testing. The clinical interview and testing were used to gather details of the nature and history of distress and perfectionism; childhood, current family, and social history; defensive and coping structures; and nature and quality of relationships, strengths, and vulnerabilities. Both content and process-related information from the interview were considered, along with the psychometric data, in constructing the working formulation. The initial interview is important not only to gather and quantify clinical data relevant to the formulation and treatment, but also is an important opportunity to establish a therapeutic alliance or connection with the patient (see Hilsenroth & Cromer, 2007). The connection was observed especially after the provision of individual feedback and the explanation of the CRP.

The selection of instruments for the psychometric testing battery served several purposes including instruments that aid in the development of the working formulation for the patient (e.g., levels of various manifestation of perfectionistic behavior, interpersonal problems), providing an indication and benchmark for degree of distress and symptom level (e. g., depression, anxiety), and level of dysfunction (e.g., work and social adjustment, satisfaction with life). Moreover, the specific selection was based on several criteria that were considered and balanced. First, the psychologist chose all measures based on the established reliability and validity of the measures in clinical samples and that have been used in clinical and research work. An important consideration was the demonstrated reliability and validity of the measures for the cultural groups that would be, potentially, represented in the treatment group and the psychologist ensured that the instruments chosen were appropriate in this respect. Thus, the instruments selected by the psychologist had been evaluated and chosen based on good psychometric properties and norms for the cultural groups. Second, the instruments were chosen with the appreciation for the demands on the patient in terms of their ability to concentrate, fatigue, and the time commitment. The patients, during the first assessment session, after completing the clinical interview, completed the psychometric testing. Consideration was given to the degree to which the patient may be taxed in this process and an explanation as to the need for depth and comprehensiveness so as to provide the best care was provided to each patient. All patients completed the interview and testing with breaks when needed to aid in recruiting their participation in the process. Moreover, patients were informed from the start that the information was gathered is used to have a deep understanding of their difficulties and to develop and enhance treatment. It was explained that the formulation that arises from the assessment will be shared with and explained to the patient in a feedback session where the patient will work with the clinician to discuss results and to work on setting appropriate goals for their treatment. More generally, the formulation is used in several ways including to further establish a therapeutic connection to the patient wherein the clinician, hopefully, communicates a depth of understanding of the patient's struggles. Second, the formulation aids in specifying treatment goals, drawing the clinicians' attention to transference patterns that are likely to manifest in the patient's interactions in the group, and, third, in predicting specific reactions of the person in the treatment (e.g., feeling the need to terminate early, not participate, and so forth).

The core test battery that has been used previously is extensive (Hewitt et al., 2015). Because the psychologist was not conducting a large research project but rather preparing a group to provide training and clinical services, she chose directly relevant measures and she chose short form versions of the main measures (the ones with demonstrated appropriate psychometric properties) to use which reduced the time commitment for the patients. These measures are presented in Table 5.8.

Following the first assessment session, a second session with the individual patient involved provision of feedback from the interview and testing material. The clinician

Table 5.8 Outcome and Process Measures in Administered in Case Study 2

Measures	Administered
Transdiagnostic Measures	
Multidimensional Perfectionism Scale-Short Form (Hewitt & Flett, 1991)	Pre, Post
Perfectionistic Self Presentation Scale-Short Form (Hewitt et al., 2003)	Pre, Post
Perfectionistic Cognitions Inventory-Short Form (Flett et al., 1998)	Pre, Post
Symptoms & Distress	
Beck Anxiety Inventory-Short Form (Beck et al., 1961)	Pre, Post
Beck Depression Inventory-Short Form (Beck et al., 1988)	Pre, Post
Inventory of Interpersonal Problems-32 (Horowitz et al., 2000)	Pre, Post
Outcome Rating Scale (Miller et al., 2003)	Pre, Post
Functioning	
Work and Social Adjustment Scale (Mundt et al., 2002)	Pre, Post
Process	
Therapeutic Factors Inventory (MacNair-Semands et al. 2010)	Session 3, 9
Group Session Rating Scale (Duncan et al., 2003)	Every Session

summarized the assessment results, usually in terms of areas of concern and areas of strength. The findings were discussed using percentile rankings (e.g., "you scored higher than 87 percent of people on anxiety") and the patient and clinician discussed the CRP with the patient and ways in which the patient's dynamics may manifest in the course of group treatment. For example, one patient scored above the 90th percentile for two components of perfectionism involving extreme avoidance of any display of behavior that is less than perfect and extreme avoidance of any disclosure of any imperfection (Hewitt et al., 2003). As these elements have been shown to interfere with personal relationships, therapeutic alliance, and eventual outcome (see Hewitt et al., 2008, 2021) these findings were discussed with the patient in terms of how they might arise in the group treatment and how they might negatively influence the benefit the person could receive. The clinician also discussed particular goals the patient had for the treatment and worked to specify three specific goals.

The clinicians noted that the patients uniformly appreciated this feedback information and the provision of the formulation in a simplified manner seemed to have improved the working alliance. Patients often commented that the clinician had a real grasp on their own unique personal issues. In addition, each patient was provided an overview of how group therapy works and, using the individual's formulation as a guide, the clinician and patient worked on articulating particular goals the patient has for treatment and issues that might arise for the patient in the treatment itself. Finally, it was discussed that the therapists will be monitoring different elements of the person's functioning over the course of treatment by measuring relevant variables that will be used as indications of therapeutic change and therapeutic benefit. Prior to the commencement of the treatment, the clinical formulation for each patient was discussed among the therapists and the psychologist in preparation for the treatment.

Pre-Group Orientation

Prior to commencement of the treatment, the therapists and patients met as a group and patients received a pre-treatment orientation to group psychotherapy (see Tasca et al., 2021). This pre-group preparation was aimed at enhancing participation and described the benefits that should accrue from the group treatment (Yalom & Leszcz, 2020). The focus of these sessions included what to expect in group psychotherapy, how to benefit most in treatment, rules and expectations, and information on the nature and outcomes of perfectionism. One week following this pre-group orientation, the group treatment proper commenced. Following each session, the GSRS, the four-item measure of the therapeutic alliance as described earlier in this volume, was administered to each patient. Clinicians reviewed the scores for each patient over the course of the treatment to monitor alliance and gain a sense of each patient's connection to the group and level of group cohesion.

Session 3 Assessment

At session 3, following the group therapy meeting, patients were asked to complete the Therapeutic Factors Inventory (TFI-19) (Joyce et al., 2011; MacNair-Semands et al., 2010) to measure factors such as level of hope in good outcome, emotional expression, and relational impact with the group (see Chapter 3). The group therapists used the results of the TFI-19 as an indication of level of involvement and presence of particular process factors that can have a positive impact on the effectiveness of the treatment. Moreover, in consultation with the psychologist during supervision, the therapists discussed potential ways to enhance the factors for this particular group.

During the scoring of the TFI-19 it was clear that one patient, Imani, endorsed being quite disconnected from the group. Imani scored very highly on Socially Prescribed Perfectionism, perceiving that others consistently required perfection of her (Hewitt & Flett, 1991) and she was often exhausted with the perceived demands for perfection she experienced. In general, Imani's perfectionism had a significant effect on relationships wherein she would take responsibility for others' emotional states and would work extremely hard to take care of their feelings. This often led to Imani being taken advantage of by others. Although in group she seemed to be working hard at engaging with others in the group and gave the appearance of being connected and caring for others, her self-report measure of emotional expression and connection indicated otherwise. Double checking on her endorsement of the GSRS revealed similarly that she felt disconnected from the group. The therapists, in consultation with the psychologist, decided that one of the therapists should meet individually with Imani to discuss this feeling of disconnection with her. Imani responded very well to the meeting with the therapist and both concluded that this was a good example of how her perfectionism was influencing her behavior in the group. Imani expressed relief with the discussion and revealed that she had been considering leaving the group. The therapist encouraged her to reveal some of what she was feeling in the group which she eventually did. In this situation, it was the self-report measure that was instrumental in alerting the therapists about what had not been observed in the therapy itself. It is impossible to tell whether the person would have left the group without the individual with the therapist; however, the fact that the issue of feeling disconnected came up from the self-report measure allowed the therapists to work with her to enhance her connection. Her scores on the measure at Session 9 and the GSRS indicated a gradual increase in ratings of connection and she attended all sessions.

Session 6 Midpoint Assessment

At Session 6, the patients were asked complete the perfectionism, symptom, interpersonal problem, and work and social adjustment measures. These were scored for each person and a brief feedback session was booked individually for each patient to review the findings and to discuss progress that may have been made to that point. This also allowed a revisiting of the goals and CRP for each patient. The clinicians noted that although they did not ask specifically whether any patient wanted to modify their goals, nobody requested such modifications. The psychologist thought that it might be appropriate in future groups to ask patients directly whether they wished to make change to their goals at this stage.

Session 11 Assessment

At Session 11, the TFI-19 was again administered to assess therapeutic factors and an indication of changes in levels of the factors over the course of treatment.

Post-Treatment Assessment

After Session 12, the patients were again administered the perfectionism, symptom, interpersonal problem, and work and social adjustment measures. These were scored for each person and a detailed feedback session was booked for each patient to review the findings and to discuss overall progress that was made over the course of treatment. The findings were presented to patients in terms of RCI as discussed in the Singapore case example and patients were also asked to review the progress on the goals they had for treatment. That is, each person's change on each of the outcome measures was reviewed with the patient in terms of the degree of reliable change that was observed. Moreover, the clinicians used the patients scores from the TFI-19 and the trajectory of scores from the GSRS to aid in understanding elements that might have contributed to that particular patient's outcome. Patients were also asked to indicate which, if any, elements of the treatment were particularly helpful or particularly unhelpful and discussed with the therapist their progress with respect to the goals they had set for the treatment. This information was gathered in order to inform the psychologist of potential refinements to the treatment protocol that might be implemented in future groups.

Overall Outcome of the Group

The psychologist, therapists, and the clinic management were all interested in the overall outcome of this group and the psychologist wanted to present a cohesive and straightforward picture of the overall outcome. Although there are a number of sophisticated analytic techniques that are very powerful but complex that can be used in group psychotherapy outcome, the psychologist had limited ability to work with such statistics. She chose to use a clinically relevant statistic that was relatively easy to use, the RCI as discussed previously. Moreover, because she would be presenting the overall results to the clinic management, she wished to present the findings in an easily understandable manner. Her use of the RCI was both straightforward and easily understood by all. She presented average levels of RCI for each outcome variable (i.e., measures of the perfectionism components, depression and anxiety symptoms, interpersonal problems, and work and social functioning) indicating the overall average degree of positive changes on the variables as well as the number of people who reliably scored above a clinical cutoff for the measures. For example, she reported that seven of eight patients showed reliable clinical improvement on at least one perfectionism measures and seven of eight patients also showed reliable clinical improvement on the symptom and functioning measures. As well she indicated that one of the eight patients showed a clinical deterioration based on the RCI. The findings were presented as consistent with past work on clinical improvements.

Using the data from the measures, the psychologist was able to demonstrate powerfully that not only were symptoms markedly reduced, but that reductions in the transdiagnostic vulnerability variables were also evident for by far the majority of patients. Moreover, the psychologist was able to present changes in the therapeutic factors of the treatment that were significant as well as factors that did not seem to change much over the treatment. She discussed the latter findings in terms of needing to refine some elements of the treatment and perhaps extend the number of sessions for patients. For example, it was noted that two patients who scored very highly on Other Oriented Perfectionism, which entails requiring others to be perfect and externally directed critical recriminations (Hewitt & Flett, 1991), had somewhat lower RCI's than others with different perfectionism issues. She was considering either increasing the number of sessions for those with Other Oriented Perfectionism or perhaps have a group specifically dealing with individuals with excessive Other Oriented Perfectionism.

An evaluation of dropouts indicated that one patient dropped out just prior to the first session of group treatment. Although Hewitt et al. (2021) indicated that pre-treatment meetings (i.e., feedback and pre-group preparation) can potentially mitigate dropouts, the one dropout was consistent with literature. A comparison of scores from the pre-treatment measures indicated that the patient who dropped scored extremely high on one trait measure of perfectionism, namely, Self-Oriented Perfectionism which involves the requirement of perfection of the self (Hewitt & Flett, 1991). Moreover, when the patient dropped out, she had left a message that although she was very interested in attending the group treatment, the pressures of work commitments was overwhelming and she needed to dedicate her time to these commitments. The psychologist noted that in future, when conducting the assessment feedback with such individuals, that reasons for not continuing treatment due to feeling overwhelmed with work or other commitments needs to explored with the person as well as fears about committing to treatment needs to covered with potential group members.

Conclusion

In this chapter we presented two examples of measurement-based care for group psychotherapy in two separate settings. In the examples, we focused on the treatment of core or transdiagnostic vulnerability factors, namely Interpersonal styles/problems and Perfectionism, and how measurement-based care can be used in development, planning, and completion of group treatment protocols. It is hoped that the reader will appreciate that the use of psychometric instruments and techniques can not only be used to evaluate the effectiveness of treatment for the individual patient and patient groups but that they can be utilized in refining and fine-tuning treatments for specific treatment settings or patient groups. Lastly, the gathering of the data can also be invaluable in the evaluation of treatment programs, used to support requests for resources and for potential changes in policy. The use of psychometrically sound instruments and methods in measurement-based care can facilitate the benefit to benefit to patients at an individual level and at both resource allocation and policy levels.

Notes

1 Individuals who obtained a high score on this scale tends to too gullible, easily taken advantaged by others and exploitable. Assertive acts were assumed to be offensive and in order to maintain cordial relationships, these individuals avoid being assertive.
2 People high on this scale are excessively affiliative and often described for being too caring, trusting and permissive. Difficulties with setting limits and maintaining boundaries are key complaints among these individuals.
3 This scale describes individuals who has an overpowering need to be engaged with others and imposes their presence onto their attention. Common interpersonal difficulties include inappropriately disclosing personal issues, being intrusive in others' business and or taking inflated responsibility over others' problems.

References

Batch, A. (2018). Dropout in group therapy: causes and prevention strategies (Doctoral dissertation, City University of Seattle).

Bemak, F. & Chung, R. C. (2019). Race Dialogues in Group Psychotherapy: Key Issues in Training and Practice. *International Journal of Group Psychotherapy*, 69(2), 172–191. doi:10.1080/00207284.2018.1498743.

Bernard, H. et al. (2008). Clinical practice guidelines for group psychotherapy. *International Journal of Group Psychotherapy*, 58(4), 455–542. doi:10.1521/ijgp.2008.58.4.455.

Bieling, P. J., Summerfeldt, L. J., Israeli, A. L., & Antony, M. M. (2004). Perfectionism as an explanatory construct in comorbidity of axis I disorders. *Journal of Psychopathology and Behavioral Assessment*, 26(3), 193–201. doi:10.1023/B:JOBA.0000022112.27186.98.

Blatt, S. J. (2004). *Experiences of depression: Theoretical, clinical, and research perspectives*. American Psychological Association. doi:10.1037/10749-000.

Bordin, E. S. (1979). The generalizability of the psychoanalytic concept of the working alliance. *Psychotherapy: Theory, research & practice*, 16(3), 252.

Bornstein, R. F. (2005). *The dependent patient: A practitioner's guide*. American Psychological Association. doi:10.1037/0735–7028.36.1.82.

Burlingame, G. M, Strauss, B., Joyce, A., MacNair-Semands, R., MacKenzie, K., Ogrodniczuk, J. & Taylor, S. (2006). *Core Battery-Revised*. New York: American Group Psychotherapy Association.

Chen, E. C., Kakkad, D., & Balzano, J. (2008). Multicultural competence and evidence-based practice in group therapy. *Journal of Clinical Psychology*, 64(11), 1261–1278. doi:10.1002/jclp.20533.

Cheung, G. & Chan C. (2002). The Satir model and cultural sensitivity: A Hong Kong reflection. *Contemporary Family Therapy*, 24, 199–215. doi:10.1023/A:1014338025464.

Chowdhary, N. et al. (2014). The methods and outcomes of cultural adaptations of psychological treatments for depressive disorders: A systematic review. *Psychological Medicine*, 44(6), 1131–1146. doi:10.1017/S0033291713001785.

Constantino, M. J., Vîslă, A., Coyne, A. E., & Boswell, J. F. (2018). A meta-analysis of the association between patients' early treatment outcome expectation and their posttreatment outcomes. *Psychotherapy*, 55(4), 73. doi:10.1037/pst0000169.

Dies, R. R. & Dies, K. R. (1993). The role of evaluation in clinical practice: Overview and group treatment illustration. *International Journal of Group Psychotherapy*, 43(1), 77–105. doi:10.1080/00207284.1994.11491207.

Duncan, B. L. & Miller, S. D. (2007). *The group session rating scale*. Jensen Beach, FL: Author.

Garceau, C., Chyurlia, L., Baldwin, D., Boritz, T., Hewitt, P. L., Kealy, D., Sochting, I., Mikail, S. F., & Tasca, G. A. (2021). Applying the Rupture Resolution Rating System (3RS) to Group Therapy: An evidence-based case study. *Group Dynamics*, 25, 89–105. doi:10.1037/gdn0000137.

Goh, K. (2020). A qualitative study of the attitudes that most affect the decision of a Singaporean whether to seek counselling or not. *Asia Pacific Journal of Counselling and Psychotherapy*, 11(2), 181–197, doi:10.1080/21507686.2020.1808800.

Hall, G., Ibaraki, A., Huang, E., Marti, C., & Stice, E. (2016). A Meta-Analysis of Cultural Adaptations of Psychological Interventions. *Behavior Therapy*, 47(6), 993–1014. doi:10.1016/j.beth.2016.09.005.

Hawley, D. R. (1995). Assessing change with preventive interventions: The Reliable Change Index. *Family Relations: An Interdisciplinary Journal of Applied Family Studies*, 44(3), 278–284. doi:10.2307/585526.

Hewitt, P. L. (2020). Perfecting, belonging, and repairing: A dynamic-relational approach to perfectionism. *Canadian Psychology/Psychologie canadienne*, 61(2), 101. doi:10.1037/cap0000209.

Hewitt, P. L., Chen, C., Smith, M. M., Zhang, L., Habke, M., Flett, G. L., & Mikail, S. F. (2021). Patient perfectionism and clinician impression formation during an initial interview. *Psychology and Psychotherapy: Theory, Research and Practice*, 94(1), 45–62. doi:10.1111/papt.12266.

Hewitt, P. L. & Flett, G. L. (1991). Perfectionism in the self and social contexts: conceptualization, assessment, and association with psychopathology. *Journal of Personality and Social Psychology*, 60(3), 456. doi:10.1037/0022-3514.60.3.456.

Hewitt, P. L., Flett, G. L., Mikail, S. F., Kealy, D., & Zhang, L. (2018). Perfectionism in the Therapeutic Context: The Perfectionism Social Disconnection Model and Clinical Process and Outcome. In J. Stoeber (Ed.), *The Psychology of Perfectionism: Theory, Research, Applications*. New York: Routledge.

Hewitt, P. L., Flett, G. L., & Mikail, S. F. (2017). *Perfectionism: A relational approach to conceptualization, assessment, and treatment*. Guilford Publications.

Hewitt, P. L. et al. (2003). The interpersonal expression of perfection: Perfectionistic self-presentation and psychological distress. *Journal of Personality and Social Psychology*, 84(6), 1303. doi:10.1037/0022-3514.84.6.1303.

Hewitt, P. L. et al. (2003). The interpersonal expression of perfection: Perfectionistic self-presentation and psychological distress. *Journal of personality and social psychology*, 84(6), 1303. doi:10.1037/0022-3514.84.6.1303.

Hewitt, P. L. et al. (2015). Psychodynamic/interpersonal group psychotherapy for perfectionism: Evaluating the effectiveness of a short-term treatment. *Psychotherapy*, 52(2), 205. doi:10.1037/pst0000016.

Hewitt, P. L. et al. (2023). The Efficacy of Group Psychotherapy for Adults with Perfectionism: A Randomized Controlled Trial of Dynamic Relational Therapy versus Psychodynamic Supportive Therapy. *Journal of Consulting and Clinical Psychology*, 91, 29–42.

Hewitt, P. L., Mikail, S. F., Dang, S. S., Kealy, D., & Flett, G. L. (2020). Dynamic-relational treatment of perfectionism: An illustrative case study. *Journal of Clinical Psychology*, 76(11), 2028–2040. doi:10.1002/jclp.23040.

Hewitt, P. L., Qiu, T., Flynn, C. A., Flett, G. L., Wiebe, S. A., Tasca, G. A., & Mikail, S. F. (2020). Dynamic-relational group treatment for perfectionism: Informant ratings of patient change. *Psychotherapy*, 57(2), 197. doi:10.1037/pst0000229.

Hilsenroth, M. J. & Cromer, T. D. (2007). Clinician interventions related to alliance during the initial interview and psychological assessment. *Psychotherapy: theory, research, practice, training*, 44(2), 205. doi:10.1037/0033-3204.44.2.205.

Horowitz, L. M., Alden, L. E., & Wiggins, J. S. (2000). *IIP – Inventory of Interpersonal Problems Manual*. San Antonio, TX: The Psychological Corporation.

Horowitz, L. M. & Strack, S. (2010). *Handbook of interpersonal psychology*. New York: Wiley.

Jacobson, N. S. & Truax, P. (1991). Clinical significance: a statistical approach to defining meaningful change in psychotherapy research. *Journal of Consulting and Clinical Psychology, 59(1)*, 12–19. doi:10.1037/10109-042.

Jensen, H. H., Mortensen, E. L., & Lotz, M. (2014). Drop-out from a psychodynamic group psychotherapy outpatient unit. *Nordic Journal of Psychiatry*, 68(8), 594–604. doi:10.3109/08039488.2014.902499.

Joyce, A. S., MacNair-Semands, R., Tasca, G. A., & Ogrodniczuk, J. S. (2011). Factor structure and validity of the Therapeutic Factors Inventory–Short Form. *Group Dynamics: Theory, Research, and Practice*, 15(3), 201. doi:10.1037/a0024677.

Kramer. U. (2019) Personality, personality disorders, and the process of change. *Psychotherapy Research*, 29(3), 324–336, doi:10.1080/10503307.2017.1377358.

Lambert, M. J. & Shimokawa, K. (2011). Collecting client feedback. *Psychotherapy*, 48(1), 72–79. doi:10.1037/a0022238.

Leary, T. (1957). *Interpersonal diagnosis of personality: A functional theory and methodology for personality evaluation*. Ronald Press.

Lenzo, V., Gargano, M. T., Mucciardi, M., Lo Verso, G., & Quattropani, M. C. (2014). Clinical Efficacy and Therapeutic Alliance in a Time-Limited Group Therapy for Young Adults. *Research in Psychotherapy: Psychopathology, Process and Outcome*, 17(1), 9–20. doi:10.4081/ripppo.2014.151.

Liew, S. M. & Whittingham, M. (2020, March 2–7). Time-limited process groups based on Focused Brief Group Therapy in Singapore: A pilot and feasibility study [Conference presentation]. American Group Psychotherapy Association Annual Conference, New York, United States.

Lin, Y. N. (2002). The application of cognitive–behavioral therapy to Chinese. *American Journal of Psychotherapy*, 55, 46–58. doi:10.1176/appi.psychotherapy.2002.56.1.46.

Lovibond, S. H. & Lovibond, P. F. (1995). *Manual for the Depression Anxiety Stress Scales*. (2nd. Ed.) Sydney: Psychology Foundation.

MacKenzie, K. R. (1981). Measurement of group climate. *International journal of group psychotherapy*, 31(3), 287–295. doi:10.1080/00207284.1981.11491708.

MacNair-Semands, R. R., Ogrodniczuk, J. S., & Joyce, A. S. (2010). Structure and initial validation of a short form of the Therapeutic Factors Inventory. *International Journal of Group Psychotherapy*, 60, 245–281. doi:10.1521/ijgp.2010.60.2.245.

Marmarosh, C. L. & Sproul, A. (2021). Group cohesion: Empirical evidence from group psychotherapy for those studying other areas of group work. In C. D. Parks & G. A. Tasca (Eds), *The Psychology of Groups: The Intersection of Social Psychology and Psychotherapy Research* (pp. 169–189). American Psychological Association. doi:10.1037/0000201-010.

Marmarosh, C. L. & Tasca, G. A. (2013). Adult attachment anxiety: Using group therapy to promote change. *Journal of Clinical Psychology*, 69(11), 1172–1182. doi:10.1002/jclp.22044.

McLeod, J., Stiles, W. B., & Levitt, H. (2021). Qualitative research: Contributions to psychotherapy practice, theory, and policy. In M. BarkhamW. Lutz, & L. G. Castonguay (Eds), *Bergin and Garfield's Handbook of Psychotherapy and Behavior Change*. Hoboken, NJ: Wiley.

MacNair, R. R. & Corazzini, J. (1994). Client factors influencing group therapy dropout. *Psychotherapy*, 31, 352–361. doi:10.1037/h0090226.

MacNair-Semands, R. R. (2002). Predicting attendance and expectations for group therapy. *Group Dynamics: Theory, Research, and Practice*, 6, 219–228. doi:10.1037/1089-2699.6.3.219.

Mundt, J. C. et al. (2002). The Work and Social Adjustment Scale: A simple measure of impairment in functioning. *British Journal of Psychiatry*, 180, 461–464. Reproduced with the kind permission of Professor Isaac Marks. doi:10.1192/bjp.180.5.461.

Ooi, Y. P., Sung, S. C., Raja, M., Kwan, C., Koh, J. B. K., & Fung, D. (2016). Web-based CBT for the treatment of selective mutism: results from a pilot randomized controlled trial in Singapore. *Journal of Speech Pathology and Therapy*, 1(2), 112. doi:10.4172/2472-5005.1000112.

Quirk, K., Miller, S., Duncan, B., & Owen, J. (2013). "Group Session Rating Scale: Preliminary psychometrics in substance abuse group interventions": Corrigendum. *Counselling & Psychotherapy Research*, 13(3), i. doi:10.1080/14733145.2013.764658.

Ribeiro, M. D. (Ed.). (2020). *Examining social identities and diversity issues in group therapy: Knocking at the boundaries*. Routledge. doi:10.4324/9780429022364.

Rosenberg, S. A. & Zimet, C. N. (1996). Brief group treatment and managed health care. *International Journal of Group Therapy*, 45(3), 367–379,. doi:10.1080/00207284.1995.11491288.

Samaritans of Singapore. (2021, July). Singapore reported 452 suicide deaths in 2020, number of elderly suicide deaths highest record since 1991. www.sos.org.sg/pressroom/singapore-reported-452-suicide-deaths-in-2020-number-of-elderly-suicide-deaths-highest-recorded-since-1991.

Sirois, F. M. & Molnar, D. S. (Eds). (2016). *Perfectionism, health, and well-being*. New York, NY: Springer. doi:10.1007/978-3-319-18582-8_13.

Soto, A., Smith, T. B., Griner, D., Domenech-Rodríguez, M., & Bernal, G. (2018). Cultural adaptations and therapist multicultural competence: Two meta-analytic reviews. *Journal of Clinical Psychology*, 74, 1907–1923. doi:10.1002/jclp.22679.

Subramaniam, M., Abdin, E., Seow, E., Vaingankar, J. A., Shafie, S., Shahwan, S., Lim, M., Fung, D., James, L., Verma, S., & Chong, S. A. (2020). Prevalence, socio-demographic correlates and associations of adverse childhood experiences with mental illnesses: Results from the Singapore Mental Health Study. *Child Abuse & Neglect*, 103, 104447. doi:10.1016/j.chiabu.2020.104447.

Tasca, G. A., Mikail, S. F., & Hewitt, P. L. (2021). *Group psychodynamic-interpersonal psychotherapy*. American Psychological Association.

Wampold, B. E. & Imel, Z. E. (2015). *The great psychotherapy debate: The evidence for what makes psychotherapy work*. Routledge.

Weiss, P. A. (2010).Time-Limited Dynamic Psychotherapy as a Model for Short-Term Inpatient Groups. *Journal of Contemporary Psychotherapy*, 40, 41–49. doi:10.1007/s10879-009-9124-6.

Whittingham, M. (2015). Focused brief group therapy: A practice-based evidence approach. In E. Neukrug (Ed.), *The Sage Encyclopedia of Theory in Counseling and Psychotherapy* (pp. 420–423). Washington, DC: Sage Publications.

Whittingham, M. (2017). Attachment and interpersonal theory and group therapy: two sides of the same coin. *International Journal of Group Psychotherapy*, 67(2), 276–279. doi:10.1080/00207284.2016.1260463.

Whittingham, M. (2018). Innovations in group assessment: How focused brief group therapy integrates formal measures to enhance treatment preparation, process, and outcomes. *Psychotherapy*, 55 (2), 186–190. doi:10.1037/pst0000153.

Whittingham, M. (2018, August). Utilizing Assessment to Predict and Prevent Dropout: A Case from Focused Brief Group Therapy. In C. L. Marmarosh (Chair). Should I Stay or Should I Go? Preventing Dropout in Group Therapy. *Symposium conducted at the meeting of the American Psychological Association*, San Francisco, CA.

Wong, C. (2018). Transdiagnostic group Cognitive Behavioral Therapy for mood and anxiety in Singapore. Poster presented at Singapore Health and Biomedical Conference; October 2018, Singapore.

Yalom, I. D. & Leszcz, M. (2020). *The Theory and Practice of Group Psychotherapy*. London: Hachette. doi:10.1080/00207284.2021.1908831.

Appendix I

Select Examples of Measures and Additional Information

Organization and Selection of Measures

It is important to note that this book was not intended to be a comprehensive detailing of every measure available. Rather, the authors of each chapter were invited to offer some examples of measures currently in use in the field. These then serve as exemplars of the kind of instruments available while also showing how they might be used. This is also the case with *these appendices*, where some but not all of the measures mentioned in the chapters are featured. In some cases, these measures are replicated in their entirety and in other cases, copyright holders gave their permission for reproduction of select items. *Therefore, not all measures mentioned in chapters are in the appendices.*

With respect to *copying measures that are printed in this book*, significant care must be taken. In some cases, measures are entirely free and in the public domain and so can be copied from this book and used in practice. However, in many cases, permission needs to be sought or measures are proprietary and a fee must be paid to the publisher. *If seeking to use a measure, it is incumbent on the reader to check carefully in our tables (and on the links provided within those tables) to determine whether the measure is proprietary or non-proprietary and to follow ethical and legal requirements in terms of appropriate credit and/or payment.*

Critical Incidents Questionnaire

Of the events that occurred in this session, which one do you feel was the most important to/for you personally? Describe the event: what actually took place, the group members involved, and your own reaction. Why was it important for you?

_____

_____

_____

_____

_____

_____

_____

_____

_____

_____

_____

_____

_____

_____

_____

_____

_____

_____

_____

_____

MacKenzie, K. R. (1987). Therapeutic factors in group psychotherapy. *Group*, 11, 26-34
MacKenzie, K. R., Dies, R., Coche, E., Rutan, J. S., & Stone, W. N. (1987). An analysis of AGPA Institute groups. *International Journal of Group Psychotherapy*, 37, 55-74.

DEQ

Listed below are a number of statements concerning personal characteristics and traits. Read each item and decide whether you agree or disagree and to what extent. If you <u>strongly agree,</u> circle7; if you <u>strongly disagree,</u> circle 1; The midpoint, if you are neutral or undecided, is 4.

	Strongly Disagree						Strongly Agree

1. I set my personal goals and standards as high as possible.   1   2   3   4   5   6   7

2. Without support from others who are close to me, I would be helpless.   1   2   3   4   5   6   7

3. I tend to be satisfied with my current plans and goals, rather than striving for higher goals.   1   2   3   4   5   6   7

4. Sometimes I feel very big, and other times I feel very small.   1   2   3   4   5   6   7

5. When I am closely involved with someone, I never feel jealous.   1   2   3   4   5   6   7

6. I urgently need things that only other people can provide.   1   2   3   4   5   6   7

7. I often find that I don't live up to my own standards or ideals.   1   2   3   4   5   6   7

8. I feel I am always making full use of my potential abilities.   1   2   3   4   5   6   7

9. The lack of permanence in human relationships doesn't bother me.   1   2   3   4   5   6   7

10. If I fail to live up to expectations, I feel unworthy.   1   2   3   4   5   6   7

11. Many times I feel helpless.   1   2   3   4   5   6   7

12. I seldom worry about being criticized for things I have said or done.   1   2   3   4   5   6   7

13. There is a considerable difference between how I am now and how I would like to be.   1   2   3   4   5   6   7

14. I enjoy sharp competition with others.   1   2   3   4   5   6   7

15. I feel I have many responsibilities that I must meet.   1   2   3   4   5   6   7

16. There are times when I feel "empty" inside.   1   2   3   4   5   6   7

17. I tend not to be satisfied with what I have.   1   2   3   4   5   6   7

18. I don't care whether or not I live up to what other people expect of me.   1   2   3   4   5   6   7

19. I become frightened when I feel alone.   1   2   3   4   5   6   7

20. I would feel like I'd be losing an important part of myself if I lost a very close friend.   1   2   3   4   5   6   7

21. People will accept me no matter how many mistakes
    I have made.   1   2   3   4   5   6   7

22. I have difficulty breaking off a relationship
    that is making me unhappy.   1   2   3   4   5   6   7

23. I often think about the danger of losing someone
    who is close to me.   1   2   3   4   5   6   7

24. Other people have high expectations of me.   1   2   3   4   5   6   7

25. When I am with others, I tend to devalue or
    "undersell" myself.   1   2   3   4   5   6   7

26. I am not very concerned with how other people
    respond to me.   1   2   3   4   5   6   7

27. No matter how close a relationship between two people is,
    there is always a large amount of uncertainty and conflict. 1   2   3   4   5   6   7

28. I am very sensitive to others for signs of rejection. 1   2   3   4   5   6   7

29. It's important for my family that I succeed.   1   2   3   4   5   6   7

30. Often, I feel I have disappointed others.   1   2   3   4   5   6   7

31. If someone makes me an gry, I let him (her) know
    how I feel.   1   2   3   4   5   6   7

32. I constantly try, and very often go out of my way,
    to please or help people I am close to.   1   2   3   4   5   6   7

33. I have many inner resources (abilities, strengths). 1   2   3   4   5   6   7

34. I find it very difficult to say "No" to the requests of friends. 1   2   3   4   5   6   7

35. I never really feel secure in a close relationship. 1   2   3   4   5   6   7

36. The way I feel about myself frequently varies: there are times
    when I feel extremely good about myself and other times
    when I see only the bad in me and feel like a total failure 1   2   3   4   5   6   7

37. Often, I feel threatened by change.   1   2   3   4   5   6   7

38. Even if the person who is closest to me were to
    leave, I could still "go it alone."   1   2   3   4   5   6   7

39. One must continually work to gain love from another
    person: that is, love has to be earned.   1   2   3   4   5   6   7

40. I am very sensitive to the effects my words or
    actions have on the feelings of other people.   1   2   3   4   5   6   7

41. I often blame myself for things I have done or
    said to someone.   1   2   3   4   5   6   7

42. I am a very independent person.   1   2   3   4   5   6   7

43. I often feel guilty.   1   2   3   4   5   6   7

44. I think of myself as a very complex person, one who has "many sides."   1   2   3   4   5   6   7

45. I worry a lot about offending or hurting someone who is close to me.   1   2   3   4   5   6   7

46. Anger frightens me.   1   2   3   4   5   6   7

47. It is not "who you are," but "what you have accomplished" that counts.   1   2   3   4   5   6   7

48. I feel good about myself whether I succeed or fail.   1   2   3   4   5   6   7

49. I can easily put my own feelings and problems aside, and devote my complete attention to the feelings and problems of someone else.   1   2   3   4   5   6   7

50. If someone I cared about became angry with me, I would feel threatened that he (she) might leave me.   1   2   3   4   5   6   7

51. I feel comfortable when I am given important responsibilities.   1   2   3   4   5   6   7

52. After a fight with a friend, I must make amends as soon as possible.   1   2   3   4   5   6   7

53. I have a difficult time accepting weaknesses in myself.   1   2   3   4   5   6   7

54. It is more important that I enjoy my work than it is for me to have my work approved.   1   2   3   4   5   6   7

55. After an argument, I feel very lonely.   1   2   3   4   5   6   7

56. In my relationships with others, I am very concerned about what they can give to me.   1   2   3   4   5   6   7

57. I rarely think about my family.   1   2   3   4   5   6   7

58. Very frequently, my feelings toward someone close to me vary: there are times when I feel completely angry and other times when I feel all-loving towards that person.   1   2   3   4   5   6   7

59. What I do and say has a very strong impact on those around me.   1   2   3   4   5   6   7

60. I sometimes feel that I am "special."   1   2   3   4   5   6   7

61. I grew up in an extremely close family.   1   2   3   4   5   6   7

62. I am very satisfied with myself and my accomplishments.   1   2   3   4   5   6   7

63. I want many things from someone I am close to.   1   2   3   4   5   6   7

64. I tend to be very critical of myself.   1   2   3   4   5   6   7

65. Being alone doesn't bother me at all.   1   2   3   4   5   6   7

66. I very frequently compare myself to standards or goals.   1   2   3   4   5   6   7

*Blatt, S. J., Zohar, A. H., Quinlan, D. M., Zuroff, D. C., & Mongrain, M. (1995). Subscales within the dependency factor of the Depressive Experiences Questionnaire. Journal of Personality Assessment, 64, 319-339. https://dx.doi.org/10.1207/s15327752jpa6402_11

ECR-12: A Brief Version of the Experiences in Close Relationships Scale (ECR)

The following statements concern *how you generally feel in close couple relationships (i.e., with romantic/marital partners)*. Respond to each statement by indicating how much you agree or disagree with it. Write the number in the space provided, using the following rating scale:

1	2	3	4	5	6	7
Disagree Strongly	*Disagree*	*Disagree Slightly*	*Neutral/ Mixed*	*Agree Slightly*	*Agree*	*Agree Strongly*

____ 1. I feel comfortable depending on romantic partners.
____ 2. I worry that romantic partners won't care about me as much as I care about them.
____ 3. I usually discuss my problems and concerns with my partner.
____ 4. I worry a fair amount about losing my partner.
____ 5. I tell my partner just about everything. [I tell my close relationship partners just about everything.]
____ 6. I worry about being abandoned.
____ 7. I don't mind asking romantic partners for comfort, advice, or help.
____ 8. I worry about being alone.
____ 9. I don't feel comfortable opening up to romantic partners.
____ 10. I need alot of reassurance that I am loved by my partner.
____ 11.I feel comfortable sharing my private thoughts and feelings with my partner.
____ 12. If I can't get my partner to show interest in me, I get upset or angry.

Note: Items 1, 3, 5, 7, and 11 must be reverse-keyed prior to computing the following scores:

(1) The *Attachment Avoidance* score is computed by averaging the 6 odd-numbered (1, 3, 5, 7, 9, 11) items. Higher scores reflect greater avoidance.

(2) The *Attachment Anxiety* score is computed by averaging the 6 even-numbered items (2, 4, 6, 8, 10, 12). Higher scores reflect greater anxiety.

When referencing the ECR-12, please cite the following article:

Lafontaine, M-F., Brassard, A., Lussier, Y., Valois, P., Shaver, P. R., & Johnson, S. M. (2015). Selecting the best items for a short-form of the Experiences in Close Relationships questionnaire. *European Journal of Psychological Assessment, 32*(2), 140-154.http://dx.doi.org/10.1027/1015-5759/a000243

General Anxiety Disorder (GAD-7)

NAME   DATE

1. Over the last 2 weeks, how often have you been bothered by the following problems?	Not at all sure	Several days	Over half the days	Nearly every day
• Feeling nervous, anxious, or on edge	☐ 0	☐ 1	☐ 2	☐ 3
• Not being able to stop or control worrying	☐ 0	☐ 1	☐ 2	☐ 3
• Worrying too much about different things	☐ 0	☐ 1	☐ 2	☐ 3
• Trouble relaxing	☐ 0	☐ 1	☐ 2	☐ 3
• Being so restless that it's hard to sit still	☐ 0	☐ 1	☐ 2	☐ 3
• Becoming easily annoyed or Irritable	☐ 0	☐ 1	☐ 2	☐ 3
• Feeling afraid as if something awful might happen	☐ 0	☐ 1	☐ 2	☐ 3
Add the score for each column				
TOTAL SCORE *(add your column scores)*				
	Not difficult at all	Somewhat difficult	Very difficult	Extremely difficult
2. If you checked off any problem on this questionnaire so far, how difficult have these problems made it for you to do your work, take care of things at home, or get along with other people?	☐ 0	☐ 1	☐ 2	☐ 3

Scoring *Add the results for question number one through seven to get a total score.*

If you score 10 or above you might want to consider one or more of the following:

1. Discuss your symptoms with your doctor,
2. Contact a local mental health care provider or
3. Contact my office for further assessment and possible treatment.

Although these questions serve as a useful guide, only an appropriate licensed health professional can make the diagnosis of Generalized Anxiety Disorder.

A score of 10 or higher means significant anxiety is present. Score over 15 are severe.

GUIDE FOR INTERPRETING GAD-7 SCORES

Scale	Severity
0-9	None to mild
10-14	Moderate
15-21	Severe

GAD-7 developed by Dr. Robert L. Spitzer, Dr. K. Kroenke. et.al.

GCQ
Group Climate
Questionnaire

Name: _____   ID: _____   Date: _____/_____/_____

Instructions:

Read each statement carefully and as you answer the questions think of the group as a whole. For each statement select the MOST APPROPRIATE answer that best describes the group during the last four sessions.

Developed by

MacKenzie 1981
MacKenzie et al. 1987

For More Information Contact:

OQ Measures, LLC
P.O. Box 521047
Salt Lake City, UT 84152

Toll-Free USA:
1-888-MH-SCORE
(1-888-647-2673)

Phone: (801) 649-4392
Fax: (801)747-6900

Email:
INFO@OQMEASURES.COM

Website:
WWW.OQMEASURES.COM

	Not at All	A Little True	Somewhat	Moderately	Quite A Bit	A Great Deal	Extremely
1. The members liked and cared about each other.	O	O	O	O	O	O	O
2. The members tried to understand why they do the things they do, tried to reason it out.	O	O	O	O	O	O	O
3. The members avoided looking at important issues going on between themselves.	O	O	O	O	O	O	O
4. The members felt what was happening was important and there was a sense of participation.	O	O	O	O	O	O	O
5. The members depended upon the group leader(s) for direction.	O	O	O	O	O	O	O
6. There was friction and anger between the members.	O	O	O	O	O	O	O
7. The members were distant and withdrawn from each other.	O	O	O	O	O	O	O
8. The members challenged and confronted each other in their efforts to sort things out.	O	O	O	O	O	O	O
9. The members appeared to do things the way they thought would be acceptable to the group.	O	O	O	O	O	O	O
10. The members rejected and distrusted each other	O	O	O	O	O	O	O
11. The members revealed sensitive personal information or feelings	O	O	O	O	O	O	O
12. The members appeared tense and anxious.	O	O	O	O	O	O	O

OQ-GCQ-S English en-us Printable Form v092202

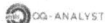 OQ-ANALYST

GROUP PSYCHOTHERAPY INTERVENTION RATING SCALE (GPIRS)

Intervention did not occur = 0; Poor = 1; Adequate = 2; Well done = 3; Excellent = 4

	0	1	2	3	4
1. Set group agendas (such as discussion topics or group activities).	☐ 0	☐ 1	☐ 2	☐ 3	☐ 4
2. Described rationale underlying treatment.	☐ 0	☐ 1	☐ 2	☐ 3	☐ 4
3. Identified and discussed fears/concerns regarding self disclosure	☐ 0	☐ 1	☐ 2	☐ 3	☐ 4
4. Discussed group rules (such as time, attendance, absences, tardiness, confidentiality, participation)	☐ 0	☐ 1	☐ 2	☐ 3	
5. Structured exercises that focus on emotional expression and exchange.	☐ 0	☐ 1	☐ 2	☐ 3	☐ 4
6. Discussed member roles and responsibility.	☐ 0	☐ 1	☐ 2	☐ 3	☐ 4
7. Discussed leader roles and responsibility.	☐ 0	☐ 1	☐ 2	☐ 3	☐ 4
8. Modeled giving personal information in the "here and now".	☐ 0	☐ 1	☐ 2	☐ 3	☐ 4
9. Modeled appropriate member-member behavior.	☐ 0	☐ 1	☐ 2	☐ 3	☐ 4
10. Modeled appropriate self disclosure.	☐ 0	☐ 1	☐ 2	☐ 3	☐ 4
11. Modeled appropriate feeling disclosure.	☐ 0	☐ 1	☐ 2	☐ 3	☐ 4
12. Maintained moderate control.	☐ 0	☐ 1	☐ 2	☐ 3	☐ 4
13. Facilitated appropriate member-member interaction.	☐ 0	☐ 1	☐ 2	☐ 3	☐ 4
14. Encouraged self disclosure without "forcing it".	☐ 0	☐ 1	☐ 2	☐ 3	☐ 4
15. Encouraged self disclosure relevant to the current group agenda.	☐ 0	☐ 1	☐ 2	☐ 3	☐ 4
16. Helped members understand that disclosed issues achieve more. resolution than undisclosed issues.	☐ 0	☐ 1	☐ 2	☐ 3	☐ 4
17. Encouraged here-and-now vs. story-telling disclosure.	☐ 0	☐ 1	☐ 2	☐ 3	☐ 4
18. Interrupted ill-timed or excessive member disclosure.	☐ 0	☐ 1	☐ 2	☐ 3	☐ 4
19. Elicited member-member feeling disclosure (versus informational disclosure).	☐ 0	☐ 1	☐ 2	☐ 3	☐ 4
20. Leader shared relevant personal experience from outside of therapy (without being judgmental or overly-intellectual)	☐ 0	☐ 1	☐ 2	☐ 3	☐ 4
21. Reframed injurious feedback (interrupting, if necessary).	☐ 0	☐ 1	☐ 2	☐ 3	☐ 4
22. Restated corrective feedback by member.	☐ 0	☐ 1	☐ 2	☐ 3	☐ 4
23. Used consensus to reinforce feedback (toward therapist or group member)	☐ 0	☐ 1	☐ 2	☐ 3	☐ 4
24. Balanced positive and corrective leader-to-member feedback.	☐ 0	☐ 1	☐ 2	☐ 3	☐ 4
25. Encouraged positive feedback.	☐ 0	☐ 1	☐ 2	☐ 3	☐ 4
26. Gave structured feedback exercise.	☐ 0	☐ 1	☐ 2	☐ 3	☐ 4
27. Helped balance positive and corrective member-to-member feedback.	☐ 0	☐ 1	☐ 2	☐ 3	☐ 4
28. Therapist helped members apply in-group feedback to out-of-group situations	☐ 0	☐ 1	☐ 2	☐ 3	☐ 4
29. Maintained balance in expressions of emotional support and confrontation.	☐ 0	☐ 1	☐ 2	☐ 3	☐ 4
30. Showed understanding of the members and their concerns.	☐ 0	☐ 1	☐ 2	☐ 3	☐ 4
31. Refrained from conveying personal feelings of hostility and anger in response to negative. member behavior (If there was no substantial negative behavior, mark 0).	☐ 0	☐ 1	☐ 2	☐ 3	☐ 4
32. Leader was not defensive when interventions failed.	☐ 0	☐ 1	☐ 2	☐ 3	☐ 4
33. Leader was not defensive when confronted by a member (If therapist was not confronted by a member, mark 0).	☐ 0	☐ 1	☐ 2	☐ 3	☐ 4
34. Maintained an active engagement with the group and its work.	☐ 0	☐ 1	☐ 2	☐ 3	☐ 4
35. Used nonjudgmental language with members.	☐ 0	☐ 1	☐ 2	☐ 3	☐ 4
36. Modeled expressions of open and genuine warmth.	☐ 0	☐ 1	☐ 2	☐ 3	☐ 4
37. Encouraged active emotional engagement between group members.	☐ 0	☐ 1	☐ 2	☐ 3	☐ 4
38. Fostered a climate of both support and challenge.	☐ 0	☐ 1	☐ 2	☐ 3	☐ 4
39. Responded at an emotionally empathic level.	☐ 0	☐ 1	☐ 2	☐ 3	☐ 4
40. Developed and/or facilitated relationships with and among group members.	☐ 0	☐ 1	☐ 2	☐ 3	☐ 4
41. Helped members recognize why they feel a certain way. (identifying underlying concerns or motives)	☐ 0	☐ 1	☐ 2	☐ 3	☐ 4
42. Prevented or stopped attacking and judgmental expressions. between members (If no opportunity for this intervention occurred, mark 0).	☐ 0	☐ 1	☐ 2	☐ 3	☐ 4
43. Assisted members in describing their emotions.	☐ 0	☐ 1	☐ 2	☐ 3	☐ 4
44. Recognized and responded to the meaning of groups members' comments.	☐ 0	☐ 1	☐ 2	☐ 3	☐ 4
45. Prevented situations in which members felt discounted, misunderstood, attacked, or disconnected (If no situation occurred, mark 0)	☐ 0	☐ 1	☐ 2	☐ 3	☐ 4
46. Involved members in describing and resolving conflict (instead of avoiding conflict)	☐ 0	☐ 1	☐ 2	☐ 3	☐ 4
47. Elicited verbal expressions of support among group members	☐ 0	☐ 1	☐ 2	☐ 3	☐ 4
48. Encouraged members to respond to other members' emotional expression (such as acceptance, belonging, empathy)	☐ 0	☐ 1	☐ 2	☐ 3	☐ 4
49. Encouraged members to respond to other members' emotional expression	☐ 0	☐ 1	☐ 2	☐ 3	☐ 4

Developed by Chris Chapman, Liz Baker, and Gary M. Burlingame.
Group Dynamics: Theory, Research, and Practice 2010, Vol. 14, No. 1, 15–31

E-MAIL: GARY_BURLINGAME@BYU.EDU

© 2010 American Psychological Association
1089-2699/10/$12.00 DOI: 10.1037/a0016628

OQ®-GRQ
Group Readiness
Questionnaire

Name: _____   ID: _____   Date: ___/___/____

	Never	Rarely	Sometimes	Frequently	Almost Always
1. When I am with a group of people who are talking about a topic I feel strong about, how likely am I to express my opinion?	O	O	O	O	O
2. I like to share my feelings with others.	O	O	O	O	O
3. I avoid talking in group.	O	O	O	O	O
4. I often feel like an outsider in group discussions.	O	O	O	O	O
5. I typically dominate group discussions.	O	O	O	O	O
6. I hardly ever say what I'm thinking when I'm with a group of people.	O	O	O	O	O
7. If I disagree with what someone is saying, I will interrupt them before they can finish what they are saying.	O	O	O	O	O
8. When I first meet someone, I like to share things about myself including quite personal information.	O	O	O	O	O
9. I am very private and hardly ever share how I feel.	O	O	O	O	O
10. I think that working in a group will really help me.	O	O	O	O	O
11. If I participate in a group, I expect to feel quite a bit better when we are finished.	O	O	O	O	O
12. I think that sharing my feelings with others will help me feel better.	O	O	O	O	O
13. I am abruptwith others if I feel strongly about what I am saying.	O	O	O	O	O
14. I tend to keep to myself in groups.	O	O	O	O	O
15. I often contribute to group discussions.	O	O	O	O	O
16. I am an open person.	O	O	O	O	O
17. I argue for argument's sake.	O	O	O	O	O
18. I am the life of aparty.	O	O	O	O	O
19. Others tend to see me as withdrawn.	O	O	O	O	O

OQ-GRQ English en-us Printable Form v092202

 OQ-ANALYST

Group Session Rating Scale (GSRS)

Name _____ Age (Yrs.): _____
ID# _____ Gender: _____
Session # _____ Date: _____

Please rate today's group by placing a mark on the line nearest to the description that best fits your experience.

Relationship

I did not feel
understood,
respected, and/or
accepted by the leader
and/or the group.
————————————————————— I
I felt understood,
respected, and
accepted by the leader
and the group.

Goals and Topics

We did *not* work on or
talk about what I
wanted to work on and
talk about.
————————————————————— I
We worked on and
talked about what I
wanted to work on and
talk about.

Approach or Method

The leader and/or the
group's approach are/is
not a good fit for me.
————————————————————— I
The leader and the
group's approach are
a good fit for me.

Overall

There was something
missing in group
today—I did not feel
like a part of the group.
————————————————————— I
Overall, today's group
was right for me—I felt
like a part of the group.

Better Outcomes Now
_____
https://betteroutcomesnow.com

Group

Therapy

Questionnaire - S

Name: _____

Date: _____

Group Leaders: _____

The Group Therapy Questionnaire is designed to help you learn more about how you might profit from group therapy and how we might be better able to help you. There are no right or wrong answers. Please respond to the questions as honestly and clearly as you can.

Counseling:

1.   Have you had previous counseling of any type?............................Yes......No.......

    A. If yes, what type?

    * Individual therapy _____
    * Group therapy   _____
    * Family therapy   _____
    * Other   _____

		(Not at all)				(Very much)		
2.	I look forward to beginning group therapy.	1	2	3	4	5	6	7
3.	I hope this group will meet my needs.	1	2	3	4	5	6	7
4.	I suspect that I will be like other group members.	1	2	3	4	5	6	7
5.	I expect I will stay with the group at least eight weeks.	1	2	3	4	5	6	7

Family:

1.   How did your parents show their caring for you?

        _____

        _____

2.   Children play different roles in their family. What role did you play in your family?

        _____

        _____

3.   How did your parents show their anger at you?

        _____

        _____

4.   How did you express your anger toward your parents?

        _____

        _____

5.   Diagram your family. It can be helpful if you use placement to depict closeness and
        size to reflect status.

6. What, if any, conflicts are arising in work or school relationships?

_____

_____

7. What role do you play in your current family or intimate relationships that contributes to difficulties?

_____

_____

8. Are there any aspects of your identity that you would like to share with the group, or that might be challenging to discuss/explore? **Aspects of identity that might be discussed include race, ethnicity, language, nationality, sex, gender identity, sexual orientation, religion, ability, and socioeconomic status**

_____

_____

_____

Health:

1. Check any of the following you experience:

   ☐ vomiting   ☐ painful menstruation
   ☐ difficulty swallowing   ☐ amnesia
   ☐ pain in legs, arms, back, joints, during urination ☐ burning sensation in sexual
   ☐ shortness of breath when not exerting oneself   organs (other than intercourse)

2. Do you have friends? (Check one)   ☐ None   ☐ Few   ☐ Many

3. Are you feeling suicidal? ☐ No   ☐ Yes, with thoughts only ☐ Yes, with intent/plan

4. Are you feeling homicidal/wanting to kill someone?

   ☐ No   ☐ Yes, with thoughts only   ☐ Yes, with a plan

5. **Please check the interpersonal problems you experience:**

☐ excessive arguments
☐ physical fights with partner
☐ physical fights with others
☐ divorce
☐ feeling too dependent on others
☐ shyness
☐ not being assertive
☐ lose my temper frequently
☐ unstable relationships
☐ lack of control of my anger
☐ feel empty and bored
☐ constantly need reassurance, approval and praise
☐ avoid social activities
☐ allow others to make my important decisions
☐ often feel uncomfortable or helpless when alone
☐ easily hurt by criticism or disapproval
☐ procrastinate
☐ often unaware of feelings or numb

☐ verbal abuse to people I care about
☐ physical fights with family
☐ separation
☐ feel isolated and lonely
☐ difficulty socializing
☐ loneliness
☐ difficulty trusting others
☐ do not enjoy or desire close relationships
☐ moods change quickly
☐ lack of personal identity
☐ feel abandoned
☐ preoccupied with feelings of envy
☐ unable to make decisions without reassurance from others
☐ difficulty initiating things on my own
☐ feel devastated when close relationships end
☐ perfectionism that interferes with task completion

6. **Are you in any kind of crisis right now?**   ☐ Yes ☐ No

   Please describe, if so:

   _____

   _____

Therapy Considerations:

1. **What are you most afraid of about group therapy?**

   _____

   _____

2. **If you could change somethingabout yourse lf as a result of group therapy, what would you change?**

   _____

   _____

3. **Specify what you believe to be your difficulties.**

   _____

   _____

   _____

4. **What are your goals for group therapy?**

   a. _____

   b. _____

   c. _____

5. **What might prevent you from reaching your goals?**

   _____

   _____

6. **Is there anything you have not told us that you believe might be helpful?**

   _____

   _____

OQ®-GQ
Group Questionnaire

Name: _____ ID: _____ Date: ___/___/___

Instructions:

Thank you for agreeing to complete the Group Questionnaire. The following questions ask about your personal experience in your therapy group. Please read each question carefully, and then select the answer that best describes how you felt during the last group session.

Developed by

Gary M. Burlingame, Ph.D.
Julie Ann Krogel, Ph.D.
Jennifer Johnson, Ph. D.

© Copyright American Professional Credentialing Services LLC.
All Rights Reserved.
License Required For All Uses

For More Information Contact:

OQ Measures, LLC
P.O. Box 521047
Salt Lake City, UT 84152

Toll-Free USA:
1-888-MH-SCORE
(1-888-647-2673)

Phone: (801) 649-4392
Fax: (801) 747-6900

Email:
INFO@OQMEASURES.COM

Website:
WWW.OQMEASURES.COM

	Not True at All	A Little True	Slightly True	Somewhat True	Moderately True	Considerably True	Very True
1. I felt that I could trust the group leaders during today's session.	O	O	O	O	O	O	O
2. I felt that I could trust the other group members during today's session.	O	O	O	O	O	O	O
3. The group leaders and I respect each other.	O	O	O	O	O	O	O
4. The other group members and I respect each other.	O	O	O	O	O	O	O
5. I feel the group leaders care about me even when I do things that they do not approve of.	O	O	O	O	O	O	O
6. I feel the other group members care about me even when I do things that they do not approve of.	O	O	O	O	O	O	O
7. The group leaders were friendly and warm toward me.	O	O	O	O	O	O	O
8. The other group members were friendly and warm toward me.	O	O	O	O	O	O	O
9. The group leaders and I agree about the things I will need to do in therapy.	O	O	O	O	O	O	O
10. The other group members and I agree about the things I will need to do in therapy.	O	O	O	O	O	O	O
11. The group leaders and I agree on what is important to work on.	O	O	O	O	O	O	O
12. The other group members and I agree on what is important to work on.	O	O	O	O	O	O	O
13. The group leaders and I have established a understanding of the kind of changes that would be good for me.	O	O	O	O	O	O	O
14. The other group members and I have established a good understanding of the kind of changes that would be good for me.	O	O	O	O	O	O	O
15. The group leaders and I are working together toward mutually agreed upon goals.	O	O	O	O	O	O	O
16. The other group members and I are working together toward mutually agreed upon goals.	O	O	O	O	O	O	O
17. Sometimes the group leaders did not seem to be completely genuine.	O	O	O	O	O	O	O

OQ-GQ English en-us Printable Form v092202

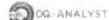 OQ-ANALYST

OQ®-GQ
Group Questionnaire

Name: _____ ID: _____ Date: ____/____/_____

Instructions:		Not True at All	A Little True	Slightly True	Somewhat True	Moderately True	Considerably True	Very True
Thank you for agreeing to complete the Group Questionnaire. The following questions ask about your personal experience in your therapy group. Please read each question carefully, and then select the answer that best describes how you felt during the last group session.	18. Sometimes the other group members did not seem to be completely genuine.	O	O	O	O	O	O	O
	19. The group leaders did not always seem to care about me.	O	O	O	O	O	O	O
	20. The other group members did not always seem to care about me.	O	O	O	O	O	O	O
	21. The group leaders did not always understand the way I felt inside.	O	O	O	O	O	O	O
	22. The other group members did not always understand the way I felt inside.	O	O	O	O	O	O	O
	23. There was friction and anger between the members.	O	O	O	O	O	O	O
	24. The members were distant and withdrawn from each other.	O	O	O	O	O	O	O
	25. There was tension and anxiety between the members.	O	O	O	O	O	O	O
	26. The members liked and cared about each other.	O	O	O	O	O	O	O
	27. The members felt what was happening was important and there was a sense of participation.	O	O	O	O	O	O	O
	28. We cooperate and work together in group.	O	O	O	O	O	O	O
	29. Even though we have differences, our group feels secure to me.	O	O	O	O	O	O	O
	30. The group members accept one another.	O	O	O	O	O	O	O

Developed by

Gary M. Burlingame, Ph.D.
Julie Ann Krogel, Ph.D.
Jennifer Johnson, Ph. D.

For More Information
Contact:

OQ Measures, LLC
P.O. Box 521047
Salt Lake City, UT 84152

Toll-Free USA:
1-888-MH-SCORE
(1-888-647-2673)

Phone: (801) 649-4392
Fax: (801) 747-6900

Email:
INFO@OQMEASURES.COM

Website:
WWW.OQMEASURES.COM

OQ-GQ English en-us Printable Form v092202

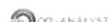 OQ-ANALYST

Inventory of Interpersonal Problems-32 (IIP-32) Sample Questions

It is hard for me to:

- Understand another person's point of view
- Be firm when I need to be

The following are things that you do too much:

- I try to control other people too much.
- I tell personal things to other people too much.

Multi-Group Ethnic Identity Measure

MEIM1.   I have spent time trying to find out more about my ethnic group, such as its history, traditions, and customs. (Choose one)

1   Strongly Disagree
2   Disagree
3   In the Middle
4   Agree
5   Strongly Agree
8   Refuse to Answer

MEIM2.   I am active in organizations or social groups that include mostly members of my own ethnic group. (Choose one)

1   Strongly Disagree
2   Disagree
3   In the Middle
4   Agree
5   Strongly Agree
8   Refuse to Answer

MEIM3.   I have a clear sense of my ethnic background and what it means for me. (Choose one)

1   Strongly Disagree
2   Disagree
3   In the Middle
4   Agree
5   Strongly Agree
8   Refuse to Answer

MEIM4.   I think a lot about how my life will be affected by my ethnic group membership. (Choose one)

1   Strongly Disagree
2   Disagree
3   In the Middle
4   Agree
5   Strongly Agree
8   Refuse to Answer

MEIM5.   I am happy that I am a member of the group I belong to. (Choose one)

1   Strongly Disagree
2   Disagree
3   In the Middle
4   Agree
5   Strongly Agree
8   Refuse to Answer

MEIM6.   I have a strong sense of belonging to my own ethnic group. (Choose one)

1   Strongly Disagree
2   Disagree
3   In the Middle
4   Agree
5   Strongly Agree
8   Refuse to Answer

MEIM7.　　I understand pretty well what my ethnic group membership means to me. (Choose one)

　　　　　1　Strongly Disagree
　　　　　2　Disagree
　　　　　3　In the Middle
　　　　　4　Agree
　　　　　5　Strongly Agree
　　　　　8　Refuse to Answer

MEIM8.　　In order to learn more about my ethnic background, I have often talked to other people about my ethnic group. (Choose one)

　　　　　1　Strongly Disagree
　　　　　2　Disagree
　　　　　3　In the Middle
　　　　　4　Agree
　　　　　5　Strongly Agree
　　　　　8　Refuse to Answer

MEIM9.　　I have a lot of pride in my ethnic group. (Choose one)

　　　　　1　Strongly Disagree
　　　　　2　Disagree
　　　　　3　In the Middle
　　　　　4　Agree
　　　　　5　Strongly Agree
　　　　　8　Refuse to Answer

MEIM10.　　I participate in cultural practices of my own group, such as special food, music, or customs. (Choose one)

　　　　　1　Strongly Disagree
　　　　　2　Disagree
　　　　　3　In the Middle
　　　　　4　Agree
　　　　　5　Strongly Agree
　　　　　8　Refuse to Answer

MEIM11.　　I feel a strong attachment towards my own ethnic group. (Choose one)

　　　　　1　Strongly Disagree
　　　　　2　Disagree
　　　　　3　In the Middle
　　　　　4　Agree
　　　　　5　Strongly Agree
　　　　　8　Refuse to Answer

MEIM12.　　I feel good about my cultural or ethnic background. (Choose one)

　　　　　1　Strongly Disagree
　　　　　2　Disagree
　　　　　3　In the Middle
　　　　　4　Agree
　　　　　5　Strongly Agree
　　　　　8　Refuse to Answer

Outcome Questionnaire (OQ®-45.2 English)

Name: _____   ID: _____   Date: ____/____/_____

Developed by

Michael J. Lambert, Ph.D.
and
Gary M. Burlingame, Ph.D.

© Copyright American
Professional Credentialing
Services LLC.

All Rights Reserved.
License Required For All
Uses

For More Information
Contact:

OQ Measures, LLC
P.O. Box 521047
Salt Lake City, UT 84152

Toll-Free USA:
1-888-MH-SCORE
(1-888-647-2673)

Phone: (801) 649-4392
Fax: (801) 747-6900

Email:
INFO@OQMEASURES.COM

Website:
WWW.OQMEASURES.COM

Instructions:

Looking back over the last week, including today, help us understand how you have been feeling. Read each item carefully and fill the circle completely under the category which best describes your current situation. For this questionnaire, work is defined as employment, school, housework, volunteer work, and so forth.

	Never	Rarely	Sometimes	Frequently	Almost Always
1. I get along well with others.	O	O	O	O	O
2. I tire quickly.	O	O	O	O	O
3. I feel no interest in things.	O	O	O	O	O
4. I feel stressed at work/school.	O	O	O	O	O
5. I blame myself for things.	O	O	O	O	O
6. I feel irritated.	O	O	O	O	O
7. I feel unhappy in my marriage/significant relationship.	O	O	O	O	O
8. I have thoughts of ending my life.	O	O	O	O	O
9. I feel weak.	O	O	O	O	O
10. I feel fearful.	O	O	O	O	O
11. After heavy drinking, I need a drink the next morning to get going. (If you do not drink, mark "never").	O	O	O	O	O
12. I find my work/school satisfying.	O	O	O	O	O
13. I am a happy person.	O	O	O	O	O
14. I work/study too much.	O	O	O	O	O
15. I feel worthless.	O	O	O	O	O
16. I am concerned about family troubles.	O	O	O	O	O
17. I have an unfulfilling sex life.	O	O	O	O	O
18. I feel lonely.	O	O	O	O	O
19. I have frequent arguments.	O	O	O	O	O
20. I feel loved and wanted.	O	O	O	O	O
21. I enjoy my spare time.	O	O	O	O	O
22. I have difficulty concentrating.	O	O	O	O	O
23. I feel hopeless about the future.	O	O	O	O	O
24. I like myself.	O	O	O	O	O
25. Disturbing thoughts come into my mind that I cannot get rid of.	O	O	O	O	O

OQ®-Analyst Document: OQ-45.2 English en-us Printable Form v092202.docx   OQ·ANALYST

Outcome Questionnaire (OQ®-45.2 English)

Name: _____   ID: _____   Date: ____/____/_____

	Never	Rarely	Sometimes	Frequemtly	Almost Always
26. I feel annoyed by people who criticize my drinking (or drug use) (If not applicable, mark "never").	O	O	O	O	O
27. I have an upset stomach.	O	O	O	O	O
28. I am not working/studying as well as I used to.	O	O	O	O	O
29. My heart pounds too much.	O	O	O	O	O
30. I have trouble getting along with friends and close acquaintances.	O	O	O	O	O
31. I am satisfied with my life.	O	O	O	O	O
32. I have trouble at work/school because of drinking or drug use (If not applicable, mark "never").	O	O	O	O	O
33. I feel that something bad is going to happen.	O	O	O	O	O
34. I have sore muscles.	O	O	O	O	O
35. I feel afraid of open spaces, of driving, or being on buses, subways, and so forth.	O	O	O	O	O
36. I feel nervous.	O	O	O	O	O
37. I feel my love relationships are full and complete.	O	O	O	O	O
38. I feel that I am not doing well at work/school.	O	O	O	O	O
39. I have too many disagreements at work/school.	O	O	O	O	O
40. I feel something is wrong with my mind.	O	O	O	O	O
41. I have trouble falling asleep or staying asleep.	O	O	O	O	O
42. I feel blue.	O	O	O	O	O
43. I am satisfied with my relationships with others.	O	O	O	O	O
44. I feel angry enough at work/school to do something I might regret.	O	O	O	O	O
45. I have headaches.	O	O	O	O	O

OQ®-Analyst Document: OQ-45.2 English en-us Printable Form v092202.docx   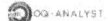 OQ-ANALYST

Outcome Rating Scale (ORS)

Name _____Age (Yrs.): ___ Gender: _____
Session # ____ Date: _____
Who is filling out this form? Please check one: Self_____   Other_____
If other, what is your relationship to this person? _____

Looking back over the last week, including today, help us understand how you have been feeling by rating how well you have been doing in the following areas of your life, where marks to the left represent low levels and marks to the right indicate high levels. *If you are filling out this form for another person, please fill out according to how you think they are doing.*

Individually
(Personal well-being)

I———————————————————————I

Interpersonally
(Family, close relationships)

I———————————————————————I

Socially
(Work, school, friendships)

I———————————————————————I

Overall
(General sense of well-being)

I———————————————————————I

Better Outcomes Now

https://www.betteroutcomesnow.com

© 2000, Scott D. Miller and Barry L. Duncan

Brief Perceived Ethnic Discrimination Questionnaire-Community Version (Brief PEDQ-CV)

Think about your **ethnicity/race**. What group do you belong to? **Do you think of yourself as**: Asian?
Black? Latino? White? Native American? American? Caribbean? Irish? Italian? Korean? Another
group?

Your Ethnicity/Race: _____

How often have any of the things listed below ever happened to you, because of your ethnicity?

BECAUSE OF YOUR ETHNICITY/RACE…

A. **How often . . .**

1. Have you been treated unfairly by teachers, principals, or other staff at school?

2. Have others thought you couldn't do things or handle a job?

3. Have others threatened to hurt you (ex: said they would hit you)?

4. Have others actually hurt you or tried to hurt you (ex: kicked or hit you)?

5. Have policeman or security officers been unfair to you?

6. Have others threatened to damage your property?

7. Have others actually damaged your property?

8. Have others made you feel like an outsider who doesn't fit in because of your dress, speech, or other characteristics related to your ethnicity?

9. Have you been treated unfairly by co-workers or classmates?

10. Have others hinted that you are dishonest or can't be trusted?

11. Have people been nice to your face, but said bad things about you behind your back?

12. Have people who speak a different language made you feel like an outsider?

13. Have others ignored you or not paid attention to you?

14. Has your boss or supervisor been unfair to you?

15. Have others hinted that you must not be clean

16. Have people not trusted you?

17. Has it been hinted that you must be lazy?

If you would like to tell us more about your experiences of discrimination, please write your story here:
_____
_____
_____

Patient Health Questionnaire-9

Introduction

The Patient Health Questionnaire (PHQ) is a self-report version of the Primary Care Evaluation of Mental Disorders (PRIME-MD) diagnostic tool for common mental disorders. The PHQ-9 is a brief, 9-item scale that includes only the depression-related items from the PHQ. The PHQ-9 has been validated for use in primary care settings and can be used to make a tentative diagnosis of depression and to monitor depression severity and response to treatment in the past 2 weeks.

Patient Health Questionnaire-9
(PHQ-9)

Over the last 2 weeks, how often have you been bothered by any of the following problems? *(Use a check mark to indicate your answer)*	Not at all	Several days	More than half the days	Nearly every day
1. Little interest or pleasure in doing things	0	1	2	3
2. Feeling down, depressed, or hopeless	0	1	2	3
3. Trouble falling or staying asleep, or sleeping too much	0	1	2	3
4. Feeling tired or having little energy	0	1	2	3
5. Poor appetite or overeating	0	1	2	3
6. Feeling bad about yourself – or that you are a failure or have let yourself or your family down	0	1	2	3
7. Trouble concentrating on things, such as reading the newspaper or watching television	0	1	2	3
8. Moving or speaking so slowly that other people could have noticed? Or the opposite – being so fidgety or restlessthat you have been moving around a lot more than usual	0	1	2	3
9. Thoughts that you would be better off dead or hurting yourself in some way	0	1	2	3

FOR OFFICE CODING   _____ + _____ + _____ + _____

= Total Score: _____

If you checked off any problems, how difficult have these problems made it for you to do your work, take care of things at home, or get along with other people?

Not difficult at all	Somewhat difficult	Very difficult	Extremely difficult
☐	☐	☐	☐

Assessor Severity Ratings for Target Objectives

DURATION: When this problem occurs, how long does it last? (Symptoms only: e.g., depression, anxiety, OCD)

(0) None
(1) A few minutes − trivial
(2) An hour − minor
(3) 4 hours − moderate
(4) 8 hours − considerable
(5) 12+ hours − extreme

FREQUENCY: How often does this problem occur?

(0) Not at all - none
(1) Less than 1 time per week − seldom − trivial
(2) 1–2 times per week − once in a while − <half the time − minor
(3) Once a day - sometimes − half the time − 3–4 times per week − moderate
(4) Several times per day − fairly often − >half the time − considerable
(5) All the time − most of the time − always − extreme

INTENSITY: How strong or uncomfortable are your feelings about this problem? Do you get into a panic or try to avoid the situation or the feelings?

(0) Not at all − none
(1) Almost no problem − minimal − slight − trivial
(2) Low key - minor strength − not too strong − minor
(3) Fairly strong − moderate strength − moderate
(4) Some panic − strong − try to avoid − considerable
(5) Overwhelming − extreme

PERVASIVENESS: How many areas of your life (work, family/home, social/leisure) does this problem affect in a negative way?

(0) None
(1) Rarely affects one area − trivial
(2) Occasionally affects one area − isolated − minor
(3) Occasionally affects 2 areas or regularly affects 1 area − moderate
(4) Regularly affects 1 area and occasionally affects another − considerable
(5) Regularly affects 2+ areas − extreme

DISRUPTIVENESS: Consider the most affected area. How much does this problem interfere with performing or enjoying activities in this area? Does it take a lot of effort to control?

(0) No problem − none
(1) Almost no problem − trivial
(2) Good to mediocre effort to control − minor
(3) Moderate effort - in the middle − moderate
(4) Very uncomfortable − considerable effort
(5) Nonfunctional − absence of activities – extreme

TARGET OBJECTIVES SCALE*

OBJECTIVES	SEVERITY

1.

D=
F=
I=
P=
D=

2.

D=
F=
I=
P=
D=

3.

D=
F=
I=
P=
D=

* C. C., Imber, S. D., Hoehn-Saric, R., Stone, A. R., Nash, E. R., & Frank, J. D. (1966). Target complaints as criteria of improvement. *American Journal of Psychotherapy, 20*, 184-192. https://dx.doi.org/10.1176/appi.psychotherapy.1966.20.1.184

<u>TARGET OBJECTIVES: PRE-THERAPY FORMULATION AND RATINGS</u>

By now you probably have had several occasions to discuss your problems. At this time, please describe in your own words the problems or goals you most want help with in group therapy, that is, your objectives for treatment. Be specific and describe each with a sentence or two.

1.

2.

3.

RATING THE OBJECTIVES

Consider each of the objectives that have been formulated. You are asked to do three different things with each objective.

First, indicate how severe (disruptive) the problem associated with each objective has been for you during the last month by placing a number in the appropriate column according to the following:

1	2	3	4	5
Slight Severity	Minor Severity	Moderate Severity	Considerable Severity	Extreme Severity

Second, indicate how important each objective is to you by placing a number in the appropriate column, according to the following:

1	2	3	4	5
Slight Importance	Minor Importance	Moderate Importance	Cosiderable Importance	Extreme Importance

Remember, severity and importance refer to two different things (e.g., a problem may be of considerable severity but only of minor importance to you, or a problem may only be of minor severity yet be of extreme importance to you).

Third, indicate how much improvement you expect for each problem by the end of psychotherapy, by placing a number in the appropriate column, according to the following:

1	2	3	4	5	6
Extreme Worsening	Considerable Worsening	Moderate Worsening	Minor Worsening	Slight Worsening	No Change

7	8	9	10	11
Slight Improvement	Minor Improvement	Moderate Improvement	Considerable Improvement	Extreme Improvement

OBJECTIVE	SEVERITY	IMPORTANCE	EXPECTED IMPROVEMENT
1.			
2.			
3.			

<u>TARGET OBJECTIVES: POST-THERAPY RATINGS</u>

Please consider each of the objectives that were formulated before therapy began. You are asked to do three different ratings with each objective.

First, indicate how severe (disruptive) the problem associated with each objective has been for you during the last month by placing a number in the appropriate column according to the following:

0	1	2	3	4	5
No Severity	Slight Severity	Minor Severity	Moderate Severity	Considerable Severity	Extreme Severity

Second, indicate how important (relevant) each objective is to you by placing a number in the appropriate column, according to the following:

0	1	2	3	4	5
No Importance	Slight Severity	Minor Importance	Moderate Importance	Considerable Importance	Extreme Importance

Remember, severity and importance refer to two different things (e.g., a problem may be of considerable severity but only of minor importance to you, or a problem may only be of minor severity yet be of extreme importance to you).

Third, indicate the type of change that occurred for each problem since therapy began by placing a number in the appropriate column, according to the following:

1	2	3	4	5	6
Extreme Worsening	Considerable Change	Moderate Worsening	Minor Worsening	Slight Worsening	No Change

7	8	9	10	11
Slight Improvement	Minor Improvement	Moderate Improvement	Cosiderable Improvement	Extreme Improvement

OBJECTIVE	SEVERITY	IMPORTANCE	OBSERVED IMPROVEMENT
1.			
2.			
3.			

Therapeutic Factors Inventory-19

Please rate the following statements as they apply to your experience in your group by circling the corresponding number, using the following scale:

1= Strongly Disagree to 7= Strongly Agree

1. Because I've got a lot in common with other group members, I'm starting to think that I may have something in common with people outside group too.   1 2 3 4 5 6 7

2. Things seem more hopeful since joining group.   1 2 3 4 5 6 7

3. I feel a sense of belonging in this group.   1 2 3 4 5 6 7

4. I find myself thinking about my family a surprising amount in group.   1 2 3 4 5 6 7

5. It's okay for me to be angry in group.   1 2 3 4 5 6 7

6. In group I've really seen the social impact my family has had on my life.   1 2 3 4 5 6 7

7. My group is kind of like a little piece of the larger world I live in; I see the same patterns, and working them out in group helps me work them out in my outside life.   1 2 3 4 5 6 7

8. Group helps me feel more positive about my future.   1 2 3 4 5 6 7

9. It touches me that people in group are caring toward each other.   1 2 3 4 5 6 7

10. In group sometimes I learn by watching and later imitating what happens.   1 2 3 4 5 6 7

11. In group, the members are more alike than different from each other.   1 2 3 4 5 6 7

12. It's surprising, but despite needing support from my group, I've also learned to be more self-sufficient.   1 2 3 4 5 6 7

13. This group inspires me about the future.   1 2 3 4 5 6 7

14. Even though we have differences, our group feels secure to me.   1 2 3 4 5 6 7

15. By getting honest feedback from members and facilitators, I've learned alot about my impact on other people.   1 2 3 4 5 6 7

16. This group helps empower me to make a difference in my own life.   1 2 3 4 5 6 7

17. I get to vent my feelings in group.   1 2 3 4 5 6 7

18. Group has shown me the importance of other people in my life.   1 2 3 4 5 6 7

19. I can "let it all out" in my group.   1 2 3 4 5 6 7

Therapeutic Factors Inventory-Short Form

Please rate the following statements as they apply to your experience in your group by circling the corresponding number, using the following scale:

1= Strongly Disagree to 7= Strongly Agree

1. Because I've got a lot in common with other group members, I'm starting to think that I may have something in common with people outside group too.   1 2 3 4 5 6 7

2. Things seem more hopeful since joining group.   1 2 3 4 5 6 7

3. I feel a sense of belonging in this group.   1 2 3 4 5 6 7

4. I find myself thinking about my family a surprising amount in group.   1 2 3 4 5 6 7

5. Sometimes I notice that in group I have the same reactions or feelings as I did with my sister, brother, or a parent in my family.   1 2 3 4 5 6 7

6. In group I've learned that I have more similarities with others than I would have guessed.   1 2 3 4 5 6 7

7. It's okay for me to be angry in group.   1 2 3 4 5 6 7

8. In group I've really seen the social impact my family has had on my life.   1 2 3 4 5 6 7

9. My group is kind of like a little piece of the larger world I live in: I see the same patterns, and working them out in group helps me work them out in my outside life.   1 2 3 4 5 6 7

10. Group helps me feel more positive about my future.   1 2 3 4 5 6 7

11. It touches me that people in group are caring toward each other.   1 2 3 4 5 6 7

12. I pay attention to how others handle difficult situations in my group so I can apply these strategies in my own life.   1 2 3 4 5 6 7

13. In group sometimes I learn by watching and later imitating what happens.   1 2 3 4 5 6 7

14. This group helps me recognize how much I have in common with other people.   1 2 3 4 5 6 7

15. In group, the members are more alike than different from each other.   1 2 3 4 5 6 7

16. It's surprising, but despite needing support from my group, I've also learned to be more self-sufficient.   1 2 3 4 5 6 7

17. This group inspires me about the future.   1 2 3 4 5 6 7

18. Even though we have differences, our group feels secure to me.   1 2 3 4 5 6 7

19. By getting honest feedback from members and facilitators, I've learned a lot about my impact on other people.   1 2 3 4 5 6 7

20. This group helps empower me to make a difference in my own life.   1 2 3 4 5 6 7

21. I get to vent my feelings in group.   1 2 3 4 5 6 7

22. Group has shown me the importance of other people in my life.   1 2 3 4 5 6 7

23.   I can "let it all out" in my group.   1 2 3 4 5 6 7

Therapeutic Reactance Scale

PsycTESTS Citation:
Dowd, E. T., Milne, C. R., & Wise, S. L. (1991). Therapeutic Reactance Scale [Database record]. Retrieved from PsycTESTS. doi: https://dx.doi.org/10.1037/t09859-000

Instrument Type:
Rating Scale

Test Format:
The measure's 28 items are rated on a 4-point Likert scale anchored from strongly agree to strongly disagree.

Source:
Supplied by author.

Original Publication:
Dowd, E. Thomas, Milne, Christopher R., & Wise, Steven L. (1991). The Therapeutic Reactance Scale: A measure of psychological reactance. Journal of Counseling & Development, Vol 69(6), 541-545. doi: https://dx.doi.org/10.1002/j.1556-6676.1991.tb02638.x

Permissions:
Test content may be reproduced and used for non-commercial research and educational purposes without seeking written permission. Distribution must be controlled, meaning only to the participants engaged in the research or enrolled in the educational activity. Any other type of reproduction or distribution of test content is not authorized without written permission from the author and publisher. Always include a credit line that contains the source citation and copyright owner when writing about or using any test.

PsycTESTS™ is a database of the American Psychological Association

The Therapeutic Reactance Scale

Instructions: Please answer each item by marking the appropriate letter. Use the following categories to record your answer.

A= strongly disagree   B=disagree   C=agree   D=strongly agree

1. If I receive a lukewarm dish at a restaurant, I make an attempt to let that be known.
2. I resent authority figures who try to tell me what to do.
3. I find that I often have to question authority.
4. I enjoy seeing someone else do something that neither of us is supposed to do.
5. I have a strong desire to maintain my personal freedom.
6. I enjoy playing "Devil's Advocate" whenever I can.
7. In discussions I am easily persuaded by others.
8. Nothing turns me on as much as a good argument
9. It would be better to have more freedom to do what I want on a job.
10. If I am told what to do, I often do the opposite.
11. I am sometimes afraid to disagree with others.
12. It really bothers me when police officers tell people what to do.
13. It does not upset me to change my plans because someone in the group wants to do something else.
14. I don't mind other people telling me what to do.
15. I enjoy debates with other people.
16. If someone asks a favor of me, I will think twice about what this person is really after.
17. I am not very tolerant of others' attempts to persuade me.
18. I often follow the suggestions of others.
19. I am relatively opinionated.
20. It is important to me to be in a powerful position relative to others.
21. I am very open to solutions to my problems from others.
22. I enjoy "showing up" people who think they are right.
23. I consider myself more competitive than cooperative.
24. I don't mind doing something for someone even when I don't know why I'm doing it.
25. I usually go along with others' advice.
26. I feel it is better to stand up for what I believe than to be silent.
27. I am very stubborn and set in my ways.
28. It is very important for me to get along well with the people with whom I work.

WHOQOL-BREF[1]

About You

Before you begin we would like to ask you to answer a few general questions about yourself by circling the correct answer or by filling in the space provided.

1. What is your gender   Male   Female

2. What is your date of birth?   _____ /_____ /_____
                                                          Date   Month   Year

3. What is the highest education you   None at all
   received?   Elementary School
                                              High School
                                              College

4. What is your marital status?   Single   Separated
                                         Married   Divorced
                                         Living as Married   Widowed

5. Are you currently ill?   Yes   No

6. If something is wrong with
   your health, what do you
   think it is?   illness/problem
                                         _____

Instructions

This questionnaire asks how you feel about your quality of life, health, or other areas of your life. Please answer all the questions. If you are unsure about which response to give to a question, please choose the one that appears most appropriate. This can often be your first response.

Please keep in mind your standards, hopes, pleasures and concerns. We ask that you think about your life in the last two weeks. For example, thinking about the last two weeks, a question might ask:

For office use		*(Please circle the number)*				
		Not at all	A little	Moderately	Mostly	Completely
	Do you get the kind of support from others that you need?	1	2	3	4	5

You should circle the number that best fits how much support you got from others over the last two weeks. So you would circle the number 4 if you got a great deal of support from others.

For office use		*(Please circle the number)*				
		Not at all	A little	Moderately	Mostly	Completely
	Do you get the kind of support from others that you need?	1	2	3	(4)	5

You would circle number 1 if you did not get any of the support that you needed from others in the last two weeks.

For office use		*(Please circle the number)*				
		Not at all	A little	Moderately	Mostly	Completely
	Do you get the kind of support from others that you need?	(1)	2	3	4	5

Please read each question, assess your feelings, and circle the number on the scale that gives the best answer for you for each question.

For office use			*(Please circle the number)*				
			Very poor	Poor	Neither poor no ood	Good	Very Good
G1 / G1.1	1.	How would you rate your quality of life?	1	2	3	4	5

For office use			*(Please circle the number)*				
			Very dissatisfied	Dissatisfied	Neithe satisfied nor dissatisfied	Satisfied	ery satisfied
G4 / G2.3	2.	How satisfied are you with your health?	1	2	3	4	5

The following questions ask about **how much** you have experienced certain things in the last two weeks.

For office use			*(Please circle the number)*				
			Not at all	A little	A moderate amount	Very much	An extreme amount
F1.4 / F1.2.5	3.	To what extent do you feel that physical pain prevents you from doing what you need to do?	1	2	3	4	5
F11.3 / F13.1.4	4.	How much do you need any medical treatment to function in your daily life?	1	2	3	4	5
F4.1 / F6.1.2	5.	How much do you enjoy life?	1	2	3	4	5
F24.2 /	6.	To what extent do	1	2	3	4	5
For office use F29.1.3		you feel your life to be meaningful?	1	2	3	4	5

For office use			*(Please circle the number)*				
			Not at all	Slightly	A Moderate amount	Very much	Extremely
F5.2 / F7.1.6	7.	How well are you able to concentrate?	1	2	3	4	5
F16.1 / F20.1.2	8.	How safe do you feel in your daily life?	1	2	3	4	5
F22.1 / F27.1.2	9.	How healthy is your physical environment?	1	2	3	4	5

The following questions ask about **how completely** you experience or were able to do certain things in the last two weeks.

For office use			*(Please circle the number)*				
			Not at all	A little	Moderately	Mostly	Completely
F2.1 / F2.1.1	10.	Do you have enough energy for everyday life?	1	2	3	4	5
F7.1 / F9.1.2	11.	Are you able to accept your bodily appearance?	1	2	3	4	5
F18.1 / F23.1.1	12.	Have you enough money to meet your needs?	1	2	3	4	5
F20.1 /	13.	How available to	1	2	3	4	5

For office use F25.1.1		(Please circle the number)				
		Not at all	A little	Moderately	Mostly	Completely
F20.1 /	13. How available to you is the information that you need in your day-to-day life?	1	2	3	4	5
F21.1 / F26.1.2	14. To what extent do you have the opportunity for leisure activities?	1	2	3	4	5

For office use		(Please circle the number)				
		Very poor	Poor	Neither poor nor well	Well	Very well
F9.1 / F11.1.1	15. How well are you able to get around?	1	2	3	4	5

The following questions ask you to say how **good** or **satisfied** you have felt about various aspects of your life over the last two weeks.

For office use		(Please circle the number)				
		Very dissatisfied	Dissatisfied	Neither satisfied nor dissatisfied	Satisfied	Very satisfied
F3.3 / F4.2.2	16. How satisfied are you with your sleep?	1	2	3	4	5
F10.3 / F12.2.3	17. How satisfied are you with your ability to perform your daily living activities?	1	2	3	4	5
F12.4 / F16.2.1	18. How satisfied are you with your capacity for work?	1	2	3	4	5
F6.4 / F8.2.2	19. How satisfied are	1	2	3	4	5

For office use		(Please circle the number)				
		Very dissatisfied	Dissatisfied	Neither satisfied nor dissatisfied	Satisfied	Very satisfied
	you with your abilities?					
F13.3 / F17.2.3	20. How satisfied are you with your personal relationships?	1	2	3	4	5
F15.3 / F3.2.1	21. How satisfied are you with your sex life?	1	2	3	4	5
F14.4 / F18.2.5	22. How satisfied are you with the support you get from your friends?	1	2	3	4	5

For office use		*(Please circle the number)*				
		Very dissatisfied	Dissatisfied	Neither satisfied nor dissatisfied	Satisfied	Very satisfied
F17.3 / F21.2.2	23. How satisfied are you with the conditions of your living place?	1	2	3	4	5
F19.3 / F24.2.1	24. How satisfied are you with your access to health services?	1	2	3	4	5
F.23.3 / F28.2.2	25. How satisfied are you with your mode of transportation?	1	2	3	4	5

The follow question refers to **how often** you have felt or experienced certain things in the last two weeks.

For office use		*(Please circle the number)*				
		Never	Seldom	Quite often	Very often	Always
F8.1 / F10.1.2	26. How often do you have negative feelings, such as blue mood, despair, anxiety, depression?	1	2	3	4	5

Did someone help you to fill out this form? *(Please circle Yes or No)*   Yes   No

How long did it take to fill out this form?   _____

THANK YOU FOR YOUR HELP

Y-OQ®-30.2PR English Name: _____ **ID:** _____ **Date:** ____/____/____
Youth Outcome Questionnaire
Parent Form

PURPOSE:

The Y-OQ® 30.2 is designed to describe a wide range of situations, behaviors, and moods that are common to children and adolescents. You may discover that some of the items do not apply to your current situation. If so, please do not leave these items blank but mark the "Never or almost never" category. When you begin to complete the Y-OQ® 30.2 you will see that you can easily make your child look as healthy or unhealthy as you wish. Please do not do that. If you are as accurate as possible it is more likely that you will be able to receive the help that you are seeking.

DIRECTIONS:
• Read each statement carefully.
• Decide how true this statement is during the **past 7 days**.
• Select the answer that most accurately describes the past week.
• Select only one answer for each statement and erase unwanted marks clearly.

Developed by
Gary M. Burlingame, Ph.D., M. Gawain Wells, Ph.D., Michael J. Lambert, Ph.D., & Curtis W. Reisinger, Ph.D.

© Copyright American Professional Credentialing Services LLC.
All Rights Reserved.
License Required For All Uses

For More Information Contact:
OQ Measures, LLC
P.O. Box 521047
Salt Lake City, UT 84152

Toll-Free USA:
1-888-MH-SCORE
(1-888-647-2673)
Phone: (801) 649-4392
Fax: (801) 747-6900

Email:
INFO@OQMEASURES.COM

Website:
WWW.OQMEASURES.COM

	Never	Rarely	Sometimes	Frequently	Almost Always
1. My child has headaches or feels dizzy.	O	O	O	O	O
2. My child doesn't participate in activities that used to be fun.	O	O	O	O	O
3. My child argues or speaks rudely to others.	O	O	O	O	O
4. My child has a hard time finishing assignments or does them carelessly.	O	O	O	O	O
5. My child's emotions are strong and change quickly.	O	O	O	O	O
6. My child has physical fights (hitting, kicking, biting, scratching) with family or others his/her age.	O	O	O	O	O
7. My child worries and can't get thoughts out of his/her mind.	O	O	O	O	O
8. My child steals or lies.	O	O	O	O	O
9. My child is has a hard time sitting still (or has too much energy).	O	O	O	O	O
10. My child uses alcohol or drugs.	O	O	O	O	O
11. My child seems tense and easily startled (jumpy).	O	O	O	O	O
12. My child is sad or unhappy.	O	O	O	O	O
13. My child has a hard time trusting friends, family members, or other adults.	O	O	O	O	O
14. My child thinks that others are trying to hurt him/her even when they're not.	O	O	O	O	O
15. My child has threatened to, or has run away from home.	O	O	O	O	O
16. My child physically fights with adults.	O	O	O	O	O
17. My child's stomach hurts or feels sick more than others his/her age.	O	O	O	O	O
18. My child doesn't have friends or doesn't keep friends very long.	O	O	O	O	O
19. My child thinks about suicide or feels s/he would be better off dead.	O	O	O	O	O
20. My child has nightmares, trouble getting to sleep, oversleeping, or waking up too early.	O	O	O	O	O
21. My child complains or questions rules, expectations, or responsibilities.	O	O	O	O	O

OQ-30.2 PR English en-us Printable Form v092202

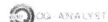 OQ ANALYST

Y-OQ®-30.2PR English   Name: _____   ID: _____   Date: ___/___/_____
Youth Outcome Questionnaire
Parent Form

PURPOSE:

The Y-OQ®30.2 is designed to describe a wide range of situations, behaviors, and moods that are common to children and adolescents. You may discover that some of the items do not apply to your current situation. If so, please do not leave these items blank but mark the "Never or almost never" category. When you begin to complete the Y-OQ® 30.2 you will see that you can easily make your child look as healthy or unhealthy as you wish. Please do not do that. If you are as accurate as possible it is more likely that you will be able to receive the help that you are seeking.

DIRECTIONS:
• Read each statement carefully.
• Decide how true this statement is during the **past 7 days.**
• Completely fill the circle that most accurately describes the past week.
• Fill in only one answer for each statement and erase unwanted marks clearly.

Developed by Gary M. Burlingame, Ph.D., M. Gawain Wells, Ph.D., Michael J. Lambert, Ph.D., & Curtis W. Reisinger, Ph.D.

© Copyright American Professional Credentialing Services LLC. All Rights Reserved. License Required For All Uses

For More Information Contact: OQ Measures, LLC P.O. Box 521047 Salt Lake City, UT 84152

Toll-Free USA: 1-888-MH-SCORE (1-888-647-2673) Phone: (801) 649-4392 Fax: (801) 747-6900

Email: INFO@OQMEASURES.COM

Website: WWW.OQMEASURES.COM

	Never	Rarely	Sometimes	Frequently	Almost Always
22. My child breaks rules, laws, or doesn't meet others expectations on purpose.	O	O	O	O	O
23. My child feels irritated.	O	O	O	O	O
24. My child gets angry enough to threaten others.	O	O	O	O	O
25. My child gets into trouble when he/she is bored.	O	O	O	O	O
26. My child destroys property on purpose.	O	O	O	O	O
27. My child has a hard time concentrating, thinking clearly, or sticking to tasks.	O	O	O	O	O
28. My child withdraws from family and friends.	O	O	O	O	O
29. My child acts without thinking & doesn't worry about what will happen.	O	O	O	O	O
30. My child feels like s/he doesn't have any friends and that no one likes them.	O	O	O	O	O

OQ-30.2 PR English en-us Printable Form v092202   OQ-ANALYST

Appendix II

Group Therapy: Often the Ideal Assistance
Here's Why…

"Just What is Group Therapy Anyway?"

In group therapy, approximately six to ten individuals meet face-to-face with two group counselors and talk about what is troubling them. Members also give feedback to each other by expressing their own feelings about what someone says or does. This interaction gives group members an opportunity to try out new ways of behaving and to learn more about the way they interact with others. What makes the situation unique is that it is a closed and safe system. The content of the group sessions are confidential; what people talk about or disclose is not discussed outside the group.

The first few sessions of a group usually focus on the establishment of trust. During this time, members usually work to establish a level of trust that allows them to talk personally and honestly. Group trust is enhanced when all members make a commitment to the group.

"Why Does Group Therapy Work?"

When people come into a group and interact freely with other group members, they usually recreate those difficulties that brought them to group therapy in the first place. Under the skilled direction of a group therapist, the group is able to give support, offer alternatives, or gently confront the person. In this way the difficulty becomes resolved, alternative behaviors are learned, and the person develops new social techniques or ways of relating to people. During group therapy, people begin to see that they are not alone. Many times people feel they are unique in their problems, and it is encouraging to hear that other people have similar difficulties. In the climate of trust provided by the group, people feel free to care about and help each other.

"What Do I Talk About When I Am In Group Therapy?"

Talk about what brought you to Counseling and Psychological Services (CAPS) in the first place. Tell the group members what is bothering you. If you need support, let the group know. If you think you need confrontation, let them know this also. It is important to tell people what you expect of them.

Unexpressed feelings are a major reason people experience difficulties. Revealing your feelings—self-disclosure—is an important part of group and affects how much you will be helped. The appropriate disclosures will be those that relate directly to your present difficulty. How much you talk about yourself depends upon what you are comfortable with. If you have questions about what might or might not be helpful, you can always ask the group.

Common Misperceptions About Group Therapy

1.   **"I will be forced to tell all of my deepest thoughts, feelings, and secrets to the group."**

     You control what, how much, and when you share with the group. Most people find that when they feel safe enough to share what is troubling them, a group can be very helpful and affirming. We encourage you not to share what you are not ready to disclose. However, you can also be helped by listening to others and thinking about how what they are saying might apply to you.

2. **"Group therapy will take longer than individual therapy because I will have to share the time with others."**

Actually, group therapy is often more efficient than individual therapy for two reasons. First, you can benefit from the group even during sessions when you say little but listen carefully to others. You will find that you have much in common with other group members, and as they work on a concern, you can learn more about yourself. Secondly, group members will often bring up issues that strike a chord with you, but that you might not have been aware of or brought up yourself.

3. **"I will be verbally attacked by the leaders and by other group members."**

It is very important that group members feel safe. Group leaders are there to help develop a safe environment. Feedback is often difficult to hear. As group members come to trust and accept one another, they generally experience feedback and even confrontation as positive, as if it were coming from their best friend. One of the benefits of group therapy is the opportunity to receive feedback from others in a supportive environment. It is rare to find friends who will gently point out how you might be behaving in ways that hurt yourself or others, but this is precisely what group can offer. This will be done in a respectful way, so that you can hear it and make use of it.

4. **"Group therapy is second-best to individual therapy."**

Group therapy is being recommended to you because your intake counselor believes that it is the best way to address your concerns. We do not put people into group therapy because we don't have space in individual therapy, or because we want to save time. We recommend group when it is the most effective method to help you. Your intake counselor can discuss with you why group is what we recommend for you.

5. **"I have so much trouble talking to people; I'll never be able to share in a group."**

Most people are anxious about being able to talk in a group. Almost without exception, within a few sessions people find that they do begin to talk in the group. Group members remember what it is like to be new to the group, so you will most likely get a lot of support for beginning to talk in the group

This text was developed by Jack Corazzini, with modifications to accommodate UNC Charlotte groups.

How to Get the Most Out of Group Counseling

1   You will develop personal goals with your group leader(s) about what *you* want to work on in group, which may be revised over time. If the group is not moving in the direction you would like it to move, please let people know how you would like it to change.

2   You are encouraged to talk about your feelings and experiences, particularly in areas that are emotionally uncomfortable or risky for you. You will make the most progress if you allow yourself to experience and discuss your true feelings and reactions to others.

3   It is normal to feel some anxiety as you talk about your personal feelings, thoughts, and experiences with others. Share these difficulties or concerns at a pace that is comfortable for you rather than forcing yourself to disclose too quickly in group.

4   You will be challenged to relate to each other without superficial conversation, social amenities, and other forms of social distancing in order to be as direct, frank, and spontaneous with your thoughts as possible. Questions should be rare, but the thoughts and feelings behind your question will be important to explore.

5 When you have reactions to something another member says it is helpful to share those feelings in group directly with the person. A good way to do this is to use "I-statements," such as "I can relate to what you are saying because I also feel afraid when …, " etc. Giving advice, labeling someone, or criticizing is generally not productive in group.

6 As group leaders, we are committed to creating a welcoming and respectful environment within our groups. We encourage group members to share aspects of their personal identity that are meaningful to them and to be supportive of this sharing by others. Aspects of identity that might be discussed include race, ethnicity, language, nationality, sex, gender identity, sexual identity, religion, ability, and socioeconomic status.

7 Confidentiality is mandatory; it is extremely important in order to help you feel safe discussing personal issues in group. You may not discuss other people or reveal the identity of other group members to those outside of the group.

8 We ask that you not have social relationships outside the group with other group members or connect with one another on social media. All members are encouraged to let the group know if you have had a conversation outside of group with another member. This helps to keep the group relationships therapeutic.

9 We make every effort to begin and end on time. We also ask that you to be on time to the sessions, and if you have to be late or miss a session due to an emergency, please contact the group leader(s) ahead of time to inform about your absence.

10 You are making a commitment to participate for the entire length of the group when you join. Your attendance is vital in order to keep the group feeling safe and cohesive. If you decide you need to leave the group before it ends, please inform the group and give the group as much time as possible to discuss this termination. It will be important for you to come and say goodbye to the other group members.

11 If you begin to have suicidal thoughts or are in need of extra support, we ask that you share this either within the group or with the group leader(s) between sessions or before or after group sessions. You should work with your group leader for a list of the best supportive and crisis referrals and safety plan arrangements that meet your specific needs. Your leader is available to discuss other treatment options and continued referrals depending upon your desires and needs.

I agree to these responsibilities as a group member: _____

Signature

This text was developed together with Jack Corazzini and UNC Charlotte Counseling and Psychological Services.

Group Therapy ContractAgreement (Sample)

Group therapy is often the treatment of choice for people who experience troubled relationships, loneliness, depression, anxiety, grief/loss, and low self-esteem. People who participate in groups that focus on the above issues have the opportunity to benefit from sharing personal experiences, giving and receiving support/constructive feedback, and experimenting with new interpersonal behaviors. In order for group to work, a safe environment must be created and expectations for members and co-leaders must be understood by the participants. Our experience with group supports that the best way to create a safe environment for personal growth is for you to understand and to agree to these guidelines.

(I) *Confidentiality*

Sharing in group can be anxiety-provoking; therefore, we ask that you keep all information discussed in this group confidential. This agreement means that you may not discuss any information shared or the reactions of any member of this group with anyone outside of the group. You may talk about your own personal reactions and are even encouraged to do so outside of group. We ask that you never disclose others' identifying information.

(II) *Attendance*

Group members are expected to make a commitment to attend group for the entire term, although we understand that making this commitment may be difficult. Members also agree to come on time every week. If you are running late or have an emergency/illness that prohibits you from coming to group, please contact the leader(s) and to inform them of the situation. If you know ahead of time that you will miss a later group session, we ask that you share the date of your absence with the group beforehand. Group will always end on time, no matter what is being discussed. Coming back the next week will allow you to continue the discussion.

   Members often feel anxious about participating in groups and should understand the positive results of your engagement can sometimes take time. If you are thinking of leaving group, we encourage you to share your concerns with the leaders and other members. If you do decide to leave group, please come back to the group to say good-bye. Members will begin to care about one another, and others may feel uneasy or unresolved if you leave without any explanation.

(III) *Relationships with Other Members*

Group is not a place to make social friends, and if you use it this way, you may not have the desired benefits you want out of your experience. Group is a chance to have therapeutic relationships in which you learn more about yourself and the ways in which you relate to others. You may have strong feelings toward some members of the group, as you do with people in your life; however, group can be a safe environment to explore those feelings and how you act on them. If you do have contact with someone outside of group (e.g., see someone in a store), please share all contacts outside of group with the group at the next meeting.

(IV) *Active Participation*

Members are not required to talk in group, but we know that the more you share in the group, the more benefits you will receive. The only time that we ask that you do speak is when a new member is added to the group and introductions and goals for group are shared. We will encourage you to talk primarily about feelings as opposed to only sharing details of stories that occurred outside of group. We will ask you to do this because not everyone can relate to a life experience, but everyone can understand feelings (e.g., fear, happiness, anger, etc.). We realize that asking you to focus on your feelings and thoughts can be frustrating at times, but group is a place to learn new ways of making deeper connections with others.

Signature of Participant_____ Date _____
Printed Name _____
Signature of Leader _____ Date _____

This example is based on contracts found online, developed by certified group therapists.

Group Confidentiality Agreement

Confidentiality, a trust of privacy or secrecy of communication and information, is special in a group setting, and is the shared responsibility of all group members and their leader(s). Although a group leader will not disclose client communications or information except as provided by law or in other limited circumstances, group members' communications and information are not protected. Thus, this agreement is an attempt to provide you and your fellow group members with as much confidentiality protection as possible.

What Is Not Permissible:

I will not disclose to anyone outside the group any information that may help to identify another group member. This includes, but is not limited to, names, physical description, biographical information, and specifics of content of interactions with other group members.

What Is Permissible:

I understand that I am free to disclose to people that I choose the fact that I am a group member and attending this group. By my choice, I also may disclose personal information about myself with respect to group experience. This includes *my* personal reactions (feelings and thoughts) to *my* group experience, feedback from other members concerning myself, and any personal information about myself such as new skills I have learned and changes I have made.

By my signature below, I indicate that I have read carefully and understand this Agreement and that I agree to its terms and conditions. I have asked and had answered any questions I have concerning the Agreement and am aware that signing of the Agreement is required for admission to the group. I am also aware that my refusal to sign this Agreement will exclude my participation in the group, and that if I breach confidentiality, I may be asked to leave the group.

_____   _____
Signature   ID #

_____
Date

From MacNair-Semands (2005)

Informed Consent for Telehealth Services (Sample)

Telehealth involves the use of electronic communications to enable us to connect with individuals and groups using interactive video and audio communications. Telehealth includes the practice of mental health care delivery, diagnosis, consultation, treatment, and referral to resources, education, and the transfer of medical and clinical data. I understand that I have the rights with respect to telehealth, for myself:

1. The laws that protect the confidentiality of my personal information also apply to telehealth. As such, I understand that the information disclosed by me during my sessions is generally confidential. However, there are both mandatory and permissive exceptions to confidentiality, including, but not limited to, reporting child, elder, and dependent adult abuse; expressed threats of violence toward an ascertainable victim; and when I make my mental or emotional state an issue in a legal proceeding. I also understand that the dissemination of any personally identifiable images or information from the telehealth interaction to other entities shall not occur without my written consent.

2. I understand that I have the right to withhold or withdraw my consent to the use of telehealth in the course of my care at any time, without affecting my right to future care or treatment.

3. My group therapist utilizes secure, encrypted audio/video transmission software to deliver telehealth. I understand that there are risks and consequences from telehealth, including, but not limited to, the possibility, despite reasonable efforts on the part of the counselor, that: the transmission of my personal information could be disrupted or distorted by technical failures, the transmission of my personal information could be interrupted by unauthorized persons, and/or the electronic storage of my personal information could be unintentionally lost or accessed by unauthorized persons.

4. I understand that if my Provider believes I would be better served by another form of intervention (e.g., face-to-face services), I will be referred to a mental health professional associated with any form of mental health services, and that despite my efforts and the efforts of my Provider, my condition may not improve, and in some cases may even get worse.

5. I understand the alternatives to mental health services through telehealth as they have been explained to me, and in choosing to participate in telehealth, I am agreeing to participate using video conferencing technology. I also understand that at my request or at the direction of my Provider, I may be directed to "face-to- face" mental health services.

6. I understand that I may expect the anticipated benefits such as improved access to care and more efficient evaluation and management from the use of telehealth in my care, but that no results can be guaranteed or assured.

7. I understand that my healthcare information may be shared with other individuals for scheduling and billing purposes.

8. I understand that I will need to keep my space private during sessions and protect the confidentiality of the group.

By signing this document, I agree that certain situations, including emergencies and crises, are inappropriate for audio-/video-/computer-based mental health services. If I am in crisis or in an emergency, I should immediately call 9-1-1 or seek help from a hospital or crisis-oriented health care facility in my immediate area. 11. I understand that different states have their own regulations for the use of telehealth. My Providers will follow all guidelines for <u>STATE YOU RESIDE IN</u> and their respective licensing boards.

I have read and understand the information provided above regarding telehealth, have discussed it with my Provider, and all my questions have been answered to my satisfaction. I have read this document carefully and understand the risks and benefits related to the use of telehealth services. I hereby give my informed consent to participate in the use of telehealth services for treatment under the terms described herein. By my signature below, I hereby state that I have read, understood, and agree to the terms of this document.

_____   _____

Patient Name Parent/Guardian Name

_____   _____

Patient or Parent/Guardian Signature Date

Index

Note: *Italic* page number refer to *figures* and **Bold** page number refer to **tables.**

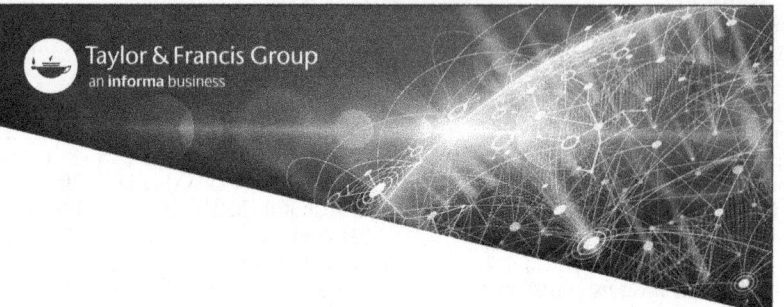
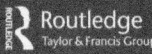
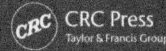